W9-ACH-122

CLINICAL ANESTHESIA IN NEUROSURGERY

CLINICAL ANESTHESIA IN NEUROSURGERY

Edited by

Elizabeth A.M. Frost, M.B., Ch.B

Professor of Anesthesiology, Albert Einstein College of Medicine, Bronx, New York

With 15 contributing authors

Foreword by H.L. Rosomoff, M.D.
Chairman, Department of Neurological Surgery, University of Miami School of Medicine, Miami, Florida

BUTTERWORTH PUBLISHERS
Boston • London
Sydney • Wellington • Durban • Toronto

Every effort has been made to ensure that the drug dosage schedules
within this text are accurate and conform to standards accepted at time
of publication. However, as treatment recommendations vary in light of
continuing research and clinical experience, the reader is advised to
verify drug dosage schedules herein with information found on product
information sheets. This is especially true in cases of new or infrequently
used drugs.

Library of Congress Cataloging in Publication Data
Main entry under title:

Clinical anesthesia in neurosurgery.

Includes index.
1. Nervous system—Surgery. 2. Anesthesia in neurology.
I. Frost, Elizabeth A.M. [DNLM: 1. Nervous system—Surgery.
2. Anesthesia. WO 200 C641]
RD593.C53   1984   617'.96748   83-15208
ISBN 0-409-95102-1

Butterworth Publishers
80 Montvale Avenue
Stoneham, MA 02180

10 9 8 7 6 5 4 3 2 1

Printed in the United States of America.

I'm môrleidr Cymraeg nad ydyw'r cariad iddo'n mynd ymaith erioed.

CONTRIBUTING AUTHORS

Steven J. Allen, M.D.
Neuroanesthesia Fellow, Department
of Anesthesiology, The University
of Texas Medical School at Houston,
Houston, Texas

I. Cary Andrews, M.D.
Associate Professor of
Anesthesiology, Albert Einstein
College of Medicine,
Bronx, New York

Carlos U. Arancibia, M.D.
Associate Professor, Department of
Anesthesiology, University of
Oklahoma Health Science Center,
Oklahoma City, Oklahoma;
Chief Anesthesiologist, Oklahoma
Memorial Hospital,
Oklahoma City, Oklahoma

Robert F. Bedford, M.D.
Associate Professor of
Anesthesiology and Neurological
Surgery, University of Virginia
School of Medicine,
Charlottesville, Virginia

Richard Brennan, Esq.
Stanley & Fisher
Counselors-at-Law
Newark, New Jersey

Jack M. Fein, M.D.
Associate Professor of Neurological
Surgery, Albert Einstein College of
Medicine,
Bronx, New York

Philip L. Gildenberg, M.D., Ph.D.
Clinical Professor of Neurosurgery,
The University of Texas Medical
School at Houston,
Houston, Texas

Betty L. Grundy, M.D.
Professor and Chairman,
Department of Anesthesiology, Oral
Roberts University School of
Medicine,
Tulsa, Oklahoma

George B. Jacobs, M.D.
Chairman, Department of
Neurosurgery,
Hackensack Medical Center,
Hackensack, New Jersey;
Associate Professor of Neurological
Surgery, Albert Einstein College of
Medicine,
Bronx, New York

Dennis R. Kopaniky, M.D., Ph.D
Assistant Professor of Neurosurgery,
The University of Texas Medical
School at Houston,
Houston, Texas

Michael E. Miner, M.D., Ph.D.
Professor and Chairman, Division
of Neurosurgery, The University of
Texas Medical School at Houston,
Houston, Texas

Robert C. Rubin, M.D.
Associate Professor of Neurological
Surgery, Albert Einstein College of
Medicine,
Bronx, New York

Kenneth Shapiro, M.D.
Associate Professor of Neurological
Surgery, Albert Einstein College of
Medicine,
Bronx, New York

Kamran Tabaddor, M.D.
Associate Professor of Neurological
Surgery, Albert Einstein College of
Medicine,
Bronx, New York

**Somasundaram Thiagarajah, M.D.,
F.R.A.R.C.S.**
Assistant Professor of Clinical
Anesthesiology, Mount Sinai School
of Medicine,
New York, New York

CONTENTS

FOREWORD

Anesthesiology, like Surgery, has fallen prey to the irrepressible forces of evolution. The explosion of knowledge, the complexity of twentieth century technology, have caused the brain of man to compress, to focus within the microcosm of speciality interest; the "man for all seasons" is no more.

Anesthesia of the eighties ordains that the technique for production of insensibility be circumscribed while responsibility expands beyond the surgical theatre to encompass preoperative and postoperative intensive care. Beyond lies perhaps an even greater role—in the physiological laboratory of intensive care for injured nervous tissue, where sustenance of perfusion, respiration and metabolism becomes the responsibility of those most precisely and extensively trained in life-support systems. The induction of sleep, always the province of anesthesiology, becomes further refined for management of the unnatural unconsciousness caused by disease or trauma: an immobile body must be nurtured through a seemingly endless period of laborious, tedious care if survival and restoration are to be achieved past the god-like fleeting act of heroism called surgery.

This newly recognized supporting cast of specialty anesthesiologists now erupts from the darkened amphitheatres to the glaring recognition of clinical care and interaction with patient, family, performing surgeon, and other medical colleagues. From the servile administration of laughing gas emerges the sophistication of neuroanesthesia and supportive care medicine. Just as neurological surgery declared its freedom from the hierarchy of the surgical guild a half century ago, the past decade has seen neuroanesthesia's successful quest for independence. The collegium of neurological surgeon and anesthesiologist has supplanted the unionism of anesthesiology. Technically the neurosurgeon still stands at the head, but it is the neuroanesthetist and critical care physician who provide the supportive stage upon which the head can act.

Gone is the silent masked partner whose invoice did present, but who was hardly more recognizable than the furtive black-shrouded Chinese prop man. In his place stands a full partner, equal in importance, armed with the tools of investigation, the inquiry of physiology, the manipulation of pharmacology, the technique of clinician, and an even more unusual new and, perhaps, still uncomfortable role of societal ecclesiastic.

Neuroanesthesia has come of age and, with it, the need for a definitive text. It no longer suffices to explore the complexities of the heart, lung and kidneys. Enter now the labyrinthine central nervous system with its own unique and varied roles. Arteries autoregulate; blood gases dictate control, remotely or locally. Vasoparalysis, not neural paralysis, may derange the functional brain. Collaterals exist, they do not form, but our newly founded team now augments them with surgical bypass. Aerobic consumption demands full and constant supply; anaerobic oxidation cannot sustain viability. The third circulation meanders a circuitous path within its rigid confinement. The political sound of the Monro-Kellie doctrine compartmentalizes brain substance, blood and cerebrospinal fluid liquor. Compliance no longer reflects only lung's function. Distant venous obstruction transmits disaster. Pharmacological and hormonal controls of pressure and fluid movement weave the threads of life. Anesthetic choice and technique become weighty occult parameters of surgical outcome. More monitors appear to confound the applicant, clutter the room and jangle the atmosphere. The physics of nervous system electricity are superimposed on the graph of the heart. Brain, visual, brainstem and spinal waveforms interpret the patient's status.

Recognition is the role of the observer anesthetist, for the surgeon fixes on the operative field. The placement and manipulation of catheters and needles become his responsibility when adversity causes reaction, shock and failure towards death. The stage must be set and kept stable for the actor surgeon to strut. The environment may need control, hot or cold, pressure up, pressure down. The airway accesses the essence of life, the drugs of somnolence and transmission of forces, good or pernicious. Their understanding evokes reflexive acts by the master craftsman, else life expires.

All this and more is the stuff of which neuroanesthesia is made. Long hours of dedicated observation, strenuous training, and honed reaction and judgment are the keystones of this guild. Years of battle will bring the accolade, but the jousts are difficult and brutally demanding.

This player has been privileged to take the field on many an occasion through the years with Elizabeth Frost, master of neuroanesthesia. These experiences, then and beyond, shape the tome that follows. She is ably assisted by her collaborators for the presentation of this definitive premier text. There will be others, as technique and knowledge expand through this century and next. All truths are self-evident; so is the importance of this work.

Hubert L. Rosomoff, M.D.

PREFACE

Just as there is no standard central nervous system lesion, there is no single best choice in neuroanesthesia. Rather, over the years, there has been a gradual evolution, albeit rather peripatetic, in neuroanesthetic care, dictated in part by neurosurgical advances. Early craniotomies were performed without any anesthesia. Subsequent local anesthetic techniques employed ice, ether as a spray jet, and cocaine. Toward the end of the nineteenth century, a balanced technique using an inhalation anesthetic (chloroform) and a narcotic (morphine) was in vogue. Increased understanding of intracranial dynamics led to the adoption of intravenous anesthesia, a technique that was less likely to increase intracranial pressure. More recently, with the growing awareness of the possible deleterious effects of nitrous oxide and the development of better agents, the trend again is to use an inhalational agent (isoflurane) combined with a narcotic (sufentanil).

The state of the art in neurosurgery is such that operative intervention of many more and complex disease processes is possible. Intracranial function is influenced not only by anesthetic agents and techniques but is also acutely sensitive to abnormalities of other organ systems. Thus, optimal outcome after any neurosurgical procedure must depend on a team approach. Careful preoperative evaluation and stabilization of multisystem disease are essential. With a knowledge of the pathology involved and the operative approach and requirements, the anesthesiologist can then make a rational and appropriate choice of technique.

This book is a collaborative effort by anesthesiologists and neurosurgeons to collate their experiences and survey the extensive literature that has flooded the academic scene of the neurosciences over the past few years. The intent has not been to advocate rigid management plans for each situation but rather to present the pathology involved and suggest rational approaches to anesthetic care. Both anesthesiologist and neurosurgeon should be aware, for example, of the hazards of anesthesia in the patient with peripheral nerve trauma who has just eaten, or the difficulty of intubating a patient with cervical spine injury. The chapters describing seizure surgery, percutaneous ablative procedures, and stereotactic techniques might suggest a limited role for the anesthesiologist. These topics have been included, however, since in many parts of the world, many of these procedures are either done under general anesthesia or actually performed by the anesthesiologist.

For the most part, neurosurgical disease processes have been considered in separate chapters. Supratentorial tumors and adult hydrocephalus are characterized mainly by raised intracranial pressure; since the anesthetic management involves principles rather than specific care, these diseases have been covered in Chapter 3, Physiology of Intracranial Pressure.

The section on intensive care is not intended as a reference for the intensivist but rather as a guide for the practitioner who, as part of a team, must see the patient through a critical period following trauma or surgery.

Finally, from two disciplines, neither of which allows room for compromise, the views from both sides of the ether screen have been presented in the belief (to paraphrase Antoine de Saint Exupéry) that "Progress does not consist in gazing at each other but in looking outward together in the same direction."

The author thanks the contributors for their patience, Carolyn Burke Giles for her secretarial help, and Nancy Megley of Butterworths for her advice and encouragement.

E.A.M.F.

CHAPTER 1

Introduction
Elizabeth A.M. Frost

It can be argued that all anesthesia is neuroanesthesia in that it concerns itself with the interruption within the central nervous system of the perception of pain by higher cortical centers. Some might say that anesthesia for neurologic surgery is only part of the larger field of anesthesiology and is not very different from other types of anesthesia.

This latter statement could be made only by someone who has not been involved to any extent in the administration of anesthesia for intracranial procedures. In essence, a patient with preexisting neurologic disease is undergoing neurosurgical intervention under the influence of centrally acting depressant anesthetic drugs. Clearly, an appreciation of the situation and an ability to balance all three factors are essential for the successful outcome of any neurosurgical operation. It quickly becomes apparent that there are major problems unique to neurosurgery that must be fully understood and solved by anesthesiologists.

UNIQUE PROBLEMS OF NEUROANESTHESIA

The primary neuroanesthetic problem is the regulation of brain volume and pressure. Whether this is done by the regulation of respiratory patterns and blood gas tensions, by the administration of diuretic or hypotensive agents, by the drainage of cerebrospinal fluid, or by any other means, changes critical to the successful outcome of a case are realized immediately.

The second major problem is the control of hemorrhage. This also can be profoundly influenced by the anesthesiologist either by choice of anesthetic agents or by control of blood pressure and ventilation.

The third critical area unique to neuroanesthesia lies in the protection of nervous tissue from ischemic and surgical injury. The regeneration of the central nervous system is slow and limited. Apart from Purkinje cells, no new cells are formed. Limited repair facilities are available. There is no hypertrophy of existing neurons. Whereas skin, bone, or liver will regenerate and hypertrophy, the central nervous system cannot do this, and requires extreme efforts to protect existing tissue.

The brain does, however, appear to have a certain redundancy of circuitry and plasticity of function that become lost as the organ matures. Perhaps it is because the brain has so little ability for repair that it is so uniquely protected, both physically and physiologically. It has its own container, the skull, and it is biochemically isolated by a barrier, the blood-brain barrier. The brain also most probably has its own waste disposal system in the cerebrospinal fluid circulation. Some of these are mixed blessings, as when the skull is confining the swollen brain and intracranial pressure increases, or the cerebrospinal fluid passages are blocked and hydrocephalus results. But this uniquely controlled environment permits the central nervous system to function and in turn to monitor and control the environment of the rest of the organ system. The responsibility for the maintenance of this stable environment during any neurosurgical experience and well into the postoperative period rests with the anesthesiologist.

Of course, numerous smaller problems also arise during neurosurgical anesthesia, such as the inaccessibility of the head, the tendency for the airway to become obstructed by position, temperature control, fluid and electrolyte balance, and the uncommonly painstaking techniques, initiated by Halsted and widely practiced by Cushing, that often result in greatly prolonged operative and thus anesthetic time. It would appear inevitable, therefore, that neuroanesthesia would appeal to a relatively small number of anesthesiologists of unusual patience who possess an almost pathologic adherence to meticulous detail in technique, for there is no room for compromise.

DEVELOPMENT OF NEUROLOGIC SUPPORTIVE CARE

With the introduction of diathermy and later of the operating microscope, many procedures that were not previously feasible are now commonplace. Many of these operations result in real or potentially reversible brain damage, which requires the same exacting postoperative care and maintenance of a stable environment as was evidenced during the operative phase. Added to these situations are the increased number of head trauma and spinal cord injury victims who, because of increased awareness and availability of resuscitation and transport mechanisms, survive major trauma. As only about 20% of these patients require surgical intervention, the emphasis in neurologic surgery is thus seen to be shifting rapidly away from the operating room only and into the realm of neurologic supportive care. Success in such an area clearly is dependent on the team approach, but the anesthesiologist with his detailed knowledge of respiratory and cardiac physiology and his understanding of fluid and electrolyte balance and of intracranial dynamics is the logical physician to lead, or even in some instances to pioneer, the neurosurgical intensive care unit.

NEUROANESTHESIA SOCIETIES

In an attempt to initiate research and teaching in the field of neuroanesthesia, a Commission of Neuroanesthesia was founded on July 9, 1960, in Antwerp, Belgium (1). The Commission comprised a group of anesthesiologists from nine different countries. Since then, several other societies in different parts of the world have been established to study this speciality. Among them is the Society of Neuroanesthesia and Neurologic Supportive Care, founded in the United States in 1973. This Society, which is recognized both by the American Society of Anesthesiologists and by the American Association of Neurological Surgeons, participates actively in the respective annual meetings and sponsors its own annual meeting.

HISTORICAL BACKGROUND

Earliest Times

Perhaps rather obviously, the development of neuroanesthesia is closely linked to the development of neurosurgery itself. Some types of neurosurgical procedures have been performed for thousands of years. The first discovery of trephined neolithic skulls, estimated to be between 4000 and 5000 years old, was received with considerable skepticism (2). Subsequent discoveries, however, confirmed that holes frequently were made in skulls using flintstones to release evil spirits and cure headache. The ancient Egyptians (circa 3000 BC) apparently had knowledge of the function of the brain and spinal cord, but no mention is made of surgical intervention in the Ebers or Edwin Smith papyri of any procedures apart from wound approximations. "Carotid artery" is derived from the Greek word meaning the artery of sleep, and it is possible that pressure or even ligation of this vessel was used as a means of producing insensibility (3). On the other hand, it may just have been that the Greeks observed that cutting the carotid artery usually resulted in unconsciousness and death from hemorrhage.

In the second century AD, Areteus, in outlining the treatment of seizures, recommended perforation of the skull with a trepan "when the meninx there is found black." If cleansing could be enacted of the putrefaction (i.e., release of a subdural clot), cure was to be expected. Apparently he recognized little need for anesthesia, as "the habit of such persons renders them tolerant of pains and their goodness of spirits and good hopes renders them strong in endurance" (4). Ancient trephined skulls have also been found in Peru, dating from about this time, when cocoa leaves (from which cocaine was purified by Nieman in 1860) were known and used for centuries to produce insensibility during procedures requiring cutting by the knife.

No mention is made in any of the other ancient writings of other kinds of intracranial surgery. The great medical work of ancient China, *The Yellow*

Emperor's Classic of Internal Medicine, was started about 2697 BC and rewritten several times between then and the Sui Dynasty (589–618 AD) (5). It consisted of two parts, the Huang Ti Nei Ching Su Wen, which is simple discussions between the Emperor and his chief physician, Ch'i Po, and the Nei Ching Ling Shu Ching, a 91-chapter treatise on acupuncture. Almost no mention was made of the use of any surgery. The Chinese felt that the superiority of internal therapy made unnecessary all operations and even all knowledge of anatomy. Probably even more important were the Confucian tenets of the sacredness of the body, which countered any tendency to the practice of surgery. Epilepsy, palsies, and many mental derangements were graphically described, but the therapy was herbal or needling of appropriate points to reestablish the balance of the meridians. Chinese medical history did record two eminent surgeons. The first was named Pien Ch'iao, and he was said to have been so skillful in his use of anesthesia that he was able to operate completely painlessly. The first heart transplant was ascribed to him during the second century BC. The other surgeon, Hua T'o, became famous for his writings on surgery and anesthesia about 200 AD. He achieved general anesthesia by means of a drug dissolved in wine. The components of this drug, ma-fei-san (literally, "bubbling drug medicine"), are not known. Dr. Erich Hauer, the sinologist, was of the opinion that ma-fei referred to opium (5).

With the fall of the Roman Empire, the Church became more influential in the practice of medicine. Headaches, attributed often to punishment or the presence of evil, were treated by trephination. The first report of any other type of neurosurgical procedure being performed appeared first in Hindu writings. In 927 AD two surgeons anesthetized the King of Dhar with a drug called *samohini*. They then opened the skull, removed a tumor, and closed the wound with sutures. A reversal agent that was specified only as a stimulant also was used (1).

Middle Ages

The use of the trephine was well described in the fourteenth century by Roland de Parme in his book *La Chirurgia*. An elderly man, head shaven, was shown sitting placidly, hands crossed in his lap, while a man of the Church drilled a hole in his head (Fig. 1.1). A pre-Columbian tumi made of champi (an alloy of copper, gold, and silver) belonged to the same period (1300 AD). The figures on the end of the instrument depicted its use (Fig. 1.2). While one man held the patient, the other man trephined the skull. About 100 years later, in 1465 AD, Charaf-ed Din in his book *La Chirurgie des Ilkhani* showed the treatment of a child with hydrocephalus (Fig. 1.3). The child was held by an assistant while the surgeon, using a bistoury, cut off the excess head. About this time (thirteenth century), Theodoric recommended that anesthesia be induced by a "spongia somnifera," a sponge impregnated with spirituous extracts of various narcotic substances. This was to be held to the nostrils of the patient until sleep was induced. After operation the patient was aroused by application of a second sponge containing vinegar and other nasal irritants such as fenugreek (6).

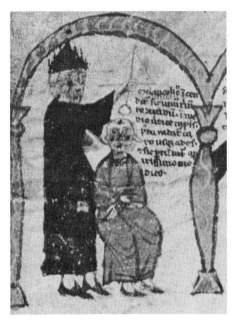

Figure 1.1 Skull operation performed by means of a trephine. From *La Chirurgia* by Roland de Parme, fourteenth century. (Biblioteca Casanatense, Rome.) (Courtesy of Richardson-Merrell, Inc.)

Renaissance

During the great revival of art, literature, and learning that began in Italy in the fourteenth century and spread throughout Europe during the fifteenth and sixteenth centuries, the ban on human dissection was lifted. There was outstanding work by such great anatomists as Vesalius, Eustachius, and Sylvius. Morgagni demonstrated remarkable developments in the understanding of the central nervous system. Despite all this activity, no further intracranial surgery was described.

That neurosurgery was practiced widely in the sixteenth century is evidenced by the surgeon's case of Ambroise Paré, surgeon to the King of France during the 1560s. Of 13 surgical instruments, 5 were trephines (Fig. 1.4).

At the beginning of the seventeenth century, one of the first medical textbooks written in English appeared, *The Physician's Practice*, "wherein are contained all inward Diseases from the Head to the Foot by that famous and worthy Physician, Walter Bruel." This book described in great anatomic detail headaches, palsies, paralyses, brain inflammations, and all the causes thereof. Surgery was not recommended. The reader was advised instead to bleed the nose to let the evil out and to use rosemary flowers and the roots of elecampany as an opiate (7). Further, bathing the patient in water prepared from flayed foxes and their whelps was guaranteed to produce results. Horse leeches applied to the temporal artery, diuretics, and cathartics were strongly recommended as means of reducing increased intracranial pressure. Gross humors could be abated and turned into vapors by holding a red-hot frying pan over the patient's shaven head.

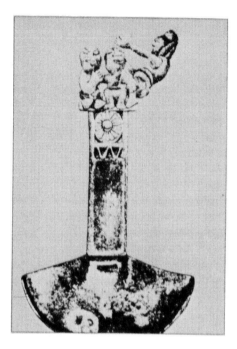

Figure 1.2 Pre-Columbian *tumi* used for trephination. Sculpture on the handle end depicts its use. Made of champi, an alloy of copper, gold, and silver. Northern coast of Peru, Chimu period (about 1300–1500 AD). (Courtesy of Richardson-Merrell, Inc.)

Throughout the eighteenth century, much anatomic dissection and further understanding of human anatomy and physiology were accomplished. By 1765, Cotugno had described the cerebrospinal fluid and outlined its composition and some of its function (8), but still no surgical advances were reported.

Nineteenth Century

Sir Astley Cooper, consulting surgeon to Guy's Hospital in London, published a series of lectures that he had delivered on the principles and practice of surgery within the operating theater at St. Thomas's Hospital in 1829. He stated that "trephining in concussion is now so completely abandoned that in the last four years I do not know that I have performed it once, whilst 35 years ago I would have performed it five or six times a year." Instead, he recommended frequent bleeding, calomel purges, and leeches (9). The leeches again were to be applied to the temporal arteries. Undoubtedly, the many successes that he recounted in his lectures could only have been due to a brinksmanship reduction of intracranial pressure by hypovolemia. Anesthesia was achieved with liberal doses of wine if it was needed at all. The surgeon gaily noted that the wine was rarely necessary as the patients were either already in an obtunded state or the surgery was not painful enough (c.f. Aretaeus).

In 1846, Dr. J.F. Malgaigne from the Faculté de Médicine in Paris wrote a manual of operative surgery, including descriptions of puncture operations for

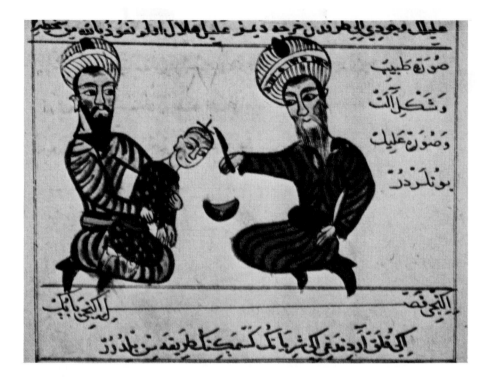

Figure 1.3   Treatment of a child's hydrocephalus. From *La Chirurgie des Ilkhani* by Charaf-ed-Din, 1465. (Bibliothèque Nationale, Paris.) (Courtesy of Richardson-Merrell, Inc.)

hydrocephalus and various types of nerve divisions for pain relief (frontal, infra-orbital, facial, and inferior dental and sciatic). A chapter on the means of diminishing pain during surgery was included. Although four years had elapsed since Crawford Long had performed the first operation under ether anesthesia, Malgaigne mentioned only the use of narcotics, animal magnetism or cutting of the nerve supply to the area (10). He also outlined James Moore's experiments with a Dupuytren's compressor to produce sufficient pressure on the nerve supplying the area to render the incised part analgesic. Other methods suggested were the use of excessive venesection as described by Wardrop or insensibility by mesmerism.

The Discovery of General Anesthesia

Sir Humphry Davy at the end of the eighteenth century had discovered the "remarkable properties exercised on the nervous system by the inhalation of nitrous oxide." Experiments were made with the gas with the hope of relieving pain during surgical operation, but they did not prove satisfactory and were abandoned except as a means of amusement (11).

In 1844, Horace Wells, a dentist in Hartford, Connecticut, inhaled nitrous oxide with the view of rendering himself insensible during the extraction of a tooth. This experiment succeeded, and he repeated it on several patients. He failed on several occasions, however, and it was a pupil and colleague of his, Dr. W.T.G. Morton, another dentist who, following the work of Dr. Crawford Long of Danielsville, Georgia, applied to the authorities of the Massachusetts General Hospital for permission to administer sulfuric ether to a man from whom Dr. J.C. Warren, a surgeon, was about to remove a tumor of the neck. So was modern anesthesia born (3).

The following year, in 1848, Dr. James Simpson of Edinburgh first used chloroform as an anesthetic agent. Chloroform had been prepared simultaneously by Liebig in Germany in 1832, by Guthrie in the United States (1831), and by Soubeiran in France in 1831. The anesthetic properties of the drug had been first described by Flourens in 1847, and it had been named *chloroform* by Alexander Dumas. The acceptance of chloroform by Queen Victoria for the delivery of her child ensured its establishment and widespread use in Great Britain.

In 1869, John Erichsen of University College Hospital in London wrote a textbook on the science and art of surgery. His summary after twenty years of general use of anesthetic techniques is as current now as it was then (6):

> The employment of anaesthetics in surgery is undoubtedly one of the greatest boons ever conferred upon mankind. To the patient it is invaluable in preventing the occurrence of pain and to the surgeon in relieving him of the stress of inflicting it. Anaesthesia is not, however, an unmixed good. Every agent by which it can be induced produces a powerful impression on the system and may occasion dangerous consequences when too freely or carelessly given; and even with every possible care, it appears certain that the inhalation of any anaesthetic agent is in some cases almost inevitably fatal. We cannot purchase immunity from suffering without incurring a certain degree of danger. There can, however, be little doubt that many of the deaths that have followed the inhalation of anaesthetics have resulted from want of knowledge or of due care on the part of the administrators. Yet, whatever precautions be taken, there is reason to fear that a fatal result must occasionally happen. This immediate result, which is but very small, is more than counterbalanced by the immunity from other dangers during operations which used formerly to occur.

On the state of the neurosurgical art at this time, Dr. Erichsen wrote that "the safest practice (for concussion) is to wrap the patient up warmly in blankets; to put hot bottles around him. Alcoholic stimulants of all kinds should be avoided" (6). Should deterioration in the general condition occur, however, purging, bleeding, and leeches were still the principal therapy. He did note a beneficial effect of opiates in general cerebral irritation to quiet the patient and induce sleep, although great care was to be taken, especially if tachycardia was apparent. In summary, he wrote: "In the treatment of injuries of the brain, little can be done after the system has rallied from the shock, beyond attention to strict antiphlogistic treatment, though this need not be of a very active kind. As much should be left to nature as possible, the surgeon merely removing all sources of irritation and excitement from his patient and applying simple local dressings." He described the operation of trephining as important but not used as much as previously. Indications for such intervention were compression and inflammation. Results were not favorable: of 45 patients described by Lente at New York Hospital, 11 recovered. Of 17 patients that Erichsen himself, along with Cooper and Liston, had treated at University College Hospital, only six recovered (6).

Several means of local anesthesia also were described by 1860. Dr. J. Arnott described a frigorific mixture of ice, snow, and salt. Dr. Richardson used a fine spray jet of ether of low specific gravity to freeze an area of skin before making the incision (6).

Sir Victor Horsley was one of the first neurosurgeons in England. He carried out extensive research at the University College Hospital in London on the functions of the brain and spinal cord to clarify his work in neurosurgery (1). Between 1883 and 1885 he investigated the different intracranial effects during surgery of chloroform, ether, and morphine sulfate. He concluded that ether caused a rise in blood pressure, increased blood viscosity, and prompted excessive bleeding, dangerous postoperative vomiting, and excitement and thus should not be used in neurosurgery. He felt that morphine was of value because of the apparent decrease in cerebral blood flow and the more readily controlled hemorrhage in the surgical field. He suggested a balanced technique using a combination of chloroform and morphine and in 1887 used this technique for the first time to remove spinal cord tumors and perform craniotomies. He later abandoned morphine because of its respiratory depressant effects. Other prominent neurosurgeons of that time, Hartley, Kenyon, and Krause, preferred to use chloroform alone (1).

In the United States, the influence of Long and Morton remained. An extremely detailed record is preserved in Lumberton, New Jersey, of Mary Catherine Anderson, age 17, shot in the head on February 7, 1887 (12). On February 22, four notable physicians, Pancoast, Spitzka, Girdner, and Spiller, crowded together in a tiny cottage and used a telephonic probe in an unsuccessful attempt to locate the bullet. Under ether anesthesia the girl's condition rapidly deteriorated, and the procedure was abandoned. Unfortunately, she died without regaining consciousness some two weeks later, and the case was referred to the judicial system.

Harvey Cushing, although a great pioneer of American neurosurgery, did not do as well as an anesthesiologist. While a second year medical student at the Massachusetts General Hospital in 1893, he anesthetized a young woman with a strangulated hernia. Cushing recorded that he had used 1/60 gr atropine, subcutaneous brandy, 1/60 gr strychnine and 1/100 gr nitroglycerine prior to etherization with the sponge. The patient died during induction (13). His future writings frequently reflected his discontent with the inadequacies of anesthesia administered by unskilled students. In 1897, working on a principle introduced by W.S. Halsted in 1885, he began to experiment with block anesthesia produced by cocaine infiltration (13). At about this time he and a classmate, Amory Codman, introduced ether charts, which quickly were developed into anesthetic

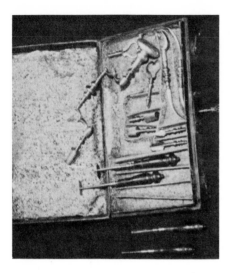

Figure 1.4 A surgeon's case, attributed to Ambroise Paré. *Bottom to top:* hand levator, bistoury, two retractors, four trephines, a punch, two double-curved levators, a brace with a fifth trephine and a key. (Museum in Laval, France.) (Courtesy of Richardson-Merrell, Inc.)

records (Fig. 1.5). Dr. Cushing is responsible also for introducing the Riva-Rocci pneumatic device for continuous recording of blood pressure during surgery. He had seen this instrument at Padua, Italy, in 1901. Despite his advances in the introduction of these safety devices for monitoring during general anesthesia, local infiltration soon became the only type of analgesia employed by Dr. Cushing and his school of neurosurgery. In fact, in 1929, a patient from whom he had removed a large intracranial cyst reported that "one of the secrets of Dr. Cushing's success is that he uses nothing except a local anesthetic which permits the normal functioning of the heart and other organs during the operation" (13). His preference was also shared by DeMartel, who in 1913 adopted local infiltration for all types of neurosurgery.

Twentieth Century Developments

Tribromethanol was synthesized by Willstaetter and Duisburg in 1923 and used as the sole anesthetic agent in neurosurgical procedures by Butzengeiger and Eichholtz in 1923. It was used rectally and described by Walter Dandy from the Johns Hopkins Hospital in 1931 as a means of reducing raised intracranial pressure (14). Leo Davidoff, finding that the effects of tribromethanol wore off too quickly, described its use in combination with local infiltration (15).

Trichlorethylene with nitrous oxide gained considerable popularity as a neuroanesthetic technique in various parts of the British commonwealth. After its description by D.E. Jackson in 1934 (16), Hewer published several successful case reports. Hershenson used low concentrations of closed-circuit cyclopropane and published reports on this method of anesthesia for neurosurgery in 1942 (17). This technique never became popular, however, undoubtedly because of the explosive hazards.

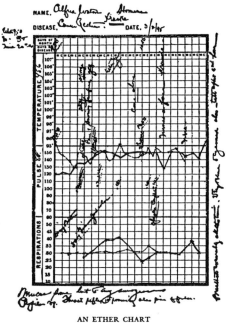

AN ETHER CHART

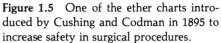

Figure 1.5 One of the ether charts introduced by Cushing and Codman in 1895 to increase safety in surgical procedures.

Thiopental was synthesized in 1930 by Volwiler and Tabern and introduced into clinical practice by Lundy and Waters in 1934. A report by Shannon and Gardner in 1946 described its use for all types of neurosurgery (18), but its popularity was short-lived. The discovery of halothane in 1951 and its introduction in 1956 by Raventos made the latter drug one of the most frequently used anesthetic in neurosurgery. In recent years, however, studies of the apparent cerebral protective effect of thiopental on the cerebral metabolic rate of oxygen utilization have caused neuroanesthesiologists to reexamine the barbiturates and narcotics.

Many other techniques developed over the past century have greatly accelerated the growth of the specialties of neurosurgery and neuroanesthesia. Mention has already been made of the cautery and the operating microscope in neurosurgery. In anesthesia, one of the most important developments has been that of endotracheal intubation, first described by Sir William Macewan in Glasgow (19) and later used routinely in surgery by Magill and Rowbotham in 1916. Finally, ventilation could be controlled, and the importance of the partial pressure of arterial blood gases in controlling cerebral blood flow was apparent.

All degrees of hypothermia, from minimal to profound, have been paraded in the neurosurgical arena. Currently the practice of extreme degrees of hypothermia using cardiopulmonary bypass techniques has been abandoned in almost all areas.

Minute control over the blood pressure by using a microinfusion of a potent hypotensive agent, such as nitroprusside, is possible. Effects can be monitored by a continuous recording from an arterial cannula and transducer. Similarly, arterial blood gas analyses may be continuously obtained using an on-line sensor. Other continuous measurements may be made of intracranial pressure, cerebral perfusion pressure, cerebral blood flow, evoked potentials, brain retractor pressures, and electroencephalographic changes. Neuroanesthesia may be unique, with the possible exception of cardiac surgery, among the anesthetic subspecialities in the degree of precision monitoring that it affords.

It can thus be seen that neurosurgery, like anesthsia, has an active and productive history of little more than 100 years. It is apparent that advances over the last century in both specialities have been truly remarkable.

The goals and principles of neuroanesthesia must rest upon three factors: the use of rapid and reversible agents, the maintenance of a stable environment, and the control of intracranial pressure. The overwhelming verity is that the brain is still irreplaceable; it is perhaps the last holdout among the organ systems. While renal and cardiac transplantation have become commonplace, and lung, liver, and pancreas replacements noteworthy but not unusual, the brain remains unsupplantable. To protect and preserve this remarkable computer, the anesthesiologist and the neurosurgeon must work as a team.

REFERENCES

1. Schapira M: Evolution of anesthesia for neurosurgery. NY State J Med 1964; June 1; 64:1301–1305.
2. Pruniérès D: Sur les crânes artificiellement perforés a l'époque des Dolmens. Bull Mem Soc Anthrop Paris 1874;9:185–205.
3. Raper HR: Man against pain, the epic of anesthesia. New York, Prentice-Hall, 1945.
4. Aretaeus, the Cappodocian. extant works, Adams F (trans). London, Syndenham Society, 1856, p 469.
5. The yellow emperor's classic of internal medicine, Veith I (trans). Baltimore, Williams & Wilkins, 1949.
6. Erichsen JE: Science and art of surgery. Philadelphia, Henry C Lea, 1869, pp 40–47, 335–337.
7. Bruel W: The physician's practice, ed 2. London, John Warton for William Sheares, 1639, pp 10, 76–89.
8. Cotugno D: De ischiade nervosa commentarius. Naples, Simoniana, 1762.
9. Cooper A: Lectures in the principles and practice of surgery. London, Westley, 1829, pp 119–129.
10. Malgaigne JF: Manual of operative surgery. London, Henry Renshaw, 1846, pp 42–43, 109–116.
11. Davy H: Researches chemical and philosophical chiefly concerning nitrous oxide. Bristol, Biggs and Cottle, 1800, pp 333–343.
12. Henderson AR: Prominent medicine convenes at Lumberton, 1887. J Med Soc NJ 1976;73:1, 18–22.
13. Fulton JF: Harvey Cushing. Springfield, Ill., Charles C Thomas, 1946, pp 69–70, 120, 578.
14. Dandy WE: Avertin anesthesia in neurologic surgery. JAMA 1931;96 (May 30):1860–1864.

15. Davidoff LM: Avertin as a basal anesthetic for craniotomy. Bulletin Neurological Institute 1934;3:544–550.
16. Jackson DE: A Study of analgesia and anesthesia with special reference to such substances as trichlorethylene and vinesthene together with apparatus for their administration. Anesth Analg (Cleve) Current Researches 1934;13:198–203.
17. Hershenson BB: Some observations on anesthesia for neurosurgery. NY State J Med 1942;42:2111–2118.
18. Shannon EW, Gardner WJ: Pentothal sodium anesthesia in neurological surgery. N Engl J Med 1946;234:15–16.
19. Macewan W: Clinical observations on the introduction of tracheal tubes by the mouth instead of performing tracheotomy or laryngotomy. Br Med J 1850;2:122–124, 163–165.

PART I

Cerebral Physiology and Evaluation

CHAPTER 2

Cerebral Hemodynamics and Metabolism
Jack M. Fein

The cerebral circulation plays a critical role in the nutrition and maintenance of the central nervous system. It delivers anesthetic and other drugs to the brain and is the origin of many disease processes requiring neurosurgical intervention. The reactions of the cerebral vasculature to chemical and physiologic stimuli can be critically affected by anesthetic and operative procedures. These dynamic changes require constant surveillance by both neurosurgeon and anesthesiologist. Cerebral circulation and cerebral metabolism have been studied extensively in laboratory experiments where invasive techniques allow for more rigid control and study of the variables affecting cerebral homeostasis. Less invasive techniques have been developed to allow limited clinical study of the cerebral circulation and cerebral metababolism.

VASCULAR ANATOMY

The nutritional needs of the brain are met by the carotid and vertebral circulations and by the superficial and deep systems of venous drainage. The left carotid and left subclavian arteries are direct branches of the aortic arch. The subclavian arteries each give origin to the vertebral arteries. The right carotid artery and right subclavian artery arise from the innominate branch of the aorta. Therefore, retrograde brachial injection of contrast material into the right subclavian artery will also fill the right common carotid artery. The common carotid artery usually divides at the level of the fourth cervical vertebrae into the internal and external carotid arteries. The carotid sinus, containing baroreceptor and chemoreceptor nerve endings, is located at the origin of the internal carotid artery. The internal carotid artery penetrates the base of the skull and the outer layer of dura, passes through the cavernous sinus lateral to the sella turcica, and then penetrates the inner layer of the dura (1) (Fig. 2.1). The proximal branches of the internal carotid artery include anastomoses with the internal maxillary artery and intracavernous branches supplying the pituitary gland and the dura. The ophthalmic artery is the first intradural branch of the internal carotid artery, passing through the optic foramen to supply the retinal and orbital circulations. Measurement of retinal artery pressure may be

region of the midbrain, posterior thalamus, choroid plexus in the lateral ventricle, medial and lateral genulate bodies, fornices, and the posterior limb of the internal capsule.

The cortical branches supply the inferior half of the inferior temporal gyrus, medial surface of the fusiform gyri and the lingual, cuneus, and quadrate gyri. The posterior occipital artery runs in the calcarine fissure to supply the posteromedial and inferior portions of the occipital lobe, particularly the lingual lobule and the cuneus.

An extensive collateral system forms anastomoses between the external and internal carotid circulations as well as between the anterior and posterior portions of the intracranial circulation (4). The external carotid artery provides collateral branches through the orbit and skull base. These include the angular branch of the external maxillary artery, the sphenopalatine and infraorbital branches of the internal maxillary arteries, and the frontal branch of the superficial temporal artery. All of these join branches of the ophthalmic artery. Around the region of the petrous bone, small branches of the external carotid artery form connections with the labyrinthine branches of the basilar artery and the tympanic branches of the internal carotid artery.

The circle of Willis forms the major intracranial anastomosis and allows communication between the right and left hemispheres and between the anterior and posterior circulations. The circle of Willis consists of the anterior communicating artery connecting both anterior cerebral arteries and the A-1 portions of the anterior cerebral arteries. The posterior communicating arteries and the segment of the internal carotid artery distal to their origin as well as the proximal portion of the posterior cerebral arteries complete the circle. There are many variations in the diameter and length of each of the components of the circle of Willis. Intracranial flow dynamics may be markedly influenced by the patency of this system in the presence of more proximal occlusive lesions (5).

The leptomeningeal extensions of the major intracranial arteries and their branches can be divided into paramedian, short circumferential, and long circumferential arteries. Paramedian arteries penetrate the cerebral parenchyma after a short course. The short circumferential arteries run further before ending in penetrating arteries, and the long circumferential arteries irrigate the surface of the cerebral hemispheres, the cerebellum, and the dorsal surface of the brain stem. The leptomeningeal arteries course along the surface of the brain and form extensive precapillary and capillary anastomoses among themselves. There are extensive connections between the anterior and middle cerebral arteries, between the middle cerebral and posterior cerebral arteries, and between the anterior and posterior cerebral arteries. These anastomoses are important in the presence of more proximal occlusions.

The venous drainage of the cortex and subcortex of the hemisphere is via the cortical veins, which drain into the veins of Trolard and Labbé laterally and inferiorly and via the superior sagittal sinus medially and superiorly (Fig. 2.2). The deep gray nuclei are drained along periependymal veins into the basal veins of Rosenthal and the vein of Galen, which makes its way to the straight sinus and

A

B

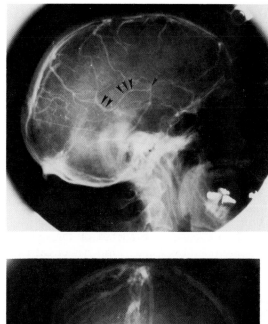

Figure 2.2 (*A*) Carotid angiogram, lateral view. During the late venous phase the cortical draining veins toward the sagittal sinus are seen. The vein of Galen (*double arrow*) and internal cerebral veins (*triple arrow*) are the major components of the deep venous drainage system, and these are also seen. The thalamostriate vein and internal cerebral vein join anteriorly to mark the position of the foramen of Monro (*single arrow*), which is posterior and superior to the sella turcica. (*B*) Carotid angiogram, anteroposterior view, late venous phase, which demonstrates some of the superficial cortical drainage to the sagittal sinus as well as components of the deep venous drainage system.

torcula to join the superior sagittal sinus. The lateral sinuses drain into the sigmoid sinus and internal jugular veins. The posterior fossa drainage is more variable, with drainage from cerebellar and basilar plexi into the sigmoid sinus.

CEREBRAL BLOOD FLOW AND METABOLISM

Measurement Techniques

Various methods are available for measuring cerebral blood flow (CBF). The most practical of these are based on the Fick principle, which is a restatement of the law of conservation of matter. As applied to CBF measurements, the amount of indicator taken up by the brain is equal to the amount brought to it less the amount carried away from it (6). Techniques have been developed to measure average CBF per unit volume of brain, total CBF, and regional CBF. Indicator dilution techniques have also been developed to measure total CBF (7). In patients, the most practical methods involve measuring the washout of an isotope that has been administered in sufficient quantity to saturate the brain. An isotope such as xenon 133, which is chemically inert, is diffusible between blood and brain at a known partition coefficient. Following administration to the patient, the rate of washout of such a material will be directly related to the rate of brain blood flow. The rate of change of concentration in the brain can be measured by external detection of radioactivity and is directly related to the blood flow rate in the field of the detector. CBF can be calculated from:

$$CBF = \lambda \frac{H}{A}$$

where λ is the tissue partition coefficient, H is the height of the concentration curve at saturation, and A is the area under the washout curve. Collimated detectors are now routinely used to measure blood flow from multiple regions of the brain. These regional studies provide information regarding the topographic distribution of blood flow rates in health and disease.

The rate of consumption or production of any metabolically active substance (X) by the brain can be calculated (8) from knowledge of the arteriovenous difference of the substance across the brain and the brain-blood flow rate, or:

$$CMR (X) = CBF [A\text{-}V (X)]$$

where CMR is the cerebral metabolic rate and A-V is arteriovenous difference. The normal CMR for oxygen ($CMRO_2$) varies from 1.33 to 1.74 μ mole per gram and that for glucose (CMR glu) from 4.48 to 6.5 mg/100 gm/min.

Consumption rates vary in different regions of the brain in relation to regional levels of electrophysiologic activity. Cerebral metabolic rates for consumption of glucose and oxygen can be measured in specific regions of the brain with positron emission tomography. This approach exploits the properties of certain positron-emitting isotopes to release oppositely directed gamma rays. Annihilation photons are recorded by a series of paired detectors that use coincidence counting and tomographic localization techniques to describe the distribution of positrons in small volumes of brain tissue (9). Local glucose consumption can be determined after the injection of 18-2-deoxy-2-fluoro-D-glucose and following of its concentration in arterial blood and in cerebral tissue over time. This substance crosses into cells and its further metabolism is arrested. Local oxygen consumption is determined from inhalation of $C^{15}O_2$ and $^{15}O_2$. The first isotope is converted to $H_2^{15}O$ in the lungs and distributed in relation to the CBF, while the second isotope is extracted from hemoglobin in relation to the rate of cerebral oxygen consumption.

PHYSIOLOGY

The physiologic responses of the cerebral circulation are based on general principles of hydrostatics and hydrodynamics. The pressure of a fluid in a rigid tube is described by Poiseuille's law of hydrodynamics, which states that

$$\Delta P = \frac{8L}{\pi r^4} \, FV$$

where ΔP is the pressure gradient, F is the flow rate, V is viscosity, L is length and r^4 is the radius of the tube. It should be noted that Poiseuille's law applies to newtonian fluids, which have a constant viscosity despite varying flow rates. Blood with its many components is not a newtonian fluid, and its viscosity varies with the flow rate as well as with changes of hematocrit, plasma proteins, and water content. The pulsatile nature of arterial flow also results in deviations from Poiseuille's law. Blood flow in vessels may be either laminar or turbulent, as described by the Reynolds number and given by the equation:

$$R = \frac{UDP}{V}$$

where U is linear velocity, D is the cross-sectional area, P is the density, and V is viscosity. At a Reynolds number between 1000 and 2000 the flow of a newtonian fluid is likely to become turbulent.

Factors Affecting CBF

CBF is directly related to the perfusion pressure across the brain and inversely related to the cerebrovascular resistance. Cerebrovascular resistance may fluctuate with changes in arterial caliber and usually is derived quantitatively from the CBF and perfusion pressure.

Perfusion Pressure

Perfusion pressure is derived clinically from the difference between arterial and venous or intracranial pressure. A small gradient normally exists between systemic and pial arterial pressures so that use of systemic pressure may overestimate the perfusion pressure (10). Since blood pressure changes continually during the cardiac cycle, mean pressure is used as an approximation.

Changes in perfusion pressure do not normally result in changes in CBF. This autoregulation of blood flow is normally effective between mean blood pressure values of 60 and 160 mm Hg. Increased perfusion pressure induces arterial vasoconstriction, and a decrease in perfusion pressure causes vasodilation. These compensatory changes of cerebrovascular resistance tend to maintain blood flow near normal (11,12). It is unclear how changes of perfusion pressure produce this effect, but increased transluminal pressure differences may induce contraction of vascular smooth muscle. If vasoparalysis occurs (e.g., vasodilation in response to carbon dioxide), then the autoregulatory mechanism becomes less effective and blood flow varies directly with perfusion pressure. Autoregulation may be impaired by many general anesthetic agents (13,14) and vasoactive drugs (15).

Moderate changes of venous or intracranial pressure normally do not influence CBF. Occasionally, venous pressure is markedly raised in conditions such as right heart failure or obstruction of the superior vena cava. This may lower cerebral perfusion pressures sufficiently to reduce CBF.

Cerebrovascular Resistance

Alterations in the proportion of solid and liquid components of blood affect its viscosity and thereby alter cerebrovascular resistance (16). Changes in arterial diameter, however, are more frequent and a more important mechanism for regulating cerebrovascular resistance and CBF. Since flow is related to the fourth power of the vessel radius, relatively small changes in vascular diameter affect the blood flow rate. Changes in arterial diameter and cerebrovascular resistance are produced by a variety of functional, chemical, neurogenic, and environmental stimuli.

Functional Activity

Regional studies have shown that CBF is responsive to the functional needs of the brain. Visual stimulation produces increases of occipital CBF (17), exercise is associated with hyperemia near the contralateral motor cortex, and sensory stimulation is followed by hyperemia in the postcentral gyrus area (18). CBF is increased in areas showing epileptic discharges on the EEG and, conversely, CBF is slightly reduced over atrophic brain adjacent to epileptogenic lesions (19).

Carbon Dioxide

Carbon dioxide is one of the most potent cerebrovasodilator agents known. Whether it acts directly on smooth muscle cells or acts by changing intracellular pH is unclear. The linear relationship of carbon dioxide and CBF was described by Reivich (20), who found that the CBF response to arterial carbon dioxide tension ($PaCO_2$) varied beween 0.95 and 1.75 ml/min/100g brain tissue/mm Hg change in $PaCO_2$. The greatest sensitivity to carbon dioxide occurs near normal $PaCO_2$ levels, and changes in CBF can be readily induced by altering ventilatory patterns. This relationship between carbon dioxide and CBF requires specification of the $PaCO_2$ level at which CBF is measured. CBF may be raised from 25 ml/100g/min at a $PaCO_2$ of 35 mm Hg to 50 ml/100g/min at a $PaCO_2$ of 45 mm Hg and to 75 ml/100g/min at a $PaCO_2$ of 55 mm Hg. If hypercapnia is maintained, CBF levels will tend to revert to normal. Carbon dioxide, therefore, influences but does not control the steady-state CBF level. Since carbon dioxide is the major byproduct of oxidative metabolism, it also provides a feedback mechanism by which the rate of blood flow is influenced by the rate of metabolism. As the metabolic rate is increased, the production of carbon dioxide in tissue induces vasodilation and increases CBF. The resulting hyperemia increases the supply of nutrients and clears lactate and hydrogen ion from the extracellular space.

Hydrogen Ion Concentration

Mild cerebral vasodilation is produced by acidosis (21), and mild vasoconstriction is produced by alkalosis (22). Patients in diabetic acidosis have a CBF 20% greater than normal despite a markedly reduced $PaCO_2$ (23). Several studies (24,25) have examined the effect of simultaneous changes in $PaCO_2$ and pH. A mild change in arterial pH may not affect cerebral hemodynamics, but a marked pH change, as in severe metabolic acidosis, will have a predominant influence on cerebrovascular tone and increase CBF.

Oxygen

Mild to moderate changes in arterial oxygen tension (PaO_2) near the physiologic range are not potent stimuli to change in CBF. Reductions in PaO_2 to levels near 50 mm Hg and arterial oxygen saturation down to 40% to 50% are required to produce arteriolar dilation and an increase of CBF. If the oxygen concentration in the inspired air mixture is reduced to 8% while maintaining constant $PaCO_2$ levels, CBF will increase by 36% (26). At these oxygen levels there is also significant alteration of cerebral glucose metabolism consisting of a 28% increase in glucose uptake, a 16% reduction in aerobic metabolism, and a 14% increase in anaerobic metabolism (27). Conversion to anaerobic metabolism may be the stimulus for increased CBF levels. There is conflicting evidence regarding the effect of moderately elevated oxygen tension on the cerebral circulation, but the effects of hyperbaric oxygen are more apparent. Thus inhalation of 85% to 100% oxygen had no significant effect on CBF (28), while oxygen at 3.5 atm reduced CBF by 25%. In another study, oxygen at 2.0 atm produced a 21% decrease in cortical blood flow (29).

The relative effectiveness with which oxygen and carbon dioxide influence the cerebral circulation varies therefore with the tension of the gas under consideration. At near normal ranges relatively small changes in $PaCO_2$ exert the predominant effect. The responses of the cerebral circulation are, however, minimal at $PaCO_2$ levels below 20 mm Hg or above 100 mm Hg. Changes in inspired oxygen between 30% and 100% result in relatively small CBF changes, while PaO_2 below 50 mm Hg or above 1 atm result in large changes of CBF (30).

Neurogenic Factors

The cerebral circulation has a rich innervation whose functional significance is still unclear. Fluorescence staining techniques and electron microscopic study have identified adrenergic nerve fibers on arterioles as small as 10 to 15 μ less in diameter. Some of these fibers, however, originate in the locus ceruleus and are independent of peripheral sympathetic ganglia that supply the extracranial carotid and vertebral arteries. Vasoconstriction appears to be mediated by norepinephrine, while α-adrenergic blocking agents eliminate this effect. Stimulation of cervical sympathetic fibers in various species have produced variable reductions of flow in the internal carotid, external carotid, and vertebral arteries (31) as well as a reduction in cortical and hypothalamic blood flow, while no change in flow occurred in the medulla and pons (32). This neural activity may also influence the response of CBF to carbon dioxide and blood pressure changes (33). Other studies indicate that sympathetic nerves limit and further modulate vasomotor responses to both carbon dioxide and oxygen (34). When the superior cervical ganglion was interrupted, CBF responses to carbon dioxide were increased, and when the parasympathetic supply was interrupted the response to carbon dioxide was decreased. Sudden surges in perfusion pressure may also be dampened by neurogenically mediated vasoconstriction. When vasodilator nerves were blocked with atropine, cerebral vasodilation did not occur with induced hypotension.

Body Temperature

When body temperature is lowered there is a corresponding fall in CBF. Several factors may contribute to this. As temperature falls, blood viscosity increases (16), and cardiac output and cerebral perfusion may simultaneously decrease. Blood pH also tends to rise because of a change in the pK of the carbonic acid equilibrium reaction (i.e., the point at which half neutralization has occurred) (35). One of the more important effects of hypothermia is to reduce the rate of cerebral oxygen consumption. This results in reduced tissue P_{CO_2}, which also will lower CBF. Increasing body temperature does not increase CBF until a temperature of 39.4°C is reached. Further increases in temperature result in increases in CBF of 30% to 50% at 42°C (36). Beyond these temperature levels, however, both CBF and $CMRO_2$ rapidly decline.

Intracranial Pressure

The difference between intraluminal pressure and intracranial pressure (ICP)—the transmural pressure difference—critically affects arteriolar tone. A rise in ICP reduces cerebral perfusion pressure in a manner equivalent to a drop in blood pressure and results in compensatory vasodilation. Studies (37) in subjects with intracranial hypertension, however, reveal that overall cerebrovascular resistance is increased. The hemodynamic responses to intracranial hypertension are further complicated by a compensatory increase in mean arterial pressure. There usually is little change in CBF levels until ICP reaches 35 mm Hg, although autoregulation already may be impaired at lower levels of ICP.

Tissue Nutrition

The transport of oxygen from hemoglobin in the capillaries to tissue is dependent on the unloading of hemoglobin and diffusion. Oxygen transport within brain tissue is limited by diffusion and therefore is dependent on the concentration gradient between arteriolar and cellular oxygen. Oxidative metabolism may be maintained in vitro with as little as 0.5 mm Hg of oxygen in the medium. While a similarly low oxygen concentration may be required in vivo, a large gradient is required to ensure these levels. In contrast, a carrier-mediated transport mechanism is involved in the transport of glucose between blood and brain tissue as well as between blood and cerebrospinal fluid (CSF). The next flux of glucose depends on the glucose concentration gradient between blood and brain, the constants for the carrier (38), and the maximal flux rate at saturation. If glucose is metabolized more quickly or the coefficients for carrier transport are changed by hormonal action, the net flux of glucose will change correspondingly.

Oxidative metabolism allows the cell to derive energy in the form of 38 moles of adenosine triphosphate (ATP) from one mole of glucose. The initial steps of glycolysis occur in the cytoplasm, where glucose is broken down to the three-carbon moiety lactate. In the presence of oxygen, lactate is converted to pyruvate, which then can undergo further oxidation to carbon dioxide and water in the mitochondria through the tricarboxylic acid cycle. This cycle regenerates oxaloacetic acid and so may provide for the oxidation of an unlimited amount of acetyl groups from pyruvate, fatty acids, amino acids, and ketone bodies. The various changes in configuration of the three-carbon moiety in the tricarboxylic acid cycle provide reducing equivalent to the mitochondrial electron transport chain. The chain is composed of a series of coenzymes, beginning with nicotinamide adenine dinucleotide (NADH), which pass these reducing equivalents along to oxygen. This orderly passage along the chain, with increases in oxidation reduction potential, allows conversion of adenosine diphosphate (ADP) to ATP at three sites. By this means, the potential energy difference between hydrogen in glucose and in water is converted to high-energy ATP. A decrease in oxygen levels below a critical threshold will reduce energy production within the mitochondria. Lactate will accumulate within the cytoplasm, leading to cellular and extracellular acidosis.

Several studies have shown that mild hypoxic insults severe enough to cause neural dysfunction may be associated with normal rates of energy metabolism and normal levels of ATP. Oxygen is required also for the production of brain monoamines. Tyrosine and tryptophan hydroxylase, which are rate-limiting enzymes in the production of brain monoamines, have 50 to 100 times less affinity for oxygen than mitochondrial coenzymes. The early disturbances of electrophysiologic function may be related to abnormalities in neurotransmitter metabolism, and neurotransmitter synthesis may be more vulnerable to mild degrees of hypoxia (39,40).

PATHOPHYSIOLOGY

The neuroanesthesiologist is called upon to deal with a variety of cerebral disorders, each of which may affect CBF and metabolism. Before describing deviations of CBF and metabolism as pathologic, certain variations from normal should be considered.

CBF normally declines from childhood to adult life. Kety (41) determined that there was a steady decline in both CBF and cerebral oxygen uptake from childhood through adult life and in the aged; however, significant decreases in both CBF and metabolism have been found in patients with evidence of dementia. When older patients were carefully selected for the absence of evidence of either dementia or cerebrovascular disease, CBF values were 860 ml/min, mean $CMRO_2$ was 3.33 ml/100g/min, and mean cerebral vascular resistance was 1.53 mm Hg/ml/100g/min (42). These values are similar to those reported for normal young adults (6). According to Lassen, Feinberg, and Lane (43), healthy elderly subjects had a 9% reduction in $CMRO_2$ but no significant reduction in CBF.

Cerebrovascular Disease

In patients with cerebrovascular disease, the effects on cerebral blood flow and metabolism depend on the severity and duration of the ischemic insult and the potential for compensatory collateral blood flow. When CBF is measured with the ^{133}Xe washout method, assumptions regarding the tissue/blood partition coefficient may be in error, and these errors may account for the disparate values for CBF obtained in different studies. In patients with transient ischemic attacks, interictal measurement of CBF usually is normal, although regional decrease in CBF has been found for up to one day following these attacks (44). In patients who survive a cerebral infarction there often are areas of focal decrease in CBF and metabolism corresponding to the areas of the infarct, while there may be enhanced perfusion in the surrounding areas. This has been consistently demonstrated after middle cerebral artery occlusion (45). This "luxury perfusion" phenomenon may be related to an accumulation of acid metabolites diffusing from ischemic tissue (46). Ischemia generally leads to failure of most cerebrovascular regulatory mechanisms. Autoregulatory mechanisms may be severely impaired, and blood flow may become pressure dependent within these areas (47). Arteries injured by the ischemic process may lose carbon dioxide reactivity. Under such conditions, attempts to augment CBF by increasing $PaCO_2$ may lead to dilation of arterioles in relatively normal areas with retained reactivity. Intracerebral steal may then develop and divert flow to a greater extent from the ischemic areas (48). Hypocapnia also has been suggested to favor flow into the ischemic areas; however, this situation produces an overall decrease in CBF (49).

Regional ischemia usually is caused by focal occlusive or stenotic arterial lesions. A generalized decrease in perfusion occasionally will result in regional ischemia in so-called watershed zones at the periphery of an arterial territory. Resulting neurologic deficits may vary from transient ischemic attacks to completed strokes, depending on the severity and duration of ischemia. Regions of the brain with higher metabolic rates are more vulnerable to ischemia than regions of lower metabolic rate. After cardiac arrest, cortical tissue (gray matter) is more severely affected than white matter, while the brain stem is relatively resistant (8). There also is selective vulnerability with regard to cell types and subcellular structures. Astrocytes show early swelling of their footplates before neuronal changes are evident and synaptic vesicles are damaged, while mitochondria remain unchanged (50). Changes in membrane transport activities are altered when the $Na^+ + K^+$-ATPase transport system is not resupplied with high-energy phosphates. Potassium may then leak into the extracellular space while sodium and chloride move intracellularly. Cerebral edema and impaired nerve conduction rapidly follow (51). Synthesis, storage release, and uptake of neurotransmitters are sensitive to ischemia. Therefore, neurotransmission between cells, and neural conduction along the soma and axons, are impaired as shown by flattening of the EEG and loss of evoked potentials. In areas of severe ischemia and infarction, the brain may autodigest by metabolizing its own lipids, keto-acids, and proteins (52).

Cerebrovascular surgical procedures are designed to reduce the risk of completed stroke in patients at risk, or to enhance recovery of neurologic function in patients who have progressive cerebrovascular insufficiency. Arteriography will identify specific occlusive lesions in either the extracranial or intracranial arteries. Carotid endarterectomy is appropriate for patients who have symptoms related to a hemodynamically significant stenosis or to an ulcerative plaque near the carotid bifurcation. Interruption of blood flow during clamping for endarterectomy is associated with a risk of cerebral ischemia. The adequacy of collateral perfusion during clamping has been assessed in a variety of ways. Sundt and co-workers (53) have described the use of ^{133}Xe washout methods to assess residual flow after carotid clamping. Simultaneous EEG studies allowed the definition of a CBF threshold of 18 to 20 ml/100 gm/min, below which EEG flattening can be predicted. We found that carotid clamping after bolus injection significantly alters the steady state required for washout techniques. EEG and stump pressure measurements have been used to assess the risks of carotid clamping and the necessity for an intraoperative shunt (54). In 52 of 380 patients subjected to endarterectomy, mean stump pressure was less than 50% of baseline pressure. EEG changes were found in 56 of 275 patients studied, but only 27 of these patients had changes considered to be of an ischemic nature. Based on EEG or stump pressure criteria, internal shunts were used in 59 patients.

Intracranial occlusive or stenotic lesions may reduce cortical artery pressure depending on the location and severity of the lesion and the contribution of collateral pathways (55). Abnormalities of NADH kinetics have been found in patients with transient ischemic attacks (56), implying that in such patients there is a limited cerebrovascular reserve during periods of increased electrophysiologic activity. Of 290 patients who had extracranial-intracranial (EC-IC) bypass, the transcranial pressure gradient between the superficial temporal artery and the cortical branch of the middle cerebral artery varied between 7 and 64 mm Hg. This gradient generally was related to the degree of perfusion of the middle cerebral territory found on a postoperative angiogram performed one week to three years postoperatively (57).

Arterial Hypertension

The effects of hypertension on the cerebrovascular systems become more significant as the disease progresses. The morphologic changes associated with hypertension include fibrinoid necrosis and lipohyalinosis of intracerebral arteries. CBF and $CMRO_2$ are not altered in the vast majority of hypertensive patients (58), although cerebral vascular resistance may be significantly elevated. In the normal brain a pressure head of 1.6 mm Hg is necessary to produce a flow of 1 ml/100g/min. In the hypertensive patient a pressure head of approximately 3 mm Hg may be required to achieve the same flow (59). Significant alteration of cerebrovascular reactivity has been found in hypertension (60). The normal relationship between pressure and flow is reset so that the lower limits of autoregulation may be raised. Measurements of cortical artery pressure in patients undergoing aneurysm surgery suggest that the critical closing pressure for pial arteries in hypertensive patients is near 40 mm Hg. In normotensive patients this is closer to 20 mm Hg (10). Decreases in flow which are significant occur before the critical closing pressure is reached.

Subarachnoid Hemorrhage

Subarachnoid hemorrhage (SAH) often is associated with major disturbances of CBF and metabolism. After SAH, vasospasm is found on angiography in 30% of patients. Under such conditions the resting level of CBF may be reduced below critical thresholds, resulting in ischemic infarction. We (61) demonstrated that autoregulation of blood flow to hypertensive stimuli was impaired and related this to the increased tone resulting from vasospasm that persists over a wider range of perfusion pressure. Significant disturbances of oxidative metabolism were found after SAH (62). A primary depression of oxidative metabolism with a secondary depression of CBF was found when ICP and perfusion pressures were normal. With increased ICP, ischemia resulted in a secondary shift to anaerobic metabolism. Ten days to two weeks after SAH, myonecrosis of medium-sized pial arteries was found (63). Grubb and associates (64) used positron emission tomography to study a group of patients after SAH. They demonstrated an increase in cerebral blood volume, probably related to a proximal pial arterial vasoconstriction.

Hydrocephalus

Acute obstructive hydrocephalus produced experimentally results in a significant decrease in CBF when CSF pressure reaches 20 to 25 mm Hg (65). This affects blood flow in the cerebral hemispheres most markedly, although the entire brain is involved. Mathew and colleagues (66) found that regional cerebral blood flow (rCBF) was focally reduced in 15 patients with normal pressure hydrocephalus, particularly in areas irrigated by the anterior cerebral arteries. The patients were then subjected to lumbar puncture. A correlation between the increases in rCBF values and clinical improvement was found. There also is evidence that both CBF and CBF reserve is limited in hydrocephalic patients (67).

Intracranial Hypertension

In a study by Grossman and associates (68), the effect of increased ICP on direct cortical response amplitude was more closely related to cerebral perfusion pressure (CPP) and CBF than to the ICP per se. Focal increases in ICP produced by a brain retractor result in flow changes in both the ipsilateral retracted hemisphere and the contralateral hemisphere (69). These effects on blood flow are thought to underlie the electrophysiologic dysfunction induced by elevated ICP. It is unclear how these blood flow changes interfere with electrophysiologic dysfunction since Schutz and co-workers (70) were unable to find deterioration of mitochondrial function even after 40 minutes of compression ischemia. Ljunggren and colleagues (71) found that complete cerebral ischemia induced by an increase in the intracranial CSF pressure produced depletion of energy-rich compounds. This was followed by complete restitution in the postischemic period when reflow was established.

Head Injury

Cerebral blood vessels undergo a wide range of responses after head injury. Resistance vessels may constrict in vasospasm or may dilate, producing vasomotor paralysis. Stasis may lead to exacerbation of cerebral edema, compression of the microcirculation, and further reduction of CBF. Dissociation of the autoregulatory response to changes in blood pressure and the response to carbon dioxide is a common finding after all types of head injury (72). Pulmonary complications are frequent and are related to intracranial damage and to inexpert first aid. Poor ventilation further decreases tissue oxygenation, and hypercapnia aggravates the effects of cerebral edema.

In pediatric patients, brain swelling associated with hyperemia is common. Bruce and co-workers (73) found a poor correlation between hemispheric CBF values and the neurologic status of comatose patients after head injury.

After most closed head injuries there also are substantial disturbances of cerebral metabolism. In a significant number of adult patients, uncoupling of CBF and metabolism occurs (74), with a CBF that is high in relation to metabolic demand. In some patients in whom blood flow is below normal, similar reduction of metabolism occurs.

NEUROANESTHESIA AND THE CEREBRAL CIRCULATION

Most anesthetic techniques profoundly affect CBF and metabolism either directly or indirectly. Anesthetic drugs may have direct vasomotor properties, while intubation may affect CBF by increasing ICP.

Volatile inhalational agents (e.g., halothane) often produce vasodilation and dissociation of CBF and $CMRO_2$, with increase of the former and decrease of the latter. In contrast, intravenous agents, such as barbiturates and Althesin, more often result in vasoconstriction and changes in CBF and $CMRO_2$, which are linked. When both types of anesthesia are used, the effects of each are modified. Combinations of nitrous oxide and 0.5% halothane preceded by induction of anesthesia with sodium thiopental, 4 mg/kg, and hypocapnia result in close association between CBF and $CMRO_2$ (13).

Intravenous Agents

Barbiturates

Barbiturates have been used in the treatment of both stroke and trauma. The suppression of electrophysiologic activity seen with barbiturates results in a decreased metabolic rate and CBF rate. Kassell and co-workers (75) determined that the optimum effects of sodium thiopental were reached when EEG burst suppression of 30 to 60 seconds was achieved. Additional barbiturates resulted in decreased blood pressure and cardiac output. Doses of 50, 150, and 250 mg of phenobarbital cause progressive reductions in $CMRO_2$ and CBF to 50% of normal (76). Hawkins and colleagues (77) described a reduction of CMRglu of 45% in anesthetized animals compared to the CMRglu in conscious animals. Siesjö found a greater reduction in CMRglu during barbiturate anesthesia (78). The specificity of action of phenobarbital was shown by selective suppression in the incorporation of 14C-labeled glucose into neuronal cells (79) while incorporation of 14C-labeled butyrate into glial cells was unaffected (80).

Fentanyl and Droperidol

Michenfelder and Theye (14) studied the effects of fentanyl and droperidol and their combination by the venous outflow technique. Droperidol was found to cause a 40% reduction in CBF but no change in $CMRO_2$. Fentanyl reduced CBF by the same amount but also produced an 18% decrease in $CMRO_2$. The combination of the two drugs reduced CBF by 50% and $CMRO_2$ by 23%. These experiments were repeated by Nilsson and Siesjö (76), who achieved the same results with regard to CBF but found that neither fentanyl nor droperidol lowered $CMRO_2$ significantly.

Ketamine

Ketamine acts by inducing a disorganized excitation of limbic and thalamocortical systems and spike-wave complexes, or even florid seizure activity, on EEG. In one experimental study, a decrease in CBF and no change in $CMRO_2$ followed ketamine administration (81); however, Dawson, Michenfelder, and Theye (82), found a transient increase of CBF to 180% of normal and of $CMRO_2$ to 116% of normal. Takeshita, Okuda, and Sari (83) found that ketamine administered to patients resulted in an increase in CBF to 170% of normal without a significant change in $CMRO_2$.

Inhalational Agents

Nitrous Oxide

When administered in a concentration of 70%, nitrous oxide provides analgesia and amnesia. The agent tends to increase ICP, and it has been suggested that the mechanism for this effect may be due to an increase in CBF. Laitinin, Johansson, and Tarkhanen (84) reported a considerable increase in the impedance amplitudes of brain when nitrous oxide is given, indicating an increased pulse amplitude of the cerebral vasculature. A marked increase in ICP occurred in patients with intracranial disorders when anesthesia was induced with 66% nitrous oxide (85).

Earlier studies by Smith and Wollman (86) showed that 70% nitrous oxide had little effect on CBF but reduced $CMRO_2$ by as much as 23%. Theye and Michenfelder (87), on the other hand, demonstrated an 11% increase in $CMRO_2$ in dogs. Carlsson, Hagerdal, and Siesjö (88) evaluated the role of stress responses when nitrous oxide is the primary agent. Using more suitable control experiments, which included a group of adrenalectomized animals and a group of animals given the beta receptor blocker propranolol, they found no significant differences in $CMRO_2$ or CBF in animals inhaling 70% nitrous oxide or 70% nitrogen.

Halothane

Halothane, a complete anesthetic, acts to depress cerebral function and metabolism in a dose-dependent fashion. In an earlier clinical study by Cohen and colleagues (89), 1% halothane was reported to reduce $CMRO_2$ by 15%. In experiments reported by McHenry and associates (90) and Christensen, Holdt-Rasmussen, and Lassen (91), 1% halothane was reported to reduce $CMRO_2$ by as much as 75%. Experimental studies have all found a reduction in $CMRO_2$, although quantitative differences were found. McDowell (92) used 0.5% and 2% halothane in 70% nitrous oxide and found that $CMRO_2$ was reduced to 70% and 80%, respectively, of resting values. Keaney and co-workers (93) found that $CMRO_2$ was reduced by 30% when halothane concentration was increased from 0.31% to 1.16%. Theye and Michenfelder (94) were able to reduce $CMRO_2$ by 17% when halothane concentration was increased from 0.1% to 0.5%. Further increases in halothane concentration were studied during cardiovascular support for extracorporeal circulation. With concentrations above 2% there was progressive lowering of $CMRO_2$—even after electrocerebral silence developed on the EEG.

Enflurane

Enflurane, developed in 1963, is compatible with catecholamines and is associated with a stable heart rhythm and excellent muscle relaxation. Although it is a widely used anesthetic, its use in neuroanesthesia is limited. EEG changes consistent with epileptiform activity occur at deeper planes of anesthesia, especially in the presence of alkalosis. In the absence of epileptiform activity, 2% to 3.2% enflurane will reduce $CMRO_2$ by 33% to 50% (86). Michenfelder and Cucchiara (95) found a reduction in $CMRO_2$ in an experimental dog preparation. With the onset of seizure activity on the EEG, however, there is a significant increase in $CMRO_2$.

Isoflurane

Isoflurane was initially introduced in 1965 but has only recently become widely available. It is nonflammable and stable, and its low solubility in blood permits the anesthetic level to be adjusted rapidly and allows rapid recovery when the anesthetic is discontinued. It does not appear to cause renal or hepatic abnormalities. At levels well below minimum alveolar concentration (MAC), isoflurane increases EEG frequency from a range of 8 to 12 Hz to greater than 15 Hz (96). As the anesthetic concentration increases to 40% of MAC, voltage fluctuations shift from posterior to anterior portions of the cerebral hemispheres. As MAC is approached, higher voltage and lower frequencies are seen. At 1.5 MAC, burst suppression appears on the EEG.

In volunteers paralyzed with d-tubocurarine and with blood pressures kept at normal levels with phenylephrine, isoflurane at concentrations of 0.6 and 1.1 MAC did not alter CBF (97). At 1.6 MAC, however, CBF doubled. One study in dogs (98) demonstrated increased blood flow. An experimental study by Cucchiara, Theye, and Michenfelder (99) showed that, as in the human studies, no changes in blood flow occurred at 1 MAC, but blood flow increased by 60% at 1.7 MAC. A decrease in $CMRO_2$ using isoflurane has been demonstrated by Murphy and co-workers (100). Isoflurane can increase CBF at higher concentrations, and an increase in ICP also may be seen. Adams and associates (101) and Schettini and Mahig (102) found that hyperventilation effectively prevented the associated increase in ICP.

Diethyl Ether

Although ether has been replaced by the agents described above, its effects on cerebral function and metabolism are of interest. Ether tends to produce a sympathomimetic effect with cerebral excitation and in sufficient concentrations may induce seizure activity on the EEG. Smith and Wollman (86) found that 2.4% ether resulted in little CBF change but produced a 34% reduction in $CMRO_2$. When ether concentration was increased to 4.5%, CBF increased and $CMRO_2$ returned toward baseline levels. The effect of 4.5% ether was related to increasing levels of circulating catecholamines.

Cyclopropane

Cyclopropane administration results in generalized EEG slowing; however, brain-stem arousal systems are activated (103). Increasing concentrations of cyclopropane (5% to 37%) produced biphasic effects on CBF. CBF decreased with concentrations of 5% to 13%, but increased with 20% and 37% cyclopropane. The role of sympathetic activation after administration of cyclopropane was clarified by Michenfelder and Theye (104), who studied varying doses of cyclopropane in control, reserpinized, or spinal anesthetic preparations. The results suggest that deep anesthesia is possible without a permanent effect on $CMRO_2$. This is in contrast to the results of Smith and colleagues (105), who found that 5% and 20% cyclopropane reduced $CMRO_2$.

Positioning during Surgery

A temporary reduction in CBF of 20% has been found when patients are moved from the supine to the standing position (106). Significant readjustments of total body blood volume are associated with these changes, including pooling of 300 to 1000 ml of blood in the legs owing to a decrease in venous return and cardiac output (107). Rapid rotation flexion or extension of the head may reduce blood flow in the carotid arteries or, more significantly, in the vertebral arteries (108).

Although most patients tolerate the sitting position, a combination of cerebrovascular disease, relative hypocapnia, and deep anesthesia may compromise CBF. Tindall, Craddock, and Greenfield (109) measured blood flow in the internal carotid artery with patients in the supine and then in the sitting position. Mean flow in the supine position was 141 ml/min. After two minutes in the sitting position there was an average flow decrease of 18% to 121 ml/min ($P < 0.05$). Cardiac output decreased from 4145 to 3401 ml/min ($P < 0.05$). The additive effects of anesthesia, hyperventilation, and the sitting position, however, resulted in an overall reduction of 36% in internal carotid flow compared to that obtained with the patient awake.

It is apparent that anesthetic agents and techniques may be appropriately manipulated to produce optimal outcome in the patient with actual or potentially altered intracranial dynamics. Clear understanding of the principles involved is essential to appropriate usage.

REFERENCES

1. Wallace S, Goldberg HI, Leeds NE: The cavernous branches of the internal carotid artery. Am J Roentgenol 1967;101:34–46.
2. Critchley M: The anterior cerebral artery and its syndromes. Brain 1930;53:120–165.
3. Thomas GI, Anderson KN, Hain RF: Significance of anomalous vertebral-basilar artery communications in operation on heart and great vessels. Surgery 1959;46: 747–757.
4. Van den Bergh R, Vander Eecken T: Anatomy and embryology of cerebral circulation, in Progress in brain research v. 30. Luyendijk W (ed): Elsevier Publishing Co., Amsterdam, 1968; pp 1–25.
5. Riggs HE, Rupp C: Variation in the form of circle of Willis. Arch Neurol 1963;8:8–14.
6. Kety SS, Schmidt CF: The nitrous oxide method for the quantitative determinations of cerebral blood flow in man: Theory, procedure and normal values. J Clin Invest 1948;27:478–483.
7. Kinsman JM, Moore JW, Hamilton WF: Studies on circulation. Injection method: Physical and mathematical considerations. Am J Physiol 1929;89:322–330.
    Himmich HE: Brain metabolism and cerebral disorders. Baltimore, Williams & Wilkins, 1951.
9. Kuhl DE, Edwards RA: Reorganizing data from transverse section scans of the brain using digital processing. Radiology 1968;91:975–983.
10. Fein J, Lipow K, Marmarou A: Cortical artery pressure measurements in normotensive and hypertensive aneurysm patients. J Neurosurg 1983;59:51–56.

11. Lassen N: Cerebral blood flow and oxygen consumption in man. Physiol Rev 1959;39:183–238.

12. Raichle ME, Stone HL: Cerebral blood flow autoregulation and graded hypercapnia. Eur Neurol 1971;6:1–5.

13. Bendtsen AO, Sorenson PM, Rosenorn J, et al. Additional reduction of CBF-$CMRO_2$ during halothane/nitrous oxide anesthesia by thiopental loading. J Cer Blood Flow Metab V1 (Suppl) 1981:409–410.

14. Michenfelder JD, Theye RA: Effects of fentanyl, droperidol and Innovar on canine cerebral metabolism and blood flow. Br J Anaesth 1971;43:630–636.

15. Heiss ND: Effects of drugs on cerebral blood flow in man. Ann Neurol 1979; 25:95–116.

16. Rand PW, Lacomebe E, Hunt HE, et al.: Viscosity of normal human blood under normothermic and hypothermia conditions. J Appl Physiol 1964;19:117–122.

17. Schmidt CF, Hendrix JP: The action of chemical substance on cerebral blood vessels. Res Publ Assoc Res Nerv Ment Dis 1938;8:229–276.

18. Olesen J: Contralateral focal increases of cerebral blood flow in man during arm work. Brain 1971;94:635–646.

19. Ingvar DH: rCBF in focal cortical epilepsy, in Langfitt T, McHenry LC, Reivich M, et al. (eds): Cerebral blood flow and metabolism. New York, Springer-Verlag, 1975, pp 361–364.

20. Reivich M: Arterial pCO_2 and cerebral hemodynamics. Am J Physiol 1964;206: 25–35.

21. Schmidt CF: The influences of cerebral blood flow on respiration. Am J Physiol 1928;84:202–259.

22. Wolff HG, Lennox WG: Cerebral circulation: The effect on pial vessels of variations in oxygen and CO_2 content of the blood. Arch Neurol Psychiatry 1930;23:1097–1120.

23. Kety SS, Polis BD, Nadler CS, et al.: The blood flow and oxygen consumption of the human brain in diabetic acidosis and coma. J Clin Invest 1948;27:500–510.

24. Harper AM, Bell RA: The effect of metabolic acidosis and alkalosis on the blood flow through the cerebral cortex. J Neurol Neurosurg Psychiatry 1963;26:341–344.

25. Lambertsen CJ, Semple SJ, Smythe MG, et al.: H+ and pCO_2 as chemical factors in respiratory and cerebral circulatory control. J Appl Physiol 1961;16:473–484.

26. Turner J, Lambersten CJ, Owens SG, et al.: Effect of .08 and .8 atmospheres of inspired PO_2 upon cerebral hemodynamics at a constant alveolar PCO_2 of 43 mm Hg. Fed Proc 1957;16:130.

27. Cohen PJ, Alexander SC, Smith TC, et al.: Effects of hypoxia and normocapnia on cerebral blood flow and metabolism in conscious man. J Appl Physiol 1967;23:183–189.

28. Kety SS, Schmidt CF: The effects of altered arterial tensions of carbon dioxide and oxygen on cerebral blood flow and cerebral oxygen consumption of normal young men. J Clin Invest 1948;27:484–492.

29. Jacobson I, Harper MB, McDowell DG: The effects of O_2 at 1 and 2 atmospheres on the blood flow and oxygen uptake of the cerebral cortex. Surg Gynecol Obstet 1964;119:737–742.

30. Noell W, Schneider H: Über die Durchblutung und die sauserstoffversorgung des Gehirns. IV. Die Rolle der Kohlensaure. Pfluegers Arch Ges Physiol 1944;247: 514–527.

31. Meyer JS, Yoshida K, Sakamoto K: Autonomous control of cerebral blood flow measured by electromagnetic flowmeters. Neurology (Minneap) 1967;17:638–648.

32.   Schmidt CF: The intrinsic regulation of the circulation in the parietal cortex of the cat. Am J Physiol 1936;114:572-585.

33.   Stone HL, Raichle ME, Hernandez M: Sympathetic innervation and carbon dioxide sensitivity, in Langfitt T, McHenry LC, Reivich M, et al. (eds): Cerebral circulation and metabolism. New York, Springer-Verlag, 1975, pp 428-430.

34.   James JM, Millar RA, Purves MJ: Observation on the extrinsic neural control of cerebral blood flow in the baboon. Circ Res 1969;25:77-93.

35.   Severinghaus J, Stupfel M, Bradley AF: Variations of serum carbonic acid pK with pH and temperature. J Appl Physiol 1956;9:197-200.

36.   Meyer JS, Handu J: Cerebral blood flow and metabolism during experimental hypothermia (fever). Minn Med 1967;50:37-44.

37.   Kety SS, Shenkin HA, Schmidt CF: The effects of increased intracranial pressure on cerebral circulatory functions in man. J Clin Invest 1948;27:493-499.

38.   Gilboe DD, Betz AL: Kinetics of glucose transport in the isolated dog brain. Am J Physiol 1970;219:774-778.

39.   Davis JN, Carlsson A: The effect of hypoxia on monoamine synthesis, levels and metabolism in rat brain. J Neurochem 1973;21:783-790.

40.   Davis JN, Carlsson A, MacMillian V, et al.: Brain tryptophan hydroxylation dependence on arterial oxygen tension. Science 1973;182:72-74.

41.   Kety SS: Human cerebral blood flow and oxygen consumption as related to aging. J Chronic Dis 1956;3:478-486.

42.   Dastur DK, et al.: Effects of aging on cerebral circulation and metabolism in man, in Birren J (ed): Human aging, a biological and behavioral study. Washington, US Department of Health, Education and Welfare, 1963.

43.   Lassen NA, Feinberg I, Lane MH: Bilateral studies of cerebral oxygen uptake in young and aged normal subjects. J Clin Invest 1960;39:491-500.

44.   Skinhoj JE, Hoedt-Rasmussen K, Paulson OB, et al.: Regional cerebral blood flow and its autoregulation in patients with transient local cerebral ischemic attacks. Neurology (Minneap) 1970;20:485-493.

45.   Paulson OB: Regional cerebral blood flow in apoplexy due to occlusion of the middle cerebral artery. Neurology (Minneap) 1970;20:63-77.

46.   Lassen NA: The luxury perfusion syndrome and its possible relation to acute metabolic acidosis localized within the brain. Lancet 1966;2:1113-1115.

47.   Fieschi CA, Agnoli A, Battistini N: Derangement of regional blood flow and of its regulatory mechanisms in acute cerebrovascular lesions. Neurology (Minneap) 1968;18:1166-1179.

48.   Fieschi CA, Agnoli A: Impairment of the regional vasomotor response of cerebral vessels to hypercarbia in vascular disease. Eur Neurol 1969;2:13-30.

49.   Christensen MS, Paulson OB, Olesen J, et al.: Cerebral apoplexy (stroke) treated with or without prolonged artificial hyperventilation. I. Cerebral circulation, clinical source and cause of death. Stroke 1973;4:568-619.

50.   Williams V, Grossman R: Ultrastructure of cortical bypass after failure of presynaptic activity in ischemia. Anat Rec 1972;166:131-141.

51.   Siesjo BK, Plum F: Pathophysiology of anoxic brain damage, in Gaull EG (ed): Biology of brain dysfunction, New York, Plenum Press, 1973, pp 319-372.

52.   Yatsu F: Membrane lipids and brain ischemia: Current concepts of cerebrovascular disease. Stroke 1974;9:5,19-22.

53.   Sundt TM Jr, Sharborough FW, Anderson RE, et al.: Cerebral blood flow

measurements and electroencephalograms during carotid endarterectomy. J Neurosurg 1974;41:310–320.

54. Fein JM: Carotid endarterectomy, in Fein J, Flamm E (eds): Cerebrovascular surgery. New York, Springer-Verlag, vol II, in press.

55. Fein JM, Lipow K: Cortical artery pressure studies in cerebrovascular occlusive disease. J Neurosurg, in press.

56. Fein JM, Olinger R: Cortical NADH kinetics in patients undergoing EC-IC bypass. Neurosurgery 1982;10:428–436.

57. Fein JM: Cortical artery pressure measurements during bypass surgery for aneurysm. Sixth International Symposium on Microsurgical Anastomoses for Cerebral Ischemia. Kyoto, Japan, Kyoto University, Sept 1982.

58. Hafkenschiel JH, Crompton CW, Friedland CK: Cerebral oxygen consumption in essential hypertension. J Clin Invest 1954;33:63–68.

59. Fazekas JF, Kleh J, Finnerty FA: Influence of age and vascular disease on cerebral hemodynamics and metabolism. Am J Med 1955;18:477–485.

60. Jones JV, Strandgaard S, MacKenzie ET, et al.: Autoregulation of cerebral blood flow in chronic hypertension, in Harper AM, Jennett WB, Miller JD, et al. (eds): Blood flow and metabolism in the brain. New York, Churchill Livingstone, 1975, pp. 510–514.

61. Fein J, Boulos R: Local cerebral blood flow in experimental middle cerebral artery vasospasm. J Neurosurg 1973;39:337–346.

62. Fein JM: Brain energetics and circulatory control after subarachnoid hemorrhage. J Neurosurg 1976;45:498–507.

63. Fein JM, Flor WJ, Cohan SM: Sequential changes in vascular ultrastructure in cerebral vasospasm: Myonecrosis of subarachnoid arteries. J Neurosurg 1974;41:49–58.

64. Grubb R, Raichle ME, Eichberg JO, et al.: Effects of subarachnoid hemorrhage on cerebral blood volume, blood flow and oxygen utilization in humans. J Neurosurg 1977;46:446–453.

65. DiMattio J, Hochwald GM, Mathan C: The effects of the hydrocephalic process on cerebral blood flow in the cat, in Langfitt T, McHenry L, Reivich M, et al. (eds): Cerebral circulation and metabolism. New York, Springer-Verlag, 1975, pp 223–227.

66. Mathew NT: The importance of CSF pressure gradients on cerebral blood flow, in Langfitt T, McHenry L, Reivich M, et al. (eds): Cerebral circulation and metabolism. New York, Springer-Verlag, 1973, pp. 238–240.

67. Salmon JH, Timperman AL: Cerebral blood flow in post-traumatic encephalopathy. The effect of ventriculo-atrial shunt. Neurology (Minneap) 1971;21:33–42.

68. Grossman RG, Turner JW, Miller JD, et al.: The relationship between cerebral electrical activity, cerebral perfusion pressure, and cerebral blood flow during increased intracranial pressure, in Langfitt T, McHenry L, Reivich M, et al. (eds): Cerebral blood flow and metabolism. New York, Springer-Verlag, 1975, pp 232–234.

69. Albin MS, Bunegin L, Helsel P, et al.: Intracranial pressure and regional cerebral blood flow responses to experimental brain retraction pressure, in Shulman K, Marmarou A, Miller J, et al. (eds): Intracranial pressure IV. New York, Springer-Verlag, 1980, pp 131–134.

70. Schutz H, Silverstein PR, Vapalahti M, et al.: The function of brain mitochondria after increased intracranial pressure, in Brock M, Dietz H (eds): Intracranial pressure. New York, Springer-Verlag, 1972, pp 96–100.

71. Ljunggren B, Granholm L, Schutz H, et al.: Energy state of the brain during and after compression ischemia, in Brock M, Dietz H (eds): Intracranial pressure. New York, Springer-Verlag, 1972, pp 90–95.

72. Enevoldsen EM, Jensen FT: Autoregulation and CO_2 responses of cerebral blood flow in patients with acute severe head injury. J Neurosurg 1978;48:689–703.

73. Bruce DA, Langfitt T, Miller JD, et al.: Regional cerebral blood flow, intracranial pressure, and brain metabolism in comatose patients. J Neurosurg 1973;38:131–144.

74. Obrist W, Generale T, Sigawa H, et al.: Uncoupling of cerebral blood flow and metabolism and acute head injury, in Gotoh F, Nagai H, Tazaki Y (eds): Cerebral blood flow and metabolism. Copenhagen, Munksgaard, 1979, pp 374–375.

75. Kassell NF, Hitchon PW, Gesh MK, et al.: High dose barbiturate therapy: 1. The effect of sodium thiopental on cerebral blood flow, oxygen metabolism and electrical activity. J Cereb Blood Flow Metab 1981;1 (suppl 1):411–412.

76. Nilsson L, Siesjö BK: The effect of phenobarbitone anesthesia on blood flow and oxygen consumption in the rat brain. Acta Anaesthesiol Scand [Suppl] 1975;57:18–24.

77. Hawkins RA, Miller AL, Cremer JE, et al.: Measurement of the rate of glucose utilization by rat brain in vivo. J Neurochem 1974;23:917–923.

78. Siesjö BK: Brain energy metabolism. New York, John Wiley & Sons, 1978, p 607.

79. Bachelard HS, Lindsay JR: Effects of neurotropic drugs on glucose metabolism in rat brain in vivo. Biochem Pharmacol 1966;15:1053–1058.

80. Strong BHC, Bacheland HS: Rates of cerebral glucose utilization in rats anesthetized with phenobarbitone, J. Neurochem 1973;20:987–996.

81. Kreuscher H, Crote J: Die Wirkung des Phencylidinderivates Ketamine auf die Durchblutung und Sauerstoffaufnahme des Gehirns beim Hund. Anaesthetist 1967; 16:304–308.

82. Dawson B, Michenfelder JD, Theye RA: Effects of ketamine on canine cerebral blood flow and metabolism. Modification by prior administration of thiopental. Anesth Analg (Cleve) 1971;50:443–447.

83. Takeshita H, Okuda Y, Sari A: The effects of ketamine on cerebral circulation and metabolism in man. Anesthesiology 1972;36:69–75.

84. Laitinin CV, Johansson GG, Tarkhanen L: The effects of nitrous oxide on pulsatile cerebral impedance and cerebral blood flow. Br J Anaesth 1967;39:781–785.

85. Henriksen HT, Jorgensen PB: The effect of nitrous oxide on intracranial pressure in patients with intracranial disorders. Br J Anaesth 1973;45:486–492.

86. Smith AL, Wollman H: Cerebral blood flow and metabolism. Anesthesiology 1972;36:378–400.

87. Theye RA, Michenfelder JD: The effect of nitrous oxide on canine cerebral metabolism. Anesthesiology 1968;29:1119–1124.

88. Carlsson C, Hagerdal M, Siesjö BK: The effect of nitrous oxide on oxygen consumption and blood flow in the cerebral cortex of the rat. Acta Anaesthesiol Scand 1976;20:91–95.

89. Cohen PJ, Wollman H, Alexander SC, et al.: Cerebral carbohydrate metabolism in man during halothane anesthesia. Anesthesiology 1964;25:185–191.

90. McHenry LC Jr, Slocum HC, Bivens HE, et al.: Hyperventilation in awake and anesthetized man. Arch Neurol 1965;12:270–277.

91. Christensen MS, Holdt-Rasmussen K, Lassen NA: Cerebral vasodilatation by halothane anesthesia in man and its potentiation by hypotension and hypercapnia. Br J Anaesth 1967;39:927–934.

92. McDowell G: The effect of clinical concentrations of halothane on the blood flow and oxygen uptake of the cerebral cortex. Br J Anaesth 1967;39:186–196.

93. Keaney NP, Pickerodt VW, McDowell DG, et al.: Cerebral circulatory and metabolic effects of hypotension produced by deep halothane anesthesia. J Neurol Neurosurg Psychiatry 1973;36:898–905.

94. Theye RA, Michenfelder JD: The effect of halothane on canine cerebral metabolism. Anesthesiology 1968;29:113–118.

95. Michenfelder JD, Cucchiara RF: Canine cerebral oxygen consumption during enflurane anesthesia and its modification during induced seizures. Anesthesiology 1974;40:575–580.

96. Clark DL, Hosick EC, Adams N, et al.: Natural effects of isoflurane (Forane) in man. Anesthesiology 1973;39:261–270.

97. Murphy FL, Jr, Kennell EM, Jober DR, et al.: The effects of Forane on cerebral blood flow and metabolism in man. New Drug Application 1975; pp 2386–2395.

98. Stulher EH, Milde JH, Michenfelder JD, et al.: The nonlinear responses of cerebral metabolism to low concentrations of halothane, enflurane, isoflurane and thiopental. Anesthesiology 1974;40:571–574.

99. Cucchiara RF, Theye RA, Michenfelder JD: The effects of isoflurane on canine cerebral metabolism and blood flow. Anesthesiology 1974;40:571–574.

100. Murphy, FL, Jr, Kennell EM, Johnstone RE, et al.: The effects of enflurane, isoflurane, and halothane on cerebral blood flow and metabolism in man, abstracted. Scientific Papers, Ann. Mtg. Amer. Soc. Anesthesiol, 1974, pp 61–62.

101. Adams RW, Cucchiara RF, Gronert GA, et al.: Isoflurane and cerebrospinal fluid pressure in neurosurgical patients. Anesthesiology 1981;54:97–99.

102. Schettini A, Mahig J: Comparative intracranial dynamic responses in dogs to three halogenated anesthetics, abstracted. Scientific Papers, Ann. Mtg. Amer. Soc. Anesthesiologists, 1973, pp 123–124.

103. Stockard J, Bickford B: The neurophysiology of anesthesia in the basis and practice of neuroanesthesia, in Gordon E (ed): Amsterdam, NY, Excerpta Medica, 1975, pp 3–46.

104. Michenfelder JD, Theye RA: Effects of cyclopropane on canine cerebral blood flow and metabolism. Modification by catecholamine suppression. Anesthesiology 1972;37:32–39.

105. Smith AL, Neigh JL, Hoffman JC, et al.: Effects of general anesthesia on autoregulation of cerebral blood flow in man. J Appl Physiol 1970;29:665–669.

106. Patterson JL, Jr, Warren JV: Mechanisms of adjustment in the cerebral circulation upon assumption of the upright position. J Clin Invest 1952;31:653.

107. Bevegard BS, Sheperd JT: Regulation of the circulation during exercise in man. Physiol Rev 1967;47:178–213.

108. Toole JF, Tucker SH: Influence of head position upon cerebral circulation. Arch Neurol 1960;2:616–623.

109. Tindall G, Craddock A, Greenfield JC: Effects of the sitting position on blood flow in the internal carotid artery of man during general anesthesia. J Neurosurg 1967; 26:383–389.

CHAPTER 3

Physiology of Intracranial Pressure
Kamran Tabaddor

Intracranial hypertension is a common complication of severe head injury and other intracranial pathologies. More than half of head trauma deaths are attributed to intracranial hypertension (1). The deleterious effect of elevated intracranial pressure (ICP) is related to a reduction of perfusion pressure and cerebral blood flow (CBF) below the critical level (60 mm Hg), resulting in ischemic brain damage (2). Successful control of ICP can significantly improve outcome (3–5).

The limited usefulness of physical findings and clinical impressions in predicting ICP level has long been known (6,7), but the clinical application of continuous ICP monitoring was not introduced until 1951 (8). Although a variety of ICP monitoring techniques have been developed, the search for an accurate and yet noninvasive method of measuring ICP has been unsuccessful. Recent studies correlating certain computed tomographic (CT) scan findings with the level of ICP have identified a group of patients in whom the risk of developing elevated pressure is decreased (9). The CT features, however, lack adequate accuracy and are unable to quantify the pressure level. Therefore, in patients at risk of developing intracranial hypertension, continuous monitoring of ICP can give an indication of the appropriate time to initiate therapy and the effectiveness of that therapy and can help determine the prognosis of the patient with head injury.

Normal ICP ranges between 5 and 15 mm Hg. Intracranial hypertension is considered mild when it ranges from 15 to 25 mm Hg, moderate when it is 25 to 40 mm Hg, and severe when it is over 40 mm Hg. These values have been commonly used to prognosticate head injury but cannot readily be applied to other conditions. Furthermore, other factors such as cerebrospinal fluid (CSF) leak and surgical decompression influence the absolute ICP values for the purpose of management and prediction of outcome.

PHYSIOLOGY OF ICP

ICP refers to CSF pressure within the cranial cavity. As long as CSF flow within the craniospinal axis is not obstructed, the CSF pressure in the recumbent position is constant along the entire system. Variation in ICP is dependent on CSF dynamics, cerebral circulation, and intracranial abnormalities. Therefore, in order to evaluate the ICP response to intracranial lesions, the role and characteristics of cerebral circulation and CSF dynamics must be considered.

Cerebral Circulation

The brain receives approximately 15% of the cardiac output. The global CBF commonly is expressed by the volume of the blood per minute per 100 gm of brain substance. Kety and Schmidt were the first to determine CBF using the Fick principle (10). They calculated global CBF to be about 53 ml/min/100 gm of brain in normal young individuals. Others have noted similar values using modifications of their techniques (11, 12). More recently, using the isotope clearance technique, the determination of CBF in discrete portions of the brain has become possible. The studies of regional CBF have shown that blood flow to different areas of the brain varies considerably. Obrist et al. (13) reported a flow of 74.5 ml/min/100 gm in the gray matter and 24.8 ml/min/100 gm in the white matter.

Measurement of cerebral blood volume (CBV) is more difficult, and its determination varies considerably from one study to another (14). Most investigators, using a freeze technique in animals, have reported the CBV to be about 2% of the intracranial volume. In vivo measurements in humans have suggested values closer to 7% (15). If this estimate is correct, an expanding mass can reach moderate size without raising ICP by displacing blood from the cranial cavity.

Cerebral circulation and ICP exert reciprocal effects (16, 17). Marked intracranial hypertension results in vasospasm and reduced CBF. As the ICP approaches the mean arterial blood pressure, cerebral circulation ceases. Cerebral vasodilation, on the other hand, leads to an increased CBV, which in turn can lead to elevation of ICP. Vasodilation may occur in both physiologic and pathologic conditions. Cerebral vessels may dilate in response to physiologic hyperactivity of the brain. This vasodilation usually is focal and produces a negligible effect on CBV. A generalized relaxation of the vascular tone is observed in hypercapnia. Carbon dioxide reduces vascular resistance, leading to an increase in CBV. The effect of carbon dioxide on cerebral vessels is independent of the factors that influence autoregulation. Within a range of 30 to 60 mm Hg in the partial pressure of carbon dioxide in arterial blood ($PaCO_2$), a change of 1 mm Hg in $PaCO_2$ is associated with 2.5% change in CBF (18). This carbon dioxide effect continues to a lesser extent beyond the above range. $PaCO_2$ no longer alters the CBF when it exceeds 80 mm Hg or falls below 15 mm Hg. During periods of severe systemic hypotension when autoregulation is abolished, the carbon dioxide effect is decreased or absent. Induced hypercapnia with 5% to 7% carbon dioxide causes an increase in CBF averaging 75%. This often is associated with a rise in systemic arterial pressure caused by peripheral vasoconstriction (19). Paradoxical peripheral vascular reaction to hypercapnia has been attributed to a massive release of catecholamines in the blood. Hypocapnia induced by active or passive hyperventilation can reduce the CBF to about one-third of the baseline in normal individuals (20,21). The effect is independent of arterial pH. The reduction in CBF in turn diminishes CBV and ICP. The ICP reduction occurs in a fraction of a minute after induced hyperventilation (Fig. 3.1). The effect of hypocapnia on ICP is more pronounced in conditions associated with cerebral swelling (22). This may be partly related to the increased ICP secondary to vasoparalysis, where the hypocapnia can be most effective. If hyperventilation is maintained for a prolonged period, the ICP gradually rises but remains at a level generally lower than the initial recording. Adaptation mechanisms responsible for the return of the pressure take about two to five hours (23), but there is considerable individual variation.

The effect of hyperventilation is best noted in hyperemic swollen brain in the early phases after brain insult. Later, when elevated ICP is related more to an increase in water content, induced hypocapnia is less effective. Hypocapnia of less than 20 mm Hg is not clinically desirable since frequently it is associated with tissue hypoxia (24) as the oxygen dissociation curve shifts to the left.

Although hyperbaric oxygenation has little effect on CBF, severe hypoxia causes marked vasodilation and increased CBF. If $PaCO_2$ is maintained, an induced deep hypoxia (7% to 8% oxygen) produces a 71% increase in CBF (10). Both severe hypercapnia and hypoxia paralyze the resistance vessels, resulting in loss of autoregulation. Clinical impairment or total loss of autoregulation is seen after

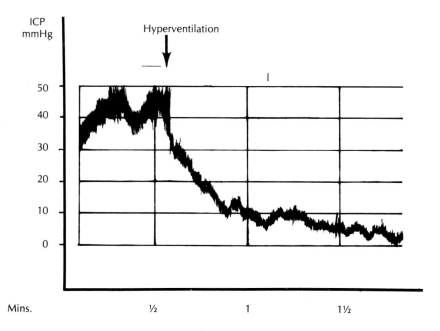

Figure 3.1 Establishment of a hyperventilatory state and hypocapnia rapidly decreases raised ICP.

cerebral insults of ischemic or traumatic origin. Loss of autoregulation is associated with increased CBV and increased ICP. Under these circumstances the CBF becomes dependent on perfusion pressure. If adequate perfusion pressure is not maintained, an additional ischemic insult will further compromise cerebral function.

CSF Physiology

A major portion of CSF is produced by the choroid plexi of the lateral ventricles (25–27). The remainder is assumed to be generated by the brain tissue and is drained into the ventricles or directly into the subarachnoid space. Ligation or removal of the choroid plexi are shown to reduce the CSF production by only about 60%. The CSF production rate ranges from 0.3 to 0.35 ml/min, which amounts to about 450 to 500 ml/day (26). Since the total CSF volume is about 150 ml in an adult, the entire CSF volume may be totally exchanged three times every day. The CSF, which is produced in ventricles, is circulated to the subarachnoid space and finally absorbed via the arachnoid villi into the sagittal sinus. The pulsatile production of CSF by the choroid plexus is the main force behind the CSF circulation (27). The rate of CSF production is constant and is not pressure dependent. That is, variations in ICP do not affect the CSF production rate.

The rate of absorption, in contrast to production, is pressure dependent and is directly enhanced by ICP elevation (26,28). This phenomenon can be explained by the pressure-regulated valve system in the arachnoid villi, which is the main site of CSF absorption (29). If the function of these valves is defective or the venous sinus pressure is increased, the CSF absorption will be impaired, leading to a rise in CSF pressure. The common sites of obstruction are at the aqueduct of Sylvius and the basal cisterns. If the flow of CSF is obstructed at any point in its pathway, an obstructive form of hydrocephalus will develop. Under physiologic conditions, transependymal absorption is negligible. In obstructive hydrocephalus, as the intraventricular pressure rises above critical levels, the transependymal pathways open and CSF is absorbed directly into the cerebral circulation.

Pressure/Volume Response

The cranium is a rigid box that restricts the free movement and expansion of the brain. The unique anatomic structure of the skull and its contents are responsible for the special hydrodynamic properties of the intracranial compartments. From a biomechanical point of view, the intracranial content is composed of three different components: brain, CSF, and blood. The total volume of these three factors in the physiologic state is constant, and an increase in one is compensated by a decrease in another (Monro-Kellie doctrine). Among the three components, brain tissue is noncompressible, and its volume is relatively constant. Some portions of the cerebral blood and CSF volume, however, are readily displaceable, compensating for additional volume introduced in the cranial cavity. As long as the intracranial volume is stable, ICP remains within physiologic ranges (pressure/volume equilibrium). In pathologic conditions, the volume of an expanding mass lesion is compensated initially by displacement of equal volumes of blood and CSF out of the cranial cavity. If the space-occupying lesion continues to expand, the compensatory mechanisms will no longer be effective, and ICP will increase. The relation of incremental expansion of volume to the resultant alteration of ICP was graphically illustrated by Langfitt and associates (30) (Fig. 3.2). This curve was generated by gradual expansion of a balloon in the supratentorial cavity. The first portion of the curve represents the compensatory capability of the system, and the steep portion of the curve represents exhaustion of this compensatory mechanism.

Lofgren et al. (31) demonstrated that the slope of the curve gradually decreases as ICP exceeds 50 mm Hg. This flattening of the curve is assumed to be

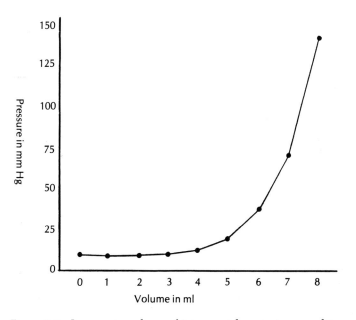

Figure 3.2   Increase in volume of intracranial contents causes little increase in pressure until a critical amount is reached. Thereafter, small additions will cause large increases in pressure. (From Langfitt TW, Weinstein JD: Vascular factors in head injury contribution to brain-swelling and intracranial hypertension, in Caveness WF, Walker AE, Head injury conference proceedings © 1966 Harper & Row, New York. Reprinted with permission of the publisher.)

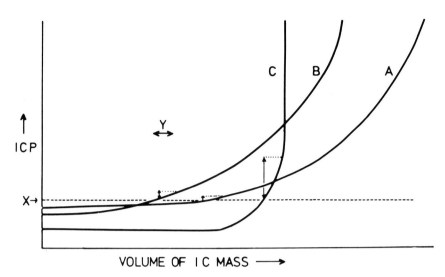

Figure 3.3 Measurement of intracranial dynamics can predict the response to increased volume. If compliance is low, pressure response is greater to small volume increases (C). If compliance is higher, with expansion of edema volume, the pressure increase will be less (A). B indicates an intermediate situation. (From Miller DJ, Leech P: Effects of manitol and steroid therapy on intracranial volume-pressure relationships in patients, J Neurosurg 1975; 42:275. Reprinted with permission.)

due to reduction in perfusion pressure and CBF beyond critical levels. The exponential property of the pressure/volume curve indicates that a similar volume increment at different points of the curve can result in a different pressure response. For example, the same amount of additional volume at point A produces a small rise in ICP, while at point B it results in marked ICP elevation. The pressure reaction to volume ($\Delta V/\Delta P$) is defined as compliance. The slope of the pressure/volume curve is dependent on factors contributing to compensatory capabilities of the system. These factors are affected by some anatomic variation, such as the size of the tentorial opening and the extensibility of the spinal dural sac or by a pathologic condition such as tentorial or foramen magnum impaction (32). In rapid expansion of increased intracranial volume, Lofgren and co-workers (31) demonstrated that the additional volume is compensated by displacement of CSF to the spinal dural sac (70%) and reduction of the cerebral venous bed (30%). In the presence of foramen magnum obstruction, the contribution of the spinal dural space is not available, and the compensatory mechanisms will be proportionately reduced. The capacity of the buffering system can be determined by the slope of the volume/pressure curve. Steepness of the slope in clinical practice is expressed as "tightness" or "stiffness" of the intracranial contents. Since the pressure/volume response varies at different pressure levels, the compliance ($\Delta V/\Delta P$) is pressure dependent. By plotting the pressure on a logarithmic axis against volume, the exponential pressure/volume curve can be converted to a linear one. The slope of this line is termed the *pressure/volume index* (33). That index numerically expresses the steepness of the slope and is defined as the volume necessary to raise the ICP by a factor of 10. As brain compliance decreases and the slope of the curve becomes steeper, the pressure/volume index value decreases. The steepness of the slope varies under different pathologic conditions or with certain pharmacologic manipulation. Figure 3.3 shows the intracranial compliance curve under three different biomechanical conditions. In these three theoretical curves, Miller and Leach (34) demonstrated that at the same resting pressure the addition of the same volume can produce different pressure responses. Therefore, it may be clinically important to measure the compliance in order to predict an impending rise in ICP. If CSF dynamic tests indicate a steep curve, it can be anticipated that any additional volume from expansion of edema volume, CBV, or a space-occupying lesion will result in critical ICP elevation. This information can be used to treat compliance before severe intracranial hypertension occurs. It has been shown that administration of osmotic diuretics and steroid therapy improve the compliance before they effectively reduce the ICP under pathologic conditions (34).

METHODS OF MONITORING ICP

Different techniques for monitoring ICP have been developed over the past decade, all of which can be classified under one of three types: epidural, subdural, and intraventricular. Each of these methods has advantages and limitations that make it suitable for specific clinical conditions. Acquaintance with these various techniques makes it possible for the clinician to select the most appropriate method of monitoring ICP in each individual patient.

Epidural Monitoring

Epidural pressure (EDP) can be monitored by pressure sensor implantation and telemetric recording (35) or by placement of a transducer directly in contact with the surface of the dura (36) (Fig. 3.4).

EDP recording obviates considerable difficulty sometimes posed by ventricular puncture in patients with small or displaced ventricles. Furthermore, the potential risk of brain cannulation and infection can be avoided. The values obtained by EDP recording commonly are higher than ventricular pressures, and the differences increase with rise in ICP (37). Change in calibration is a common problem and is estimated at the rate of 5 mm Hg per 24 hours by some investigators (38). Determination of EDP is, however, accurate enough to distinguish between mild, moderate, and severe intracranial hypertension. Although EDP recording may not give an accurate quantitative measure of ICP, it can reflect changes. In addition to the lack of quantitative accuracy, this method

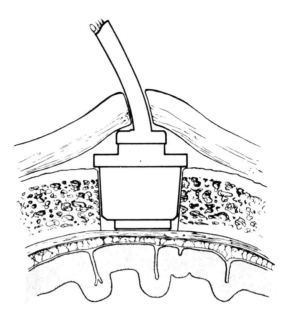

Figure 3.4 Epidural pressure may be measured by placement of a transducer directly in contact with the dura.

does not provide access to ventricular fluid, which is often drained to lower ICP or to determine intracranial compliance.

Subdural Pressure Monitoring

Vries et al. (39), in 1972, developed a system for monitoring ICP from the subdural space over the cerebral hemisphere. This system is based on a specially designed hollow screw that is threaded into the skull through a 5-mm twist drill hole (Fig. 3.5). The screw is then connected by means of saline-filled tubing to a strain-guage transducer to record ICP. Others have used miniature strain gauges applied directly over the brain surface; these cannot be calibrated against atmospheric pressure. Both techniques require specially designed burr holes to accommodate the instrumentation. The craniostomy preferably is performed over the coronal suture or immediately in front of it, at about 5 cm from midline.

Recently, a simple technique of monitoring subdural pressure without any special equipment has been described. The method consists of placing a stopcock filled with saline into the subdural space through a regular twist drill hole (Fig. 3.6). The stopcock is then connected to a transducer by saline-filled intravenous

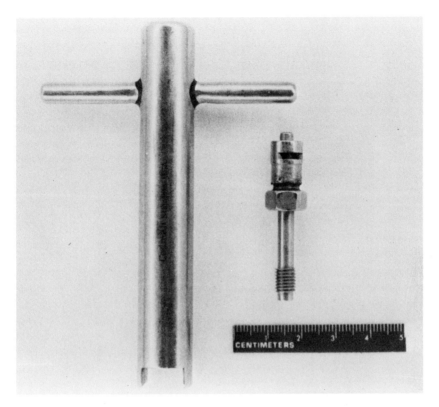

Figure 3.5 A system for monitoring subdural pressure includes a 5-mm twist drill and a hollow screw (*right*), which is threaded into the skull. (From Wilkinson HA: Intracranial pressure monitoring techniques and pitfalls, in Cooper PR (ed.), Management of head injuries © 1982, the Williams and Wilkins Co., Baltimore. Reprinted with permission of the publisher and author.)

tubing. This procedure can be simplified further by placing plastic tubing (such as a multiple-orifice soft stomach tube) directly into the twist drill hole, thus eliminating the additional connection, which can be a potential source of leakage or infection. When subdural monitoring is used because of an unsuccessful attempt at ventricular catheterization, drilling a separate hole is preferable in order to avoid herniation of the brain tissue into the tubing.

Subdural pressure monitoring is simple, but its correlation with ventricular pressure is controversial (40). Although measurements are not as reliable as those obtained by ventricular catheter, subdural pressure monitoring can be used to estimate the intracranial elastance and compliance. Disadvantages of this system include frequent clogging of the tubing, particularly after severe brain contusion, and elevated ICP (41). It also does not provide access to ventricular fluid for CSF drainage.

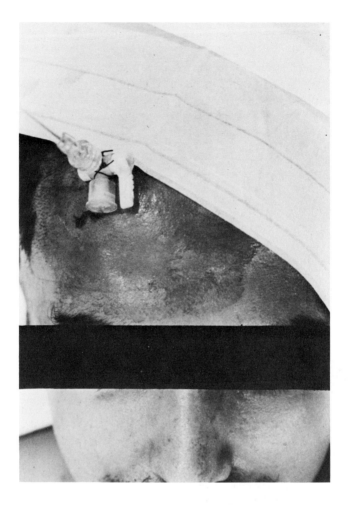

Figure 3.6   Subdural pressure may be simply and inexpensively measured by placing a three-way stopcock through a twist drill hole into the subdural space and connecting it via a fluid-filled system to a venous pressure transducer.

Ventricular Pressure Monitoring

The use of ventriculostomy for the purpose of removing CSF fluid or performing diagnostic studies is an old neurosurgical procedure. The adaptation of the ventriculostomy for continuous recording of pressure as described by Lundberg (42) remains the most reliable method of ICP monitoring.

The success rate of ventricular catheterization can be increased by using CT scan information as to the location, size, and extent of ventricular displacement.

If the lateral ventricles are collapsed and not visible on CT scanning, the patient is not a suitable candidate for ventricular pressure monitoring, and the subdural technique is the more practical alternative. The ventricle selected for catheterization is the one contralateral to the involved hemisphere. Frequently it is displaced further laterally. Several techniques of ventricular catheterization have been described, but the technique preferred here is the frontal approach (Fig. 3.7). For this bedside procedure, the patient is placed in a supine position and the forehead is prepared in a sterile fashion. A point about 5.5 cm from the nasion and 4 cm from the midline is marked, and a horizontal incision of about 1 cm is made to expose a small area of the frontal bone. The distance of the incision from the midline can be modified based on the extent of ventricular displacement. A twist drill hole is aimed in the direction of the external occipital protuberance. It must be emphasized that the direction of the twist drill is critical in the placement of the cannula since the ventricular catheter commonly follows the direction of the bony canal made by the twist drill. After the inner table of the skull is gently penetrated, the dura can be opened with a smaller twist drill bit or a needle. The ventricular catheter is then introduced until ependymal resistance is felt and the ventricle is entered. The catheter is connected to a strain-gauge pressure transducer via fluid-filled plastic tubing. The advantages of this technique include accuracy and access to the ventricular fluid for drainage purposes. Any dampen-

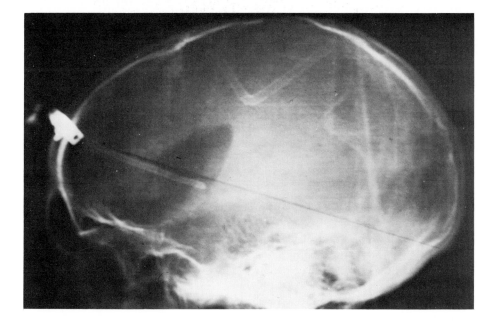

Figure 3.7   A Scott cannula placed within the ventricular system allows direct ventricular pressure monitoring, accurate intracranial compliance calculations, and easy withdrawal of CSF for rapid decrease of raised ICP.

ing of the pulse wave suggests partial obstruction of the cannula. This can easily be relieved by injection of small amounts of sterile saline (e.g., 0.5 ml).

Ventricular catheterization makes it possible to compute cerebral compliance, CSF production rate, and outflow resistance by injecting or withdrawing a small amount of fluid (43). This information can be used to predict the potential elevation of ICP and to institute appropriate therapeutic measures early. Such information is especially useful in patients with normal or mildly elevated ICP and in whom the compliance is reduced. Critical reduction of intracranial compliance suggests that all compensatory mechanisms are exhausted, and any further expansion of the space-occupying lesion will result in rapid rise of ICP and deterioration of neurologic conditions if the pressure is not promptly controlled. The information regarding CSF dynamics can be used to identify the patients with significant impairment of CSF absorption. These patients are best managed by CSF drainage with or without adjunctive therapy.

The potential risks of ventricular pressure monitoring are intracranial hemorrhage and infection. Extraparenchymal or intracerebral bleeding is rare. We have encountered only one such case in over 500 patients subjected to this procedure. This complication must be suspected when the ICP begins to rise rapidly after ventriculostomy. Infection is another potential risk of intraventricular pressure monitoring and can be minimized by careful attention to sterility at the time of insertion and avoidance of prolonged monitoring (42,44,45). The rate of infection increases after three days. If continuous monitoring is required beyond three days, a new system should be inserted, preferably in the contralateral ventricle. Other factors that increase the rate of infection are frequent irrigation or manipulation of ventricular fluid. Movement of the ventricular catheter at the skin site also may contribute to infection by contaminating the portion of the catheter that comes in contact with the skin surface, thus allowing access for organisms into the cranial cavity. Securing the hub of the catheter tightly to the skin can avoid this source. Passing the catheter under the skin and using a separate scalp opening that does not rest over the craniostomy site can reduce further the risk of infection. Attention to these details can lower the infection rate to about 1% to 3%.

CLINICAL APPLICATION OF ICP INFORMATION

Although the level at which ICP elevation becomes harmful remains controversial, most clinicians consider any ICP level above normal (15 to 20 mm Hg) to be detrimental; however, no direct relationship exists between ICP elevation and clinical neurologic impairment. For example, the marked intracranial hypertension of pseudotumor cerebri is associated with minimal neurologic dysfunction, while the moderate ICP elevations in severe head injury may prove fatal. The ICP values can provide useful information only when used in conjunction with other clinical data. The present experience with ICP monitoring in patients with head trauma has led to the identification of several factors critical in the management of intracranial hypertension.

Elevated ICP in the presence of a unilateral mass lesion is associated with a higher morbidity. As a lesion expands, it produces pressure gradients between compartments of the intracranial space, leading to structural displacement and ultimately to brain-stem compression. Structural shift is related to the location of lesions within the cranium. Frontal lobe masses commonly are associated with marked elevation of ICP before they manifest clinical signs of brain-stem compression. Monitoring ICP in these patients can provide a margin of safety before brain-stem compression occurs. On the other hand, temporal lobe lesions can result in brain-stem compression before the ICP becomes markedly elevated. The safety margin is therefore quite narrow, and any elevation of ICP requires vigorous medical or surgical treatment (46).

Since intracranial volume is constant, the introduction of any additional volume, such as a hematoma or edema fluid, is compensated by displacement of an equal volume out of the cranium. The volume compensation is accomplished by reduction of venous blood volume and/or intracranial CSF. When these compensatory mechanisms are exhausted, any additional volume results in a sharp rise in ICP. In patients with basilar skull fractures and CSF leaks, ICP does not accurately reflect the influence of an expanding lesion (47). As the volume of a mass increases, CSF is forced out of the cranium without a significant rise in ICP. The determination of intracranial compliance is no longer valid because the cranial cavity loses the property of a closed box. Under these circumstances, a normal ICP should not militate against the surgical treatment of a focal intracranial mass lesion.

PROGNOSTIC VALUE OF ICP

Although the association of severe intracranial hypertension and poor outcome after head injury has been shown by several investigators (48–50), the role of ICP monitoring as a guide in clinical management or as an index of prognosis in head injury remains controversial (3,51–54). Elevated intracranial pressures may never occur in many fatal head injuries and are occasionally observed in patients who make a good recovery from their injury. Adams and Graham (55) have shown a correlation between the extent of ICP elevation and neuropathologic signs of raised pressure. Thus, raised ICP may be responsible for pathologic changes and poor outcome. Nine of their 35 patients, however, died without either clinical or neuropathologic evidence of raised ICP, suggesting that the final outcome is not solely dependent on the degree of ICP elevation. Recent studies (53,56) indicate that in the presence of a mass lesion, outcome correlates with the extent of neurologic dysfunction, such as abnormal posturing and pupillary light reactivity, rather than absolute level of ICP. In diffuse brain injuries without mass lesions, Miller et al. (53) reported a good correlation between ICP level and outcome at the two extremes of the pressure range. Marked ICP elevation in their series was associated with poor outcome, while patients with normal pressures on admission had significantly better outcomes. The group that fell between these extremes showed poor correlations between ICP values and outcome. Johnson and Jennett (52) used the highest ICP value reached during the monitoring period in 54 head trauma patients. Fourteen of 21 patients with pressures over 40 mm Hg had a fatal outcome, while 8 of 11 patients with normal pressures succumbed to their injuries. They concluded that no clear prognostic differentiation can be made on the basis of ICP values alone. They contended, however, that the treatment of ICP elevation cannot be guided by clinical judgment and is best done by continuous monitoring. Availability of information concerning actual ICP level may obviate the need for unnecessary pharmacologic manipulation and allow the clinician to adjust therapy according to the patient's need. The critical question remains of whether treatment of ICP elevation can improve the outcome. In answering this question, the trend of ICP elevation during the course of therapy should be defined. One of the difficulties inherent in all of the studies designed to determine the effect of ICP on prognosis of injury is the lack of a clear definition of raised pressure. ICP after head trauma is no longer in a steady state, and values may vary at different times. This variation is the function of brain reaction to trauma, which is dependent on the extent of different factors such as ischemia, edema, expanding hematoma, and so forth. Also, in addition to the above pathophysiologic changes, the use of therapeutic measures makes any single pressure determination invalid in characterizing the pressure trend. Some of the therapeutic measures, like ventricular drainage and mannitol, commonly are administered intermittently, resulting in variation of ICP levels from normal to markedly abnormal during the course of a day. Some of these difficulties can be obviated by considering the ICP trend during the acute phase. Using the ICP trend and its response to management, the author has noted that all patients with intractable ICP elevations have a fatal outcome (57); but when ICP can be controlled, the outcome does not differ from that of patients who do not develop intracranial hypertension. This observation suggests that successful control of ICP may have a favorable influence. Miller et al. (53) have noted that in patients who demonstrate abnormal posture or absent pupillary light reaction, the result is poor, irrespective of ICP level. These abnormal reflexes, which are strong determinants of outcome, overshadow the prognostic value of ICP. With the popular use of CT scan, however, another parameter has been introduced, which in many cases may enhance the capability of outcome predictions (9,58).

Therapy of raised ICP is considered more fully in Chapter 15, which deals with care of the head-injured patient.

ANESTHETIC CONSIDERATIONS

The anesthetic relevance of an understanding of ICP dynamics is greatest in the management of patients with head injury (see Chapter 15) and in patients with supratentorial tumors or hydrocephalus. For this reason, anesthesia for supratentorial tumor excision and shunt placement is considered in this chapter.

Gliomas are the most common primary intracranial neoplasms. They arise from neuroglial tissue, are locally invasive, and of varying degrees of malignancy.

Astrocytomas are the slowest growing and least malignant, although they frequently undergo cystic degeneration. Glioblastomas are highly malignant and rapidly growing. Biopsy to confirm the type may be the only operative measure indicated. Meningiomas are benign tumors arising from the dura mater. Although bone may be infiltrated, the brain is compressed rather than invaded. Meningiomas are slow-growing tumors but often are highly vascular, deriving large feeding vessels from intracranial and extracranial arteries.

Tumors in and around the third ventricle cause obstruction of CSF flow and internal hydrocephalus. Such neoplasms include ependymomas (gliomas growing from the ventricular ependymal lining), papillomas of the choroid plexus, colloid cysts, and pinealomas. Tumors derived from congenital cell rests include dermoid and epidermoid lesions and craniopharyngiomas (see Chapter 8).

The clinical course of a brain tumor may be exacerbated by pregnancy. Although the incidence of tumors in pregnant patients is no higher than that observed in non-pregnant women, generalized water retention may cause greater cerebral swelling around the lesion. Mitotic activity is probably not increased. Therapy should be aimed at pharmacologic reduction of intracranial hypertension. If the patient's condition deteriorates, however, craniotomy and surgical decompression may be indicated prior to delivery. All the necessary precautions dictated by pregnancy should be adopted.

Finally, the brain is a common site for metastases from breast, bronchus, or kidneys.

Anesthetic Management

Whether the surgical approach is simply through burr holes (for diagnosis, biopsy, or drainage) or craniotomy, the main anesthetic consideration is stabilization of ICP.

As a supratentorial mass expands, venous blood and CSF are initially displaced. As the compensatory mechanisms become exhausted, there is a reduction in cerebral perfusion either globally or locally. Pressure gradients may cause herniation beneath the falx or through the tentorial hiatus or foramen magnum. If the brain is extruded through the dura during surgery, further tissue damage may occur, especially if excessive retractor pressure is necessary for exposure.

Preanesthetic evaluation must include the signs and symptoms of raised ICP, which comprise headache (often paroxysmal in nature, relieved by sitting and worsened by coughing), vomiting (usually projectile), papilledema, blurred vision, and dizziness. Steroid administration (dexamethasone, 4 mg qid) for two to three days prior to surgery is very effective in reducing the edema surrounding a tumor and decreasing ICP.

Premedication should avoid the use of narcotics that cause respiratory depression. Diazepam, 5 mg orally, usually suffices. Close physician-patient contact is very important in allaying anxiety and decreasing a preoperative hypertensive response to stress. Indeed, there is no pharmacologic substitute as effective in this respect as a careful preanesthetic visit. Antiseizure medication and supplemental steroids should be given on the morning of surgery.

A smooth induction of anesthesia is essential, using thiopental, 3 to 5 mg/kg, lidocaine, 1 mg/kg, and succinylcholine 1 mg/kg. Laryngotracheal spray (4 ml of 4% lidocaine) should be used prior to passage of the endotracheal tube. Small doses of propranolol (1 to 2 mg) have been used intravenously prior to induction in hypertensive patients. If a defasciculating dose of pancuronium bromide (1 mg) or d-tubocurarine (3 mg) is then given, marked immediate potentiation of neuromuscular blockade may be apparent. We do not use nondepolarizing agents in this manner because of the risk of drug interaction or abnormal response to muscle relaxants. Moreover, succinylcholine does not increase ICP if hypocapnia is maintained.

There is some debate as to appropriate choice of anesthetic technique for patients with space-occupying lesions. At normocapnia, halothane, methoxyflurane, and enflurane all increase ICP (60), an effect that is greater with frontal lobe tumors than with parietal lesions. With neuroleptanalgesic drugs at normocapnia, increases in ICP are much less (61). Neuroanesthetic practice uses hypocapnia with $PaCO_2$ levels at 27 to 30 mm Hg. One study indicated that under these circumstances, rises in ICP were clinically unimportant with volatile agents (62). Other investigators showed that major increases may still be seen, particularly in patients with severely raised pressure (63). Isoflurane at 1 minimal alveolar concentration (MAC) causes almost no increase in CBF, and simultaneous hyperventilation during administration of this agent is sufficient to produce a stable ICP (74). This has been our experience, even in situations of severely decreased compliance.

Fentanyl administered during hypocapnia does not cause any increase in ICP (61). Thiopental, methohexital, and Althesin all decrease ICP. The first two agents have been given by continuous infusion to supplement nitrous oxide relaxant anesthesia (65,66); however, cumulative doses of barbiturates may become excessive over many hours, and delay return to consciousness. Infusions of methohexital have the added risk of causing seizures, especially in patients with tumors, in the immediate postoperative period. Moreover, the vasoconstricting action of these drugs may have deleterious effects on areas of the brain that are marginally perfused because of tumor compression.

The rate of production and absorption of CSF is a further determinant in maintenance of stability of intracranial dynamics. Nitrous oxide has little effect on either CSF production (V_f) or absorption (V_a) (67), but both enflurane and ketamine have been shown to markedly increase V_f and thus ICP for several hours (67,68). This effect may be due to an action on choroid plexus metabolism whereby the metabolic rate for glucose is significantly increased (69). Halothane, which has no effect on glucose metabolism in the choroid plexus, decreased V_f by 30%, an effect that did not change significantly with time (70). Fentanyl in a dog model was shown to cause no significant change in V_f and V_a over the awake state (69). Consistent with these findings, it has been shown clinically that in patients with borderline or increased ICP, hyperventilation blocks any further increase in

ICP caused by halothane but fails to prevent increases caused by enflurane (62,71). Thus, in patients with increased ICP owing to impaired reabsorption of CSF, fentanyl or halothane may be preferred to anesthetics that increase CSF volume. Combination of these agents might allow optimal beneficial effect on increased ICP (i.e., decreased CBF and decreased V_f).

Diuretics frequently are used to lower ICP intraoperatively. Mannitol, 1 gm/kg of a 20% solution, is infused over 15 to 20 minutes during elevation of the bone flap. Careful attention must be paid to fluid and electrolyte balance and to maintenance of systemic blood pressure, especially in elderly patients who may already be acutely or chronically dehydrated (e.g., long-term ingestion of antihypertensive medication). A sudden increase in the circulating blood volume may be caused by the osmotic agent and increase systemic blood pressure. This should be compensated by increasing the anesthetic administration.

In critical situations, ICP may be acutely lowered by cannulation of the lateral ventricle prior to commencing the craniotomy. If necessary, this maneuver may be performed under local anesthesia.

Careful attention must be paid to fluid administration since excessive administration can lead to fluid retention and predispose to cerebral edema, which is accentuated by the increased secretion of antidiuretic hormone and decreased renal excretion of sodium that occurs postoperatively. Solutions of dextrose in water should be avoided as intravenous glucose is distributed equally throughout the body, including the brain and CSF. Subsequently, the serum glucose levels decrease more rapidly than the concentrations in the brain, and a rebound osmotic effect may cause cerebral swelling (61). Therefore, isotonic saline or Ringer's lactate solutions are recommended at a rate of 3 to 5 ml/kg/hr after compensation has been made for fluid deficits caused by fasting.

The second major anesthetic consideration for patients with supratentorial tumors is control of hemorrhage by induced hypotension. Available agents and their effects on intracranial dynamics are discussed in Chapter 6.

Following tumor surgery, some postoperative brain swelling caused by surgical cauterization and manipulation is inevitable; however, removal or at least debulking of the mass should have improved the intracranial compliance. Bucking and straining, which may increase edema, can be minimized during extubation by infusion of lidocaine, 50 mg. Ideally the patient should be awake at the conclusion of surgery. Should ICP again rise in the early postoperative period as the effects of hyperventilation and mannitol wear off, or if a hematoma or tension pneumocephalus develops, it would be detected immediately as deterioration in sensorium. Therapy requires diagnosis (CT scan), reintubation and ventilation, diuretic administration and, if necessary, reexploration.

Shunts

Obstruction to free flow of CSF may be caused by tumors compressing the third ventricle or aqueduct or a mass within the posterior fossa. Hydrocephalus may also be associated with head injury, infectious processes, degenerative disease, or unknown causes.

The principles of anesthetic management of patients with supratentorial tumors apply also to patients undergoing shunt placement. Further increases in ICP must be avoided by a smooth technique using controlled ventilation.

Bypass procedures usually involve placement of a cannula into a lateral ventricle and then passing it below the skin and inserting it into the peritoneal cavity. Careful monitoring of the electrocardiogram during initial withdrawal of CSF is important since too rapid decrease of CSF volume may cause traction on the brain stem and severe ventricular arrhythmias. Fluid should be replaced and drained more slowly. Increased depth of anesthesia and muscle relaxation are required during the abdominal incision, and appropriate adjustments should be made.

More rarely, shunts may be passed from the ventricle to the internal jugular vein and into the right atrium or from the lumbar subarachnoid space to the peritoneal cavity. In this latter approach, the patient is operated in a lateral position.

Postoperatively, the patient should be nursed supine or in a very slightly head-up position to ensure slow drainage of CSF.

REFERENCES

1. Langfitt TW: The incidence and importance of intracranial hypertension in head-injured patients, in Beks JWF, Bosch DA, Brock M (eds): Intracranial pressure. III. New York, Springer-Verlag, 1976, pp 67–72.
2. Johnston IH, Rowan JO: Raised intracranial pressure and cerebral blood flow. 3. Venous outflow tract pressures and vascular resistance in experimental hypertension. J Neurol Neurosurg Psychiatry 1974;37:392–402.
3. Marshall LF, Smith RW, Shapiro HM: The outcome with aggressive treatment in severe head injuries. Part 1. The significance of intracranial pressure monitoring. J Neurosurg 1979;50:20–25.
4. Saul TG, Ducker TB: Effect of intracranial pressure monitoring and aggressive treatment on mortality in severe head injury. J Neurosurg 1982;56:498–503.
5. Becker DP, Miller JD, Ward JD, et al.: The outcome from severe head injury with early diagnosis and intensive management. J Neurosurg 1977;47:491–502.
6. Browder J, Meyer R: Observations on behavior of the systemic blood pressure, pulse and spinal fluid pressure following craniocerebral injury. Am J Surg 1936;31:403–426.
7. Ryder HW, Rosenauer A, Penka EJ, et al.: Failure of abnormal cerebrospinal fluid pressure to influence cerebral function. AMA Arch Neurol Psychiatry 1953; 70:563–586.
8. Guillaume J, Janny P: Manométrie intracranienne continué: intérêt de la méthode et premiers résultats. Rev Neurol (Paris) 1951;84:131–142.
9. Tabaddor K, Danziger A, Wisoff HS: Estimation of intracranial pressure by CT scan in closed heat trauma. Surg Neurol 1982;18:212–215.
10. Kety SS, Schmidt CF: The effects of altered arterial tensions of carbon dioxide and oxygen on cerebral blood flow and cerebral oxygen consumption of normal young men. J Clin Invest 1948;27:484–492.
11. Lassen NA, Munk O: The cerebral blood flow in man determined by the use of radioactive krypton. Acta Physiol Scand 1955;33:40–49.

12. Novack P, Shenkin HA, Borten L, et al.: The effects of carbon dioxide inhalation upon the cerebral blood flow and cerebral oxygen consumption in vascular disease. J Clin Invest 1953;32:696–702.

13. Obrist WD, Thompson HK Jr, King CH, et al.: Determination of regional cerebral blood flow by inhalation of Xenon 133. Circ Res 1967;20:124–135.

14. Sklar FH, Burke EF Jr, Langfitt TW: Cerebral blood volume: Values obtained with $^{51}CR^-$ labeled red blood cells and RISA. J Appl Physiol 1968;24:79–82.

15. Nylin G, Hedlund S, Regnstrom O: Studies of the cerebral circulation with labeled erythrocytes in healthy man. Circ Res 1961;9:664–674.

16. Ryder HW, Espey FF, Kimbell FD, et al.: Influence of changes in cerebral blood flow on the cerebrospinal fluid pressure. AMA Arch Neurol Psychiatry 1952;68:165–169.

17. Rowan JO, Johnston IH, Harper AM, et al.: Perfusion pressure in intracranial hypertension, in Brock M, Dietz H (eds): Intracranial pressure. New York, Springer-Verlag, 1972, pp. 165–170.

18. Harper AM: The inter-relationship between a pCO_2 and blood pressure in the regulation of blood flow through the cerebral cortex. Acta Neurol Scand 1965;41 (Suppl 14):94–103.

19. Sechzer PH, Egbert LD, Linde HW, et al.: Effect of CO_2 inhalation on arterial pressure ECG and plasma cathecholamines and 17-OH corticosteroids in normal man. J Appl Physiol 1960;15:454–458.

20. Kety SS, Schmidt CF: The effects of active and passive hyperventilation on cerebral blood flow, cerebral oxygen consumption, cardiac output and blood pressure of normal young men. J Clin Invest 1946;25:107–119.

21. Alexander SC, Cohen PJ, Wollman H, et al.: Cerebral carbohydrate metabolism during hypocarbia in man. Anesthesiology 1965;26:624–632.

22. Lundberg N, Kjallgruist A, Bien C: Reduction of increased intracranial pressure by hyperventilation. A therapeutic aid in neurological surgery. Acta Psychiatr Scand 1959;34 (suppl):139.

23. Miller JD, Ledingham I.McA: Reduction of increased intracranial pressure. Comparison between hyperbaric oxygen and hyperventilation. Arch Neurol 1971;24:210–216.

24. Allen GD, Morris LE: Central nervous system effects of hyperventilation during anesthesia. Br J Anaesth 1962;34:296–305.

25. Weed LH: Certain anatomical and physiological aspects of the meninges and cerebrospinal fluid. Brain 1935;58:383–397.

26. Cutler RWP, Page LK, Galicich J, et al.: Formation and absorption of cerebrospinal fluid in man. Brain 1968;91:707–720.

27. Bering EA Jr: Circulation of the cerebrospinal fluid, demonstration of the choroid plexus as the generator of the force for flow of fluid and ventricular enlargement. J Neurosurg 1962;19:405–413.

28. Davson H, Hollingsworth G, Segal MB: The mechanism of drainage of the cerebrospinal fluid. Brain 1970;93:665–678.

29. Weed LH: The pathways of escape from the subarachnoid spaces with particular reference to the arachnoid villi. J Med Res 1941;31:51–91.

30. Langfitt TW, Weinstein JD, Kassel NF: Vascular factors in head injury contribution to brain-swelling and intracranial hypertension, in Caveness WF, Walker AE (eds): Head injury conference proceeding. Philadelphia, JB Lippincott, 1966, pp 172–194.

31. Lofgren J, von Essen C, Zwetnow NN: The pressure-volume curve of the cerebrospinal fluid space in dogs. Acta Neurol Scand 1973;49:557–574.

32. Johnson RT, Yates PO: Clinico-pathological aspects of pressure changes at the tentorium. Acta Radiol (Kbh) 1956;46:242–249.
33. Marmarou A: A theoretical model and experimental evaluation of the cerebrospinal fluid system, thesis. Drexel University, Philadelphia, 1973.
34. Miller JD, Leach P: Effects of mannitol and steroid therapy on intracranial volume-pressure relationships in patients. J Neurosurg 1975;42:274–281.
35. Foroglou G, Zander E, Favre R, et al.: Telemetric measurement of intracranial pressure with an electromagnetic detector, in Lundberg N, Ponten U, Brock M (eds): Intracranial pressure. II. New York, Springer-Verlag, 1975, p 377.
36. Mackay RS: Biomedical telemetry. New York, John Wiley & Sons, 1970, pp 138–147.
37. McGraw CP: Epidural intracranial pressure monitoring, in Lundberg N, Ponten U, Brock M (eds): Intracranial pressure. II. New York, Springer-Verlag, 1975, pp 394–396.
38. Jorgensen PB, Ritshede J: Comparative clinical studies of epidural and ventricular pressure, in Brock M, Dietz H (eds): Intracranial pressure. New York, Springer-Verlag, 1972, pp 41–45.
39. Vries JK, Becker DP, Young HF: A subarachnoid screw for monitoring intracranial pressure. J Neurosurg 1973;39:416–419.
40. Mendelow AD, Rowan JO, Murray L, et al.: A clinical comparison of subdural screw pressure measurements with ventricular pressure. J Neurosurg 1983;58:45–50.
41. Gosch HH, Kindt GW: Subdural monitoring of acute increased intracranial pressure. Surg Forum 1972;23:405–406.
42. Lundberg N: Continuous recording and control of ventricular fluid pressure in neurosurgical practice. Acta Psychiatr Neurol Scand 1960;36 (Suppl):149.
43. Marmarou A, Shulman K, LaMorgese J: Compartmental analysis of compliance and outflow resistance of the cerebrospinal fluid system. J Neurosurg 1975;43:523–534.
44. Bruce DA, Berman WA, Schut L: Cerebrospinal fluid pressure monitoring in children: Physiology, pathology and clinical usefulness. Adv Pediatr 1977;24:233–290.
45. Gucer G, Viernstein LS, Chubbuck JG, et al.: Clinical evaluation of long-term epidural monitoring of intracranial pressure. Surg Neurol 1979;12:373–377.
46. Weinstein JD, Langfitt TW, Bruno L, et al.: Experimental study of patterns of brain distortion and ischemia produced by an intracranial mass. J Neurosurg 1968;28:513–521.
47. Teasdale G, Galbraith S, Jennett B: Operate or observe? ICP and the management of the "silent" traumatic intracranial hematoma, in Shulman K, Marmarou A, Miller JD, et al. (eds): Intracranial pressure. IV. New York, Springer-Verlag, 1980, pp 36–38.
48. Becker DP, Vries JK, Young HF, et al: Controlled cerebral perfusion pressure and ventilation in human mechanical brain injury: Prevention of progressive brain swelling, in Lundberg N, Ponten U, Brock M (eds): Intracranial pressure. II. New York, Springer-Verlag, vol II, 1975, pp 480–484.
49. Vapalahti M, Troupp H: Prognosis for patients with severe brain injuries. Br Med J 1971;3:404–407.
50. Troupp H: Intraventricular pressure in patients with severe brain injuries. J Trauma 1965;5:373–378.
51. Fleischer AS, Payne NS, Tindall GT: Continuous monitoring of intracranial pressure in severe closed head injury without mass lesions. Surg Neurol 1976;6:31–34.
52. Johnson IH, Jennett B: The place of continuous intracranial pressure monitoring in neurosurgical practice. Acta Neurochir (Wien) 1973;29:53–63.
53. Miller JD, Becker DP, Ward JD, et al.: Significance of intracranial hypertension in severe head injury. J Neurosurg 1977;47:503–516.

54. Lobato RD, Rivas JJ, Protillo JM, et al.: Prognostic value of the intracranial pressure levels during the acute phase of severe head injuries. Acta Neurochir (Wien) 1979; 28:(suppl):70–73.
55. Adams H, Graham DI: The relationship between ventricular fluid pressure and the neuropathology of raised intracranial pressure, in Brock M, Dietz H (eds): Intracranial pressure. New York, Springer-Verlag, 1972, pp 250–253.
56. Miller JD, Becker DP, Rosner MJ, et al.: Implications of intracranial mass lesions for outcome of severe head injury, in Popp AJ, Bourke RS, Nelson LR, et al. (eds): Neural trauma. New York, Raven Press, 1979, pp 173–180: Seminars in Neurological Surgery.
57. Tabaddor K: Is ICP monitoring useful? Presented at the 30th annual meeting of the Congress of Neurological Surgeons, Houston, Texas, 1980.
58. Narayan RK, Greenberg RP, Miller JD, et al.: Improved confidence of outcome prediction in severe head injury. A comparative analysis of the clinical examination, multimodality evoked potentials, CT scanning, and intracranial pressure. J Neurosurg 1981;54:751–762.
59. Shnider SM, Levinson G: Anesthesia for operations during pregnancy, in SM Shnider, G Levinson (eds): Anesthesia for obstetrics. Baltimore, Williams & Wilkins, 1979, pp 312–330.
60. Campkin TV, Turner JM: Anesthesia for supratentorial surgery, in Neurosurgical anesthesia and intensive care. Boston, Butterworth, 1980, pp 129–146.
61. Misfeldt BB, Jorgensen PB, Spotoft H, et al.: The effects of droperidol and fentanyl on intracranial pressure and cerebral perfusion in neurosurgical patients. Br J Anaesth 1976;48:963–968.
62. Adams RW, Gronert GA, Sundt TM, et al.: Halothane, hypocapnia and cerebrospinal fluid pressure in neurosurgery. Anesthesiology 1972;37:510–517.
63. Fitch W, Burke J, McDowall DG, et al.: The effect of methoxyflurane on cerebrospinal fluid pressure in patients with and without intracranial space-occupying lesion. Br J Anaesth 1969;41:564–573.
64. Adams RW, Cucchiera RF, Gronert GA, et al.: Isoflurance and cerebrospinal fluid pressure in neurosurgical patients. Anesthesiology 1981;54:98.
65. Hunter AR: Thiopentone supplemented anaesthesia for neurosurgery. Br J Anaesth 1972;44:506–510.
66. Hunter AR: Methohexitone as a supplement to nitrous oxide during intracranial surgery. Br J Anaesth 1972;44:1188–1190.
67. Artru AA, Nugent M, Michenfelder JD: Enflurance causes a prolonged and reversible increase in the rate of CSF production in the dog. Anesthesiology 1978;57:779–84.
68. Mann JD, Cookson SL, Mann ES: Differential effects of pentobarbital, ketamine hydrochloride and enflurane anesthesia on CSF formation rate and outflow resistance in the rat, in Shulman K, Marmarou A, Miller JD, et al. (eds): Intracranial pressure. IV. Berlin, Springer-Verlag, 1980, pp 466–71.
69. Meyers RR, Shapiro HM: Paradoxical effect of enflurane on choroid plexus metabolism: Clinical implications, abstracted. Annual Meeting, American Society Anesthesiologists, 1978; pp 489–90.
70. Artru AA: Effects of halothane and fentanyl on the rate of CSF production in dogs. Anesth Analg 1983;62:581–815.
71. Zattoni J, Siani C, Rivano C: The effects of ethrane on intracranial pressure. Proceedings of the First European Symposium on Modern Anesthetic Agents. Anes. & Resuscitation 1975;84:272–279.

CHAPTER 4

Electrophysiologic Monitoring
Betty L. Grundy

The electroencephalogram (EEG) and sensory evoked potentials (EP) are of in terest to the anesthesiologist because they can be used to assess the function of the nervous system during anesthesia and surgery. The hope is that these electrophysiologic monitoring modalities will detect neurologic dysfunction early so that appropriate interventions can optimize function intraoperatively and decrease the chance of permanent neurologic injury. For example, EEG monitoring is employed during carotid endarterectomy (1); somatosensory evoked potentials (SEP) are used during operations on the spine or spinal cord (2); brain-stem auditory evoked potentials (BAEP) are used during operations in the posterior cranial fossa (3); and visual evoked potentials (VEP) are valuable during operations on the pituitary gland (4).

Recordings of EEG or EP also are used to identify specific neural structures or foci during stereotactic neurosurgical procedures or open craniotomy. Characteristic EEG patterns recorded from stereotactically placed depth electrodes can distinguish gray matter from white. Epileptic foci may be localized for resection by recording from electrodes placed on the surface of the cerebral cortex or within its substance. SEP recorded directly from the cortical surface accurately identify the sensorimotor strip (5). This identification is particularly important during resection of temporoparietal lesions that may both impinge upon the primary somatosensory cortex and distort the usual anatomic landmarks.

In the neurologic intensive care unit, EEG and EP are used to help assess the prognoses of comatose patients. EEG monitoring is useful in patients with drug overdose or metabolic encephalopathy. Multimodality EP recordings help to localize lesions and predict outcome in head injury (6,7).

Finally, electrodiagnostic studies done preoperatively and postoperatively in neurosurgical patients deserve the anesthesiologist's attention (8,9). These tests sometimes help to identify the possible risks of anesthesia. Comparisons of tests done before and after surgery can be used to characterize the amount of improvement or deterioration associated with the operative procedure.

MONITORING THE ELECTROENCEPHALOGRAM

Successful electrodiagnostic testing of the nervous system requires some understanding of basic neurophysiology as well as knowledge of the equipment used for recording EEG and EP and the methods and techniques by which these tiny electrical signals are captured, analyzed, and interpreted (10,11).

Characteristics of the EEG

Spontaneous EEG activity arises in the granular layer of the cerebral cortex. It represents the graded summation of excitatory and inhibitory postsynaptic potentials of the pyramidal cells, whose long dendritic trees are oriented perpendicularly to the cortical surface (Fig. 4.1). The resulting electrical field potentials can be recorded from the scalp, a single electrode reflecting activity generated within a radius of approximately 2.5 cm. Regional differences in EEG activity, like regional differences in cerebral blood flow (CBF), may be critical to accurate diagnosis and monitoring. These regional differences can be detected only when recording is in more than one channel. Additional channels increase resolution. The typical diagnostic EEG uses 16 or, in some centers, 32 channels.

The EEG traditionally is described in terms of underlying frequencies, voltages or amplitudes, degree of organization and symmetry, abnormal patterns and rhythms, and reactivity to physiologic manipulations such as eye opening, hyperventilation, and sleep. The basic EEG rhythms are alpha, beta, theta, and delta. Alpha rhythm (8 to 13 Hz) is typical of relaxed wakefulness with eyes closed and is maximal over the occiput (Fig. 4.2). This rhythm is suppressed by opening of the eyes or by focusing of attention or performance of mental arithmetic. Beta activity (from 13 to between 25 and 30 Hz) is the low-voltage, relatively fast EEG rhythm seen in alert attentive wakefulness, especially with the eyes open (Fig. 4.3). Frontal beta rhythms are produced by barbiturates or benzodiazepines and persist as long as two weeks after withdrawal of chronic therapy with long-acting drugs such as diazepam. Theta activity (4 to 8 Hz) normally is seen in infants and children, during sleep, and with some general anesthetics (Fig. 4.4). Children and

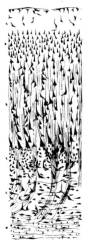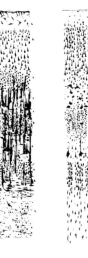

Figure 4.1 Laminations of pyramidal cells in the cerebral cortex. Left and center: Six-layered precentral and eight-layered occipital cortex, from Meynert, *Psychiatrie*, Braumuller, 1884. Right: Nine-layered calcarine cortex, from Ramon y Cajal, *Histologie du système nerveux*, vol 2, 1911. (Reproduced in Brazier MAB, Petsche H (eds): *Architectonics of the cerebral cortex*. New York, Raven Press, 1978. Reprinted with permission of the publisher.)

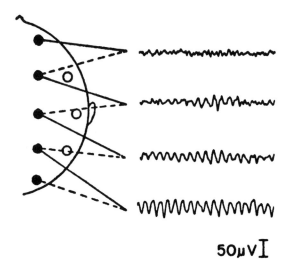

50μV I

I SEC

Figure 4.2 Normal alpha rhythm. (Modified from Spehlmann R: EEG primer. Amsterdam, Elsevier/ North Holland Biomedical Press, 1981, p 184.)

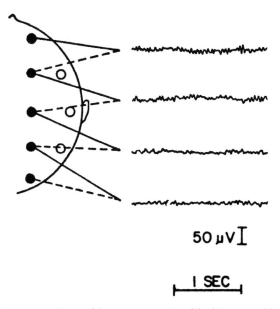

50 μV I

I SEC

Figure 4.3 Normal beta activity. (Modified from Spehlmann R: EEG primer. Amsterdam, Elsevier/North Holland Biomedical Press, 1981, p 190.)

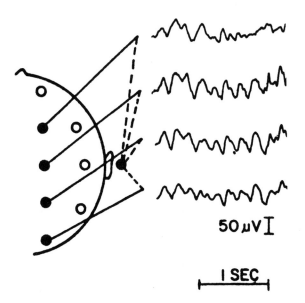

Figure 4.4   Theta rhythm. (Modified from Spehlmann R: EEG primer. Amsterdam, Elsevier/North Holland Biomedical Press, 1981, p 442.)

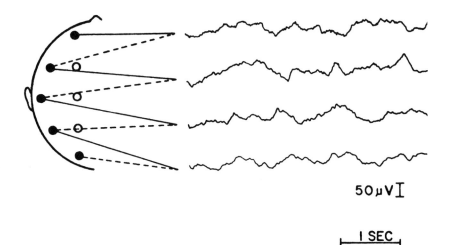

Figure 4.5   Delta rhythm. (Modified from Spehlmann R: EEG primer. Amsterdam, Elsevier/North Holland Biomedical Press, 1981, p 363.)

young adults may develop high-voltage frontal theta activity with hyperventilation. Delta activity (0 to 4 Hz) is characteristic of metabolic coma, cerebral hypoxia or ischemia, deep anesthesia, and normal deep sleep (Fig. 4.5). Underlying white-matter lesions and localized cortical injury may produce focal delta activity.

Recording the EEG

The traditional EEG is a 16-channel strip chart record of voltage on the y axis against time on the x axis. Chart speed is most often 30 mm/sec. The voltages recorded are usually 2 to 200 μV, ranging to as high as 1000 μV in the case of massive seizure activity. The usual standardization mark on the clinical EEG record represents 50 μV. (Contrast this small signal with the 1 mV standardization mark on the clinical electrocardiagram.) Recording of such small signals in an electrically hostile environment such as the operating room or intensive care unit demands both reliable equipment and meticulous attention to the technical details of signal acquisition and processing.

The interface between patient and electrode often is the weakest link in the system. Electrodes must be mechanically and electrically stable for the duration of recording. Interelectrode impedances must be low and matched, preferably 3000 ohms or less. For intraoperative recording we use silver/silver chloride disk electrodes, 7 mm in diameter, applied with collodion and filled with salt gel. Skin preparation by rubbing with an abrasive electrolyte minimizes the need for light abrasion with a blunt-tipped needle. Conductive pastes are easier to use than collodion, but they hold electrodes less securely. Needle electrodes are quick and easy to apply, but their recording characteristics are less desirable than those of disk electrodes because their surface area is smaller. Most subdermal (needle) electrodes are made of platinum. Disk electrodes are made of several metals including silver, gold, and tin. Stainless steel is an undesirable substance for EEG electrodes because of its poor recording characteristics, but it has been used in some applications because of its low cost.

Placement of EEG electrodes is critical. The International Ten–Twenty Electrode System (Fig. 4.6) allows accurate localization over specific brain areas according to a standard and universally understood pattern. Electrodes are placed according to measurements of the individual subjects' head circumference, interaural distance, and distance from nasion to inion. Once electrodes are applied, recordings can be made between different pairs of electrodes by mechanical or electronic switching. The pattern of electrodes used for a particular recording or segment of a recording is called the *electrode montage*. Typically, the recording montage is varied during the acquisition of the diagnostic EEG but kept constant during monitoring in the acute clinical situation.

The electroencephalograph amplifies and filters the tiny electrical signals detected by the electrodes. Filters are set to minimize input of frequencies below 0 to 1 Hz and above 30 to 70 Hz. Each EEG channel shows the difference in elec-

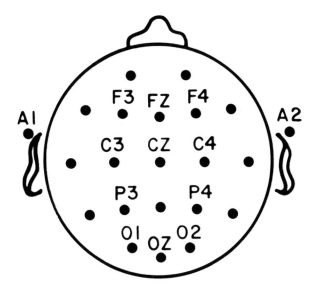

Figure 4.6 Electrode placements according to the International Ten–Twenty System. Unlabeled positions also have specific letter-number designations. Note that odd numbers are on the left, even numbers on the right. (Reprinted with permission of the publisher from Grundy BL: Electrophysiological monitoring: EEG and evoked potentials, in Newfield P, Cottrell J (eds): Manual of neuroanesthesia. Boston, Little, Brown, 1983.)

trical potential between two electrodes, with reference to a common electrode most often called a *ground electrode.* The electroencephalographer's ground electrode is not a ground to earth but rather a subject reference electrode. It allows rejection of noise that is common to the ground electrode and both active electrodes.

Devices for Processing EEG Signals

A number of signal-processing devices have been developed to simplify EEG monitoring in the operating room and critical care unit. These devices generate a variety of qualitative and quantitative displays, usually in fewer channels than the traditional strip chart EEG record. A few of the more familiar methods and devices are described.

The Cerebral Function Monitor (CFM), manufactured by Critikon, Inc. of Tampa, Florida, is a small, rugged, microprocessor-based single-channel unit. Clinical experience with this device exceeds that with all the other automated EEG monitors combined, and the currently available unit (CFM 870, Fig. 4.7) incorporates several improvements over the original version (12). The first stage of am-

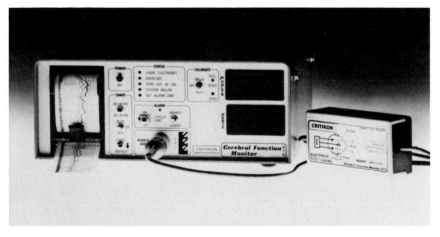

Figure 4.7   The CFM 870. (Courtesy of Critikon Inc., Tampa, Florida.)

plification is in a box mounted near the patient's head, so that noise picked up by the cable between the patient and the processor has relatively little effect on the final ratio of signal to noise. The amplified signal is heavily filtered to minimize input of signals below 2 Hz and above 17 Hz, and lower frequencies within this bandpass are filtered more heavily than faster components. The mean frequency and total microvoltage of the filtered signal are quantitatively displayed on a lighted display and plotted on a slow strip chart recorder (Fig. 4.8). Advantages of this unit include its size, reliability, simplicity, quantitative representation of data, and automatic production of a condensed paper record. Limitations include the inability to obtain the analog EEG waveform for purposes of quality control, loss of information in processing the signal, and availability of only a single channel.

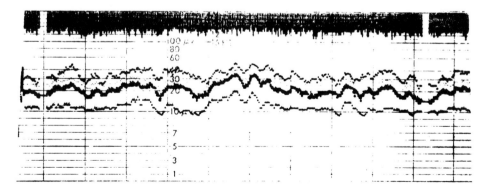

Figure 4.8   Output from CFM 870. See text for explanation. (From Grundy BL: Electrophysiologic brain monitoring, in Deutsch S (ed): ASA audio reviews in anesthesiology, 1983).

The Power Spectrum Analyzer (PSA), a similar device recently marketed by Neurologics, Inc., Nashville, Tennessee, differs from the CFM in several respects. It, too, is a small microprocessor-based unit developed for use by the nonelectroencephalographer in the operating room and critical care unit (13). Levels of EEG activity are displayed by illuminating red, yellow, or green lights for each of two channels. Provision is made for access to the analog EEG signal, but no display is provided. The two channels constitute an advantage of the PSA over the CFM. Relative disadvantages include the lack of quantitative representation of data, the lack of an automatic paper record, and the paucity of evaluative reports in the peer-reviewed literature.

The Neurometrics Monitor by Diatek (San Diego, CA) is a larger and more expensive unit, originally confined to a single channel (14). Recent versions record in two channels but still display only a single channel at one time. This device, too, has an amplifier near the patient's head. Fiberoptic transmission of signals from this amplifier to the processor eliminates noise that might be picked up by an electrical cable. The processor detects each wave in the analog EEG and represents it by a vertical line whose height is proportional to the wave's amplitude

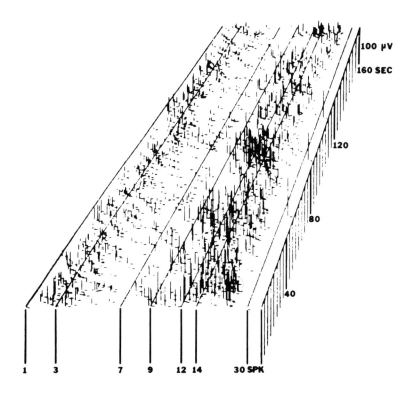

Figure 4.9 Display format from Neurometrics monitor by Diatek. See text for explanation. (From Saidman LJ, Smith NT (eds): Monitoring in anesthesia. New York, Wiley, 1978, p 311.)

(Fig. 4.9). The vertical lines are positioned on the x axis and color coded according to the frequencies of the EEG waves. An edge track shows spike activity. The entire display moves up a color television screen with time, and four minutes' data usually are displayed at once. The method of EEG analysis involves essentially no loss of data, but a proportion of the analyzed information is supresed to keep the display from becoming overcrowded. The processed data are stored on floppy disks, and paper copies can be obtained from the manufacturer. Several investigators have used this instrument to demonstrate effects of anesthetics and of global cerebral ischemia during cardiopulmonary bypass. Some quantitative representation of the data derived by this method of signal analysis eventually may prove even more useful than the presently available visual display.

A number of commercially available instruments perform power spectral analysis. These devices transform the EEG from the time domain to the frequency domain. EEG signals are then displayed in terms of voltage or power on the y axis and of frequency on the x axis. Each line in such a plot represents the EEG activity in a given epoch, or time segment, usually 4 to 32 seconds in duration. The most

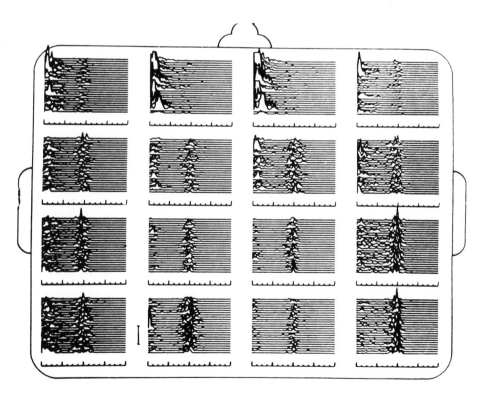

Figure 4.10 Multichannel compressed spectral array. See text. (Reprinted by permission of the author and the publisher from Bickford RG: Computer analysis of background activity, in Remond A (ed): EEG informatics. A didactic review of methods and applications of EEG data processing. Amsterdam, Elsevier/North Holland Biomedical Press, 1977.)

familiar display based on such power spectral analysis is the compressed spectral array (CSA) developed by Bickford (Fig. 4.10). A measurement derived from the CSA and found useful by some investigators is the spectral edge frequency, the frequency above which the EEG has very little energy.

The ultimate value of these computer-based instruments for EEG analysis in terms of relative cost effectiveness is not yet clear. Further evaluations comparing these devices to the standard 16-channel EEG, observed continually by an experienced EEG technologist, are needed. Regardless of the instrument used, meticulous quality control in signal acquisition is critical to successful monitoring.

Clinical Applications of EEG Monitoring

The most important application of EEG monitoring in the operating room is in detection of cerebral ischemia. Although monitoring of EEG is not universally accepted as routine during any operation, it is widely used during carotid endarterectomy (1,15) and during cardiopulmonary bypass. Some clinicians also monitor EEG during induced hypotension. The EEG usually is stable until CBF falls below 18 to 20 ml/100 gm/min, when the first changes are loss of fast activity and decreases in voltage. The dominant rhythm then progressively slows, and delta waves often are seen before the EEG becomes completely flat. With complete cessation of perfusion, as in cardiac arrest, the EEG becomes flat within seconds. At flows below about 12ml/100 gm/min, potassium begins to leak out of cells. Irreversible destruction begins when CBF is less than 10 ml/100 gm/min. The zone of flow between initial loss of EEG activity and destruction of neurons is known as the *ischemic penumbra* (16). Neurons in this low-flow zone can remain viable for many hours. Once the EEG is flat, however, it no longer can be used to determine when flows fall below the minimum required to prevent permanent neuronal damage.

EEG changes during carotid endarterectomy are used to determine which patients require bypass shunts during occlusion of the carotid artery. Some surgeons routinely use a shunt. Because the shunt itself may produce neurologic damage by artery-to-artery embolism, some surgeons restrict their use to those patients who show evidence of cerebral ischemia during test occlusion of the carotid artery. Ischemia may be detected by clinical neurologic assessment in patients operated upon under regional anesthesia (17) or by EEG monitoring in patients under general anesthesia. EEG changes are initially and most dramatically apparent in differences that develop between symmetrical channels recorded from opposite sides of the head (Fig. 4.11), particularly from electrodes placed over the watershed areas of the middle cerebral artery. Shunt malfunction can be detected with EEG monitoring, as can ischemic episodes related to embolic phenomena.

Inadequate cerebral perfusion pressure during carotid endarterectomy, cardiopulmonary bypass, or induced hypotension usually is reflected in EEG activity while neurologic dysfunction is still reversible. In such cases, timely restoration of adequate perfusion can prevent permanent neurologic injury. EEG alterations

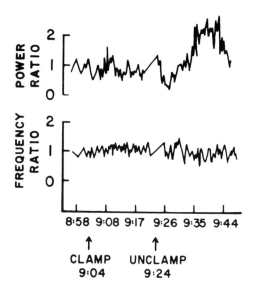

Figure 4.11 Asymmetry in EEG power after unclamping carotid artery following endarterectomy. (Reprinted with permission of the publisher from Grundy BL, Sanderson AC, Webster MW, Richey ET, Procopio PT, Karanjia P: Hemiparesis following carotid endarterectomy: comparison of monitoring methods. Anesthesiology 1981;55:462–466.)

also can warn of cortical dysfunction from causes such as hypoxia, hypoglycemia, severe anemia, or anesthetic overdose. In many instances, therapeutic intervention can avert permanent brain damage. The tragedies of permanent neurologic injury seem to occur when problems are not promptly detected.

EEG activity is altered by anesthetic agents, and varying dose-related patterns of change are produced by different anesthetic agents and adjuvant drugs (18,19). Physiologic factors such as body temperature and tensions of respiratory gases also affect the EEG, and interactions between pharmacologic and physiologic factors may be complex. EEG changes can reflect the depth of anesthesia and have even been used to provide servocontrol of anesthetic depth with agents such as thiopental and halothane. These techniques are of little use in the operating room today because deep surgical planes of anesthesia produced by a single agent have been largely displaced by combinations of agents and lighter levels of anesthesia supplemented with muscle relaxants. An EEG index of awareness during anesthesia would be valuable, but at present no such index is available. EEG monitoring of drug effects is currently useful in the intensive care unit when barbiturates are used to control intractable intracranial hypertension.

MONITORING SENSORY EVOKED POTENTIALS

Sensory evoked potentials (EP) are the electrophysiologic responses of the nervous system to sensory stimulation. The same general principles govern EP recording as govern recording of the spontaneous EEG. In addition, however, provision must be made to separate the neurophysiologic response to sensory stimulation from the ongoing background EEG. This is accomplished using a small computer to sum or average a number of individual responses that are precisely time-locked to repeated stimuli. Because spontaneous EEG activity is to some extent random, it is progressively attenuated as more and more responses to stimulation are averaged.

Characterization of EP

The usual representation of EP is as a plot of voltage against time (Fig. 4.12). The polarity of plotted waveforms has not been standardized and must be specified in each case. In this chapter, positivity at the first-named electrode is up. The duration of displayed activity varies from 10 to 500 msec or more and often is referred to as the "sweep time" of the EP. Amplitudes vary from nanovolts to microvolts and must be designated by appropriate standardization marks.

Peaks in EP waveforms are described in terms of polarity and poststimulus latency (20). The poststimulus latency is the time between stimulus onset and occurrence of the peak. Peaks are usually labeled P for positive and N for negative, with numbers representing nominal poststimulus latency. Amplitudes are measured from peak to following trough or with reference to a baseline voltage. When EP are abnormal or are altered by changes in pharmacologic or physiologic state, individual peaks may still be referred to in terms of a nominal or usual

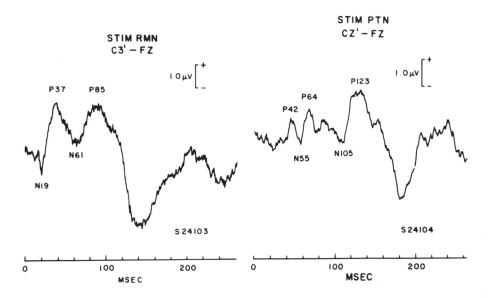

Figure 4.12 Normal somatosensory evoked potentials to stimulation of (A) median nerve at the wrist and (B) posterior tibial nerve at the ankle. (Reprinted with permission of the publisher from Grundy BL: Intraoperative monitoring of sensory-evoked potentials. Anesthesiology 1983;58:72–87.)

poststimulus latency. In some cases, other labeling is accepted by convention. The peaks in brain-stem auditory evoked potentials are assigned roman numerals.

Classification of EP

EP are classified according to (a) modes of sensory stimulation, (b) poststimulus latencies, (c) the distances separating neural generators from the recording electrodes, and (d) the neural generators of the displayed waveforms.

Modes of Sensory Stimulation

The modes of stimulation used in the operating room and intensive care unit are auditory, visual, and somatosensory (21,22). Auditory stimulation consists of pure tones or filtered clicks delivered by headphones or ear-insert transducers (Fig. 4.13). White noise (which is made up of equal parts and intensities of pure tones, harmonies and discordants throughout the range of human hearing) is

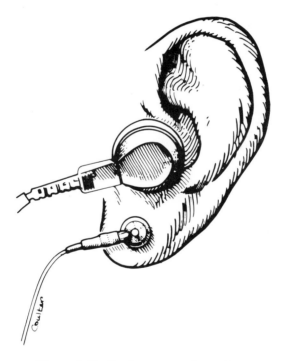

Figure 4.13 Ear-insert transducer for click stimulation during intraoperative monitoring of BAEP. (Reprinted with permission of the publisher from Grundy BL, Jannetta PJ, Procopio PT, Lina A, Boston, JR, Doyle E: Intraoperative monitoring of brain-stem auditory evoked potentials. J Neurosurg 1982; 57: 674–681.)

often used in the unstimulated ear to help minimize the effects of extraneous auditory stimuli. For intraoperative monitoring we use clicks at a sound level 60 decibels above the patient's hearing threshold and white noise 35 decibels above average hearing level.

Visual stimulation is provided by flashes from light-emitting diodes mounted in opaque goggles (Fig. 4.14). Protective eye ointment is used and the eyelids are taped closed with clear plastic tape under the stimulating goggles. Light-emitting diodes can be mounted on scleral contact lenses when these lenses are used in the surgical field to protect the eye during major craniofacial operations; however, contact lenses should not be placed in the eye during anesthesia unless the eye can be directly observed throughout the operation. The presently available goggle stimulators are convenient for transphenoidal operations but are too bulky for convenient use during low frontal craniotomy. A new design is needed.

Electrical current is used for somatosensory stimulation. Surface or subdural electrode pairs are placed over the median nerve at the wrist and the posterior tibial nerve at the ankle. Other nerves may be stimulated as necessary. We prefer subdermal electrodes for intraoperative monitoring because displacement is less likely with needle electrodes, and no pressure on the skin is needed to assure good contact. Constant-current stimulators are used to deliver 1 to 20 mA over 100 to 300 μ sec. The current is set to provide a visible motor twitch and may be increased somewhat during anesthesia.

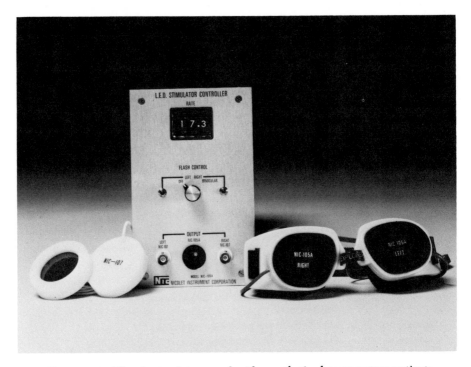

Figure 4.14   Visual stimulators used with anesthetized or comatose patients.

Poststimulus Latencies

Poststimulus latencies may be short (< 10 up to 40 msec), intermediate (20 to 120 msec) or long (100 to 500 msec). Short-latency potentials arise near the site of sensory stimulation and are relatively robust in the face of pharmacologic and physiologic manipulation. They are minimally affected by anesthetic agents. These potentials are small when recorded from the scalp because they arise at some distance from the recording electrodes. Thus, many repetitions are needed to extract the "signal" of the short-latency EP from the "noise" of the background EEG. The rate at which stimuli are repeated, however, can be more rapid with short-latency EP than with EP of intermediate or long latency. The later potentials require more time for recovery between stimuli, perhaps because more synapses are involved. EP of intermediate latency are definitely altered by anesthetics, but with appropriate anesthetic management, cortical and subcortical function can be reliably monitored. Late EP are so sensitive to drugs and to relatively subtle physiologic alterations that they are not useful in the operating room.

Distances from Neural Generators to Recording Electrodes

Electrophysiologic signals arising within approximately 2 centimeters of a recording electrode are known as *near-field potentials*. Those arising farther away but still transmitted to the electrode by volume conduction are called *far-field potentials*. Because signal strength falls as distance from the source increases, voltages of far-field EP are smaller than those of near-field potentials. For example, auditory evoked potentials of cortical origin are large enough that they can sometimes be seen at 50 μV or more in the ongoing EEG. These are near-field EP. In contrast, BAEP are much smaller than the background EEG activity. Two thousand repetitions are usually averaged to display these far-field potentials, and amplitudes measure only a few hundred nanovolts. BAEP recorded from an electrode placed on the eighth nerve during posterior fossa craniotomy (23) are, of course, near-field EP and have correspondingly higher voltage.

Neural Generators of EP

Evoked potential activity may arise in sensory receptors (e.g., electrocochleogram, electroretinogram), in peripheral or cranial nerve, in nerve plexus, in spinal cord, or in subcortical or cortical structures of the brain. The purported neural generators of specific peaks in SEP waveforms have not definitely been proved, but available evidence supports several clinically useful designations. These are described in the following sections.

Signal Processing for EP

Several manufacturers provide stand-alone systems for recording EP (Fig. 4.15). A complete EP system provides for (a) acquisition and conditioning of electro-

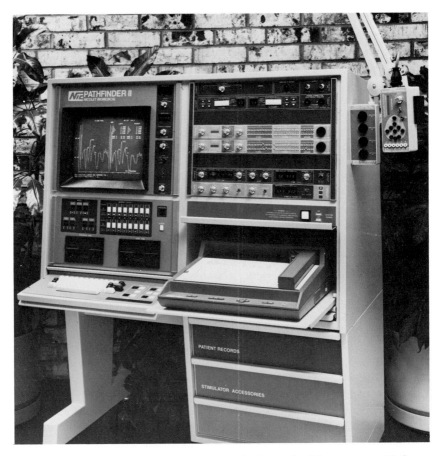

Figure 4.15 Pathfinder II. (Courtesy of Nicolet Biomedical Instruments, Madison, Wisconsin.)

physiologic signals; (b) signal processing, including summation or averaging; (c) display and measurement of EP; and (d) data storage.

The signal acquisition and conditioning segment of the EP system includes electrodes for signal acquisition, amplifiers to magnify the small voltages of EP, and filters to exclude signals outside the frequency bands of interest. At the heart of the EP system is a microprocessor, or small computer. This computer controls the sensory stimulators and precisely times the acquisition of segments of electrophysiologic activity. The amplified and filtered analog EEG is digitized, and, when a specified number of repetitions is completed, the recorded EEG segments are summed or averaged. Averaged EP are converted to analog form and displayed on an oscilloscope for precise measurement with electronic cursors, then plotted on paper to provide a permanent record. The digitized EP may also be electromagnetically stored.

Many EP systems can be programmed to automate some steps in monitoring. Most of the commercially available systems have some capability for automatically rejecting EEG segments contaminated with high-amplitude artifact, but these only partly substitute for continuous observation of the incoming signal by an experienced technologist. Manual suspension of averaging when the spontaneous EEG signal is noisy remains an important step in quality control.

EP systems can be developed in-house from hardware components that are considerably less expensive than ready-to-use systems. Even centers with outstanding engineering support, however, are likely to find the development of software lengthy and burdensome. Extensive software for EP systems has been developed by Nicolet Biomedical Instruments of Madison, Wisconsin, TECA Corporation of Pleasantville, New York, Tracor Northern of Middleton, Wisconsin, and BIK Systems, Inc. of La Jolla, California, among others.

EP Used for Monitoring in the Operating Room and Intensive Care Unit

BAEP, SEP, and VEP are used to monitor neurologic function in anesthetized and comatose patients.

Brain-stem Auditory Evoked Potentials

BAEP, in the operating room as in the diagnostic laboratory, are the simplest EP to record and interpret. The parameters used in our laboratory for stimulation and recording are shown in Table 4.1. A normal BAEP waveform (i.e., a situation in which there is no pathology in the circuit) is shown in Figure 4.16. The peaks are traditionally labeled with roman numerals, and the purported neural generators of these peaks (23–25) are shown in Table 4.2. Note that BAEP are short-latency far-field potentials of subcortical origin.

BAEP often are abnormal preoperatively in patients with vascular lesions or tumors in the posterior cranial fossa (26), but even abnormal EP are valuable for intraoperative monitoring if they are reproducible. It is important to remember that BAEP can be abnormal or absent because of audiologic abnormalities when central neurologic function is otherwise completely normal. Ideally, audiograms should be obtained preoperatively in patients who are to have intraoperative monitoring of BAEP. In any case, threshold hearing levels to the stimuli that will be used intraoperatively must be determined before induction of anesthesia. When BAEP are absent in comatose patients, an electrocochleogram should be made to rule out a peripheral audiologic abnormality.

Several observers have noted a high incidence of alterations in BAEP during operations in the posterior cranial fossa (22). Changes thought to be clinically important were seen during 37 of our first 54 cases (27). The factor most frequently associated with BAEP alteration was operative retraction in the cerebellopontine angle (Fig. 4.17). Changes were seen also with operative manipulation, with posi-

Table 4.1   Stimulus and Recording Parameters for Brain-stem Auditory Evoked Potentials

Stimulation

Insert earphones (Madsen Electronics, Inc., Buffalo, New York)
Clicks: Alternating rarefaction/condensation
Intensity: 60 dBSL*
Duration: 100 μ sec
Rate: 11.3 Hz
Contralateral masking: Wide band pseudorandom noise, 35 dBHL[†]

Recording

Channel 1: C_z-A_1[‡] (vertex to left ear)
Channel 2: C_z-A_2 (vertex to right ear)
Ground: F_pZ (midforehead)
Filters: 30–3000 Hz
Sensitivity: ±25 μV full scale
Sweep time: 10.24 msec
Sampling rate: 50,000 Hz[§]
Repetitions per average: 2000

*Sixty decibels above the patient's sensation level (hearing threshold).

[†]Thirty-five decibels above the average hearing level for the normal population.

[‡]Electrode positions according to the International Ten Twenty System (Fig. 4.6)

[§]Sampling rates as low as 10,000 to 12,500 Hz would be satisfactory.

Reprinted by permission of the publisher, from Grundy, BL: Neurosurgery, vol 11, no 4. Congress of Neurological Surgeons, 1982.

tioning of the head for retromastoid craniectomy, and with relative hypotension and hypocapnia. In 32 of the 37 cases showing BAEP alteration, changes were reversible in the operating room and hearing was preserved. The five patients who irretrievably lost BAEP had diminished hearing and markedly abnormal BAEP preoperatively. In each of these five, the eighth nerve had to be deliberately sacrificed during the course of the surgical procedure. Hearing was, of course, lost in all five cases.

In the intensive care unit, BAEP are useful indicators of brain-stem function in comatose patients (28,29). They show characteristic progressive changes with herniation of the brain stem. The degree to which BAEP may serve as indicators of less disastrous rises in intracranial pressure has not yet been determined.

BAEP provide no indication of cortical function. Extensive cortical damage can occur while BAEP remain quite stable (4). Conversely, damage to the eighth cranial nerve or brain stem, readily seen in BAEP, is not reflected in the EEG. Auditory evoked potentials of cortical origin do reflect function of both the auditory cortex and underlying auditory pathways, but little experience has been gained with monitoring of these intermediate-latency potentials in the operating room or intensive care unit.

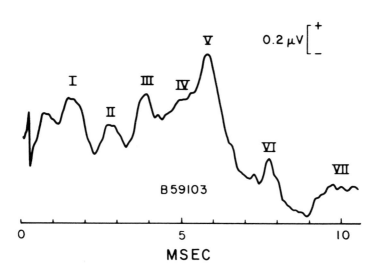

CZ−Ai

MSEC

Figure 4.16 Normal brain-stem auditory evoked potential. (Reprinted with permission of the publisher from Grundy BL: Intraoperative monitoring of sensory-evoked potentials. Anesthesiology 1983;58:72–87.)

Somatosensory Evoked Potentials

The most extensive collective experience with intraoperative monitoring of EP has been with somatosensory evoked potentials (SEP). Much of the early work was aimed at monitoring function of the spinal cord during operations on the spine (2,30) and during neurosurgical procedures on the cord itself (31). After the

Table 4.2 Purported Generators of Brain-stem Auditory Evoked Potentials*

Peak	Generator
I	Acoustic nerve
II	Intracranial acoustic nerve and/or cochlear nucleus (medulla)
III	Superior olive (pons)
IV	Lateral lemniscus (pons)
V	Inferior colliculus (midbrain)
VI	Medial geniculate (thalamus)
VII	Thalamocortical radiations

*Listed peaks are positive at the vertex. See text for references. Reprinted by permission of the publisher, from Grundy, BL: Neurosurgery, vol 11, no 4. Congress of Neurological Surgeons, 1982.

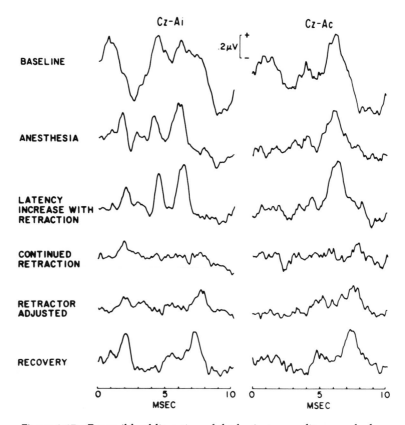

Figure 4.17 Reversible obliteration of the brainstem auditory evoked potential with retraction of the eighth cranial nerve. (Reprinted with permission from the International Anesthesia Research Society from Grundy BL, Lina A, Procopio PT, Jannetta PJ: Reversible evoked potential changes with retraction of the eighth cranial nerve. Anesth Analg (Cleve) 1981; (84:835–838.)

1975 report by MacEwen et al. (32), of neurologic injuries associated with the operative treatment of scoliosis, several orthopedic surgeons began to test the function of the cord during spinal fusion for scoliosis by awakening patients to check motor function or by monitoring SEP. More recently, SEP have been monitored during operations on the brachial plexus (33), on the dorsal roots of spinal nerves, and on the thoracic aorta. Cortical SEP have long been used to identify the sensorimotor strip during resection of adjacent lesions (5), and somatosensory central conduction times are useful for detecting cerebral ischemia during carotid endarterectomy and during induced hypotension for operations on intracranial aneurysms (34).

SEP of both short and intermediate poststimulus latency are useful in the operating room and intensive care unit. Short-latency SEP are far-field potentials when recorded from the scalp but may be near-field when recorded over

Table 4.3 Purported Generators of Short-latency Somatosensory Evoked Potentials

Peak	Generator
N9	Brachial plexus
N11	Spinal roots or dorsal columns
N13, 14	Spinal cord gray matter or dorsal columns
N14, 15	Brain stem and/or thalamus
N20	Primary somatosensory cortex

NOTE: Stimulation: median nerve; recording: clavicle, mastoid process, second cervical vertebra, primary somatosensory cortical area; reference electrode: F_2 or noncephalic. (Early positive waves are obscured in frontally referenced recordings.) See text for references.

Reprinted by permission of the publisher, from Grundy, BL: Neurosurgery, vol 11, no 4. Congress of Neurological Surgeons, 1982.

Table 4.4 Stimulus and Recording Parameters for Somatosensory Evoked Potentials

Stimulation

Sites[*]: (1) Right median nerve at wrist
(2) Right posterior tibial nerve at ankle
(3) Left posterior tibial nerve at ankle
(4) Left median nerve at wrist

Electrode pairs: Subdermal platinum electrodes (Grass Instrument Corp., Quincy, Massachusetts), 3 cm apart, cathode proximal

Constant current: Sensory threshold plus motor threshold, usually 3 to 10 mA

Duration: 250 μ sec

Rate: 0.9–1.9 Hz

Recording

Channel 1: C_3' (2 cm behind C_3)–F_z[†]

Channel 2: CV_2 (skin over 2nd cervical vertebra)–F_z

Channel 3: C_4' (2cm behind C_4)–F_z

Channel 4: C_z' (2cm behind C_z)–F_z

Ground: sternum

Filters: 1–1500 Hz

Sensitivity: ±50 μV full scale

Sweep time: 253 msec

Sampling rate: 4032 Hz

Repetitions: 128

[*]Only one site is stimulated for a given EP average.

[†]Electrode positions designated according to International Ten-Twenty System (Fig. 4.6)

Reprinted by permission of the publisher, from Grundy, BL: Neurosurgery, vol 11, no 4. Congress of Neurological Surgeons, 1982.

peripheral nerve or brachial plexus. Short-latency SEP recorded from electrodes placed in the spinal epidural space or in the ligaments of the spinal column are also near-field potentials (35). All the SEP peaks occurring earlier than 20 msec after stimulation of the median nerve at the wrist are subcortical in origin (36,37). Purported generators of these peaks are listed in Table 4.3. SEP of intermediate latency are cortical in origin and are near-field potentials when recorded from the scalp.

The parameters for stimulation and recording of SEP that we have found most convenient for intraoperative monitoring are shown in Table 4.4. A typical normal recording is shown in Figure 4.18. We stimulate each of the four extremities singly, and the same recording montage is used throughout. Electrodes placed over the brachial plexus or lumbar plexus may be required in some applications. Recording in multiple channels greatly aids the interpretation of SEP, and comparison of potentials at risk from operative manipulation to potentials not at risk from surgical perturbations helps to distinguish those changes originating at the operative site from alterations caused by anesthesia or other systemic factors.

Intraoperative alterations in SEP are seen more frequently during high-risk neurosurgical procedures than during orthopedic operations (21,30). Changes have been associated with operative manipulation, surgical retraction, hypotension (Fig. 4.19), ischemia of the spinal cord, and systemic hypoxia (Fig. 4.20). In our experience, SEP alterations reversible in the operating room have been associated with preservation of function, and irretrievable loss of SEP has been followed by functional loss in the monitored pathway (Fig. 4.21).

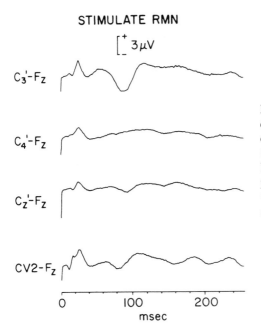

STIMULATE RMN

Figure 4.18 Normal somatosensory evoked potentials recorded simultaneously from the scalp and neck. (Reprinted with permission from Grundy BL: Monitoring of sensory evoked potentials during neurosurgical operations: methods and applications. Neurosurgery 1982; 11:556–575.)

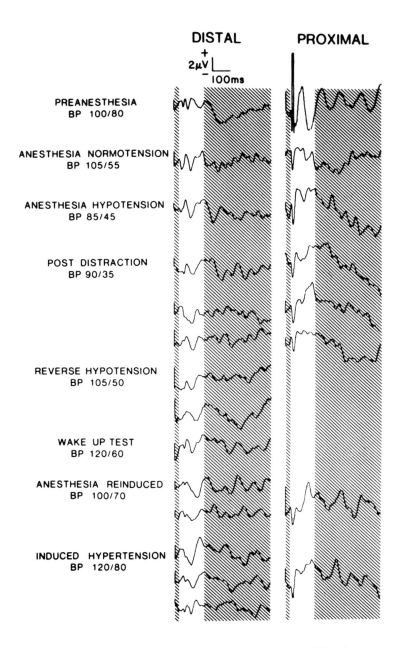

Figure 4.19 SEP changes related to manipulation of arterial blood pressure during scoliosis fusion. Unshaded areas highlight the primary specific cortical responses. (From Grundy BL, Nash CL, Brown RH: Arterial pressure manipulation alters spinal cord function during correction of scoliosis. Anesthesiol 1981;54:249–253.)

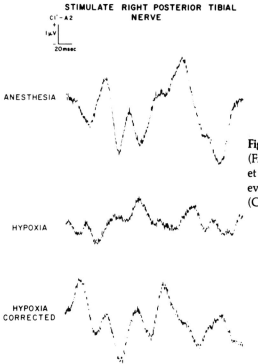

STIMULATE RIGHT POSTERIOR TIBIAL
CI'—A2   NERVE

ANESTHESIA

HYPOXIA

HYPOXIA
CORRECTED

Figure 4.20 SEP change with hypoxia. (From Grundy BL, Heros RC, Tung AS, et al.: Intraoperative hypoxia detected by evoked potential monitoring. Anes Analg (Cleve) 1981;60:437–439.)

Recording of SEP is technically complex, and some observers have encountered a number of technically inadequate studies. Although most investigators find a high degree of correlation between intraoperative SEP findings and postoperative neurologic function, this experience has not been universal. Perhaps some erroneous results were related to problems with quality control in a difficult recording environment or to alterations in SEP produced by anesthetics or other extraneous factors.

In the neurosurgical intensive care unit, SEP are used to monitor function of both spinal cord (38) and brain stem. Multimodality cortical evoked potentials, including SEP, are valuable prognostic indicators in victims of head injury (6,7). Somatosensory central conduction times are early indicators of cerebral ischemia in patients with subarachnoid hemorrhage (39).

Visual Evoked Potentials

Little is known about subcortical VEP (40), although ophthalmologists have recorded the electroretinogram (41) for a number of years. Both the pattern-reversal VEP recorded in the diagnostic laboratory and the flash-evoked potentials recorded in anesthetized and comatose patients are cortical in origin. They are near-field potentials of intermediate latency. A normal flash-evoked VEP is shown in Figure 4.22. Parameters used for stimulating and recording are shown in Table 4.5.

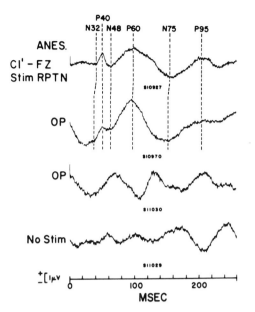

Figure 4.21 SEP elicited by stimulation of the right posterior tibial nerve. The first waveform, abnormal but reproducible, was recorded before opening the dura. The second, recorded three hours later, shows increasing loss of definition. The third waveform, recorded after five hours of intradural operation, was not distinguishable from an average recorded without stimulation. The artifact seen in the last two tracings probably stems from spontaneous EEG rhythms. Artifact of this kind is now eliminated by using pseudorandom interstimulus intervals. (Reprinted with permission of the publisher from Grundy BL, Nelson PB, Doyle E, Procopio PT: Intraoperative loss of somatosensory evoked potentials predicts loss of spinal cord function. Anesthesiology 1982;57:321–322.)

VEP have been monitored during operations on the pituitary gland and during neurosurgical procedures in the anterior cranial fossa (4,21,43). Early enthusiasts have grown disillusioned with intraoperative VEP monitoring, however. Our experience is still limited, but experience with our first six cases was encouraging. Only a single patient had changes in VEP that persisted to the end of the surgical procedure. His intraoperative improvement in VEP (Fig. 4.23) correlated well with the documented improvement in his visual fields after resection of a large recurrent pituitary tumor.

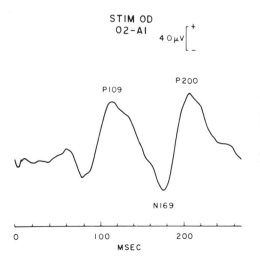

Figure 4.22 A normal flash-evoked VEP. (Reprinted with permission of the publisher from Grundy BL: Electrophysiological monitoring: EEG and evoked potentials, in Newfield P, Cottrell J, eds: Manual of Neuroanesthesia. Boston, Little, Brown, 1983.)

Table 4.5   Stimulus and Recording Parameters for Visual Evoked Potentials

Stimulation

Flash: LED array in opaque goggles over closed eyelids (Nicolet Biomedical, Inc., Madison, Wisconsin)

Duration: 5 msec

Rate: 0.9–1.9 Hz

Recording

Channel 1: O_z–A_2* (ground A_1)

Channel 2: P_z–A_2 (ground A_1)

Channel 3: 5 cm left of O_z to A_2 (ground A_1)

Channel 4: 5 cm right of O_z to A_1 (ground A_2)

Filters: 1–1500 Hz

Sensitivity: ±50 μV full scale

Sweep time: 253 msec

Sampling rate: 4032 Hz

Repetitions: 128

*Electrode positions according to the International Ten-Twenty System (Fig. 4.6).

Reprinted by permission of the publisher, from Grundy, BL: Neurosurgery, vol 11, no 4. Congress of Neurological Surgeons, 1982.

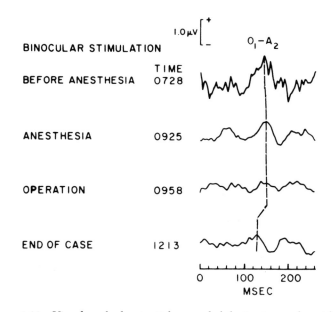

Figure 4.23   Visual-evoked potentials recorded during transsphenoidal resection of a pituitary tumor. (Reprinted with permission of the publisher from Grundy BL: Intraoperative monitoring of sensory-evoked potentials. Anesthesiology 1983;58:72–87).

The current difficulties with intraoperative monitoring of VEP may stem from technical difficulties and from the remarkable sensitivity of these waveforms to general anesthetics (43). Perhaps new techniques and protocols will lead to more sensitive and reliable monitoring methods.

CURRENT LIMITATIONS OF ELECTROPHYSIOLOGIC MONITORING

Present barriers to electrophysiologic monitoring in the operating room and critical care unit include the technical difficulties of signal acquisition in electrically hostile recording environments, difficulties in monitoring and constraining potentially confounding variables, shortages of well-trained personnel to record and interpret electrophysiologic waveforms, the paucity of well-controlled studies relating changes in EEG and EP to neurologic outcomes of monitored patients, and the costs of personnel and equipment.

Available technology and data from a number of recent clinical studies go far toward overcoming these barriers to more widespread use of electrophysiologic monitoring of the nervous system. New methods and devices for signal acquisition and processing are being introduced more rapidly than they can be compared in well-documented clinical trials. Although several of these facilitate monitoring, valuable information often is sacrificed to convenience. Clearly, howevever, technically satisfactory recordings can be obtained using standard equipment, provided meticulous attention is given to quality control. A decade from now, today's instrumentation will seem relatively primitive, but skill and experience will still be required to place and secure electrodes, to recognize artifacts and the effects of confounding variables, and to interpret intraoperative changes in electrophysiologic recordings. With the progressive accumulation of data from well-documented clinical series and from laboratory studies in humans and in animals, we will be able to define more accurately the parameters of interest in EEG and EP signals and to determine acceptable tolerance limits for these parameters. Automatic alarm functions can then be generated to warn the surgeon and the anesthesiologist of neurologic dysfunction. Given the devastating effects of permanent neurologic injury and the high costs of such injuries in both human and economic terms, it seems likely that our society will find electrophysiologic monitoring well worth its cost for patients who are at risk for serious injury to the central nervous system.

REFERENCES

1. Sundt TM Jr, Sharbrough FW, Piepgras DG, et al.: Correlation of cerebral blood flow and electroencephalographic changes during carotid endarterectomy: With results of surgery and hemodynamics of cerebral ischemia. Mayo Clin Proc 1981;56: 533–543.
2. Nash CL, Lorig RA, Schatzinger LA, et al.: Spinal cord monitoring during operative treatment of the spine. Clin Orthop 1977;126:100–105.

3. Grundy BL, Procopio PT, Lina A, et al.: Reversible evoked potential changes with retraction of the eighth cranial nerve. Anes Analg (blue) 1981;60:835–838.
4. Raudzens PA: Intraoperative monitoring of evoked potentials. Ann NY Acad Sci 1982;388:308–326.
5. Woolsey CN, Erickson TC, Gilson WE: Localization in somatic sensory and motor areas of human cerebral cortex as determined by direct recording of evoked potentials and electrical stimulation. J Neurosurg 1979;51:476–506.
6. Greenberg, RP, Mayer DJ, Becker DP, et al.: Evaluation of brain function in severe human head trauma with multimodality evoked potentials. Part 1: Evoked brain-injury potentials, methods, and analysis. J Neurosurg 1977;47:150–162.
7. Greenberg RP, Becker DP, Miller JD, et al.: Evaluation of brain function in severe human head trauma with multimodality evoked potentials. Part 2: Localization of brain dysfunction and correlation with posttraumatic neurological conditions. J Neurosurg 1977;47:163–177.
8. Chiappa KH, Ropper AH: Evoked potentials in clinical medicine. Part 1. N Engl J Med 1982;306:1140–1150.
9. Chiappa KH, Ropper AH: Evoked potentials in clinical medicine. Part 2. N Eng J Med 1982;306:1205–1211.
10. Niedermeyer E, da Silva FL: Electroencephalography: Basic principles, clinical applications and related fields. Baltimore, Urban & Schwarzenberg, 1982.
11. Cooper R, Osselton JW, Shaw JC: EEG Technology. Third edition. Boston, Butterworths, 1980.
12. Prior PF: Monitoring cerebral function: Long-term recordings of cerebral electrical activity. Amsterdam, Elsevier/North-Holland Biomedical Press, 1979.
13. String TS, Callahan A: The critical manipulable variables of hemispheric low flow during carotid surgery. Surgery 1983;93:46–49.
14. Levy WJ, Grundy BL, Smith NT: Electroencephalography and evoked potentials, in Saidman LJ, Smith NT (eds.), Monitoring in anesthesia. Edition 2. Boston, Butterworths, 1984.
15. Chiappa KH, Burke SR, Young RR: Result of electroencephalographic monitoring during 367 carotid endarterectomies. Stroke 1979;10:381–388.
16. Astrup J, Siesjö BK, Symon L: Thresholds in cerebral ischemia—the ischemic penumbra. Stroke 1981;12:723–725.
17. Steed D, Webster M, Grundy B, et al.: Causes of stroke in carotid endarterectomy. Surgery 1982;92:634–641.
18. Clark DL, Rosner BS: Neurophysiologic effects of general anesthetics: I. The electroencephalogram and sensory evoked responses in man. Anesthesiology 1973;38:564–582.
19. Rosner BS, Clark DL: Neurophysiologic effects of general anesthetics: II. Sequential regional actions in the brain. Anesthesiology 1973;39:59–81.
20. Donchin E, Callaway E, Cooper R, et al.: Publication criteria for studies of evoked potentials (EP) in man. Prog Clin Neurophysiol 1977;1:1–11.
21. Grundy BL: Monitoring of sensory evoked potentials during neurosurgical operations: Methods and applications. Neurosurgery 1982;11:556–575.
22. Grundy BL: Intraoperative monitoring of sensory-evoked potentials. Anesthesiology 1983;58:72–87.
23. Moller AR, Jannetta P, Bennett M, et al. Intracranially recorded responses from the human auditory nerve: New insights into the origin of brain-stem evoked potentials (BSEPs). Electroencephalogr Clin Neurophysiol 1981;52:18–27.

24. Achor LJ, Starr A: Auditory brainstem responses in the cat: I. Intracranial and extra-cranial recordings. Electroencephalogr Clin Neurophysiol 1980;48:154–173.

25. Achor LJ, Starr A: Auditory brainstem responses in the cat: II. Effects of lesions. Electroencephalogr Clin Neurophysiol 1980;48:174–190.

26. Stockard JJ, Rossiter VS: Clinical and pathologic correlates of brainstem auditory response abnormalities. Neurology (NY) 1977;27:316–325.

27. Grundy BL, Jannetta PJ, Lina A, et al.:Intraoperative monitoring of brain-stem audi-tory evoked potentials. J Neurosurg 1982;57:674–681.

28. Nagao S, Roccaforte P, Moody RA: Acute intracranial hypertension and auditory brain-stem responses: Part 2. The effects of brain-stem movement on the auditory brain-stem responses due to transtentorial herniation. J Neurosurg 1979;51:846–851.

29. Nagao S, Roccaforte P, Moody RA: Acute intracranial hypertension and auditory brain-stem responses: Part 3. The effects of posterior fossa mass lesions on brain-stem function. J Neurosurg 1980;52:351–358.

30. Grundy BL, Nash CL Jr, Brown RH: Deliberate hypotension for spinal fusion: Pro-spective randomized study with evoked potential monitoring. Can Anaesth Soc J 1982;29:452–461.

31. McCallum JE, Bennett MH: Electrophysiologic monitoring of spinal cord function during intraspinal surgery. Surg Forum 1975;26:469–471.

32. MacEwen GD, Bunnell WP, Sriram K: Acute neurological complications in the treat-ment of scoliosis: A report of the Scoliosis Research Society. J Bone Joint Surg [Am] 1975;57A:404–408.

33. Jones SJ: Investigation of brachial plexus traction lesions by peripheral and spinal somatosensory evoked potentials. J Neurol Neurosurg Psychiatry 1979;42:107–116.

34. Hargadine J: Evoked potentials, in Rand E (ed.): Microneurosurgery. St. Louis, CV Mosby Company, in press, 1983.

35. Hahn JF, Lesser R, Klem G, et al.: Simple technique for monitoring intraoperative spinal cord function. Neurosurgery 1981;9:692–695.

36. Jones SJ: Short latency potentials recorded from the neck and scalp following me-dian nerve stimulation in man. Electroencephalogr Clin Neurophysiol 1977;43:853–863.

37. Mauguière F, Courjon J: The origins of short-latency somatosensory evoked poten-tials in humans. Ann Neurol 1981;9:607–611.

38. Perot PL Jr: The clinical use of somatosensory evoked potentials in spinal cord in-jury. Clin Neurosurg 1972;20:367–381.

39. Symon L, Hargadine J, Zawirski M, et al. Central conduction time as an index of ischemia in subarachnoid haemorrhage. J Neurol Sci 1979;44:95–103.

40. Cracco RQ, Cracco JB: Visual evoked potential in man: Early oscillatory potentials. Electroencephalogr Clin Neurophysiol 1978;45:731–739.

41. Armington JC:Electroretinography, in Aminoff MJ(ed.): Electrodiagnosis in Clinical Neurology. New York, Churchill Livingstone, 1980, pp 305–347.

42. Allen A, Starr A, Nudleman K: Assessment of sensory function in the operating room utilizing cerebral evoked potentials: A study of fifty–six surgically anesthetized patients. Clin Neurosurg 1981;28:457–481.

43. Uhl RR, Squires KC, Bruce DL, et al.: Effect of halothane anesthesia on the human cortical visual evoked response. Anesthesiology 1980;53:273–276.

CHAPTER 5

Anesthetic Management for Neuroradiologic Diagnostic Procedures
I. Cary Andrews

From the discovery of x-ray to the introduction of computed tomography, a basic requirement for obtaining satisfactory and interpretable neuroradiologic studies is immobilization of the patient. Any motion of the patient during the examination not only interferes with the study but also increases the rate of complications through repetition of the examination and subjects the patient to unnecessary radiation exposure. Especially in apprehensive and uncooperative patients and in children, a form of general anesthesia frequently is employed for obtaining easily interpretable studies. Angiography occasionally may be painful when areas rich in pain receptors, such as the face, are studied, and these patients may require general anesthesia. Many patients have a history of allergic reactions to the iodinated contrast material, and anesthesiologists frequently are consulted to help prevent such reactions or to manage this type of individual for a neuroradiologic study. Certain procedures may require the use of hyperventilation or apnea (controlled ventilation) to slow the cerebral circulation time, to demonstrate abnormal vascularity of a brain tumor, and to relieve arterial spasm. These studies can only be performed under apnea achieved with general anesthesia (1). Therefore, it is imperative that anesthesiologists be familiar with the diagnostic tools used in neuroradiology, be aware of the various positions in which patients may be placed during the examinations, and be available to manage anaphylactic reactions to contrast material used during the studies.

Before a patient is to undergo an intracranial or intraspinal surgical procedure, it is important that diagnostic studies be done to obtain accurate information on the type and location of the lesion. Therefore, patients frequently are subjected to prolonged studies, some of which introduce appreciable difficulty. Procedures include ventriculography, angiography, pneumoencephalography (PEG), and computed tomography (CT scan) for intracranial lesions and lumbar puncture and myelography for spinal lesions. The CT scan has replaced many procedures, particular PEG and ventriculography. In many centers, however, all of these procedures are used to a varying degree. Although not all diagnostic

95

procedures are complicated or exhaustive, arteriography and PEG are particularly time-consuming and exacting and involve significant risks. In children the usual risks are increased by more frequent need of general anesthesia for procedures that most adults can tolerate under local anesthesia.

GENERAL CONSIDERATIONS

It is important to note that whether the choice is general anesthesia, intravenous sedation and local anesthesia, or monitoring either a critically ill patient or a patient with a history of untoward reactions to contrast media, the usual preoperative assessment must be done. In patients with increased intracranial pressure (ICP), the importance of ensuring a smooth course of anesthesia and avoiding cerebral vasodilator stimuli or a rise in venous pressure must be strictly adhered to. This may be more important during a radiologic investigation than during a craniotomy, since it may be more difficult to provide rapid decompressive therapy.

Occasionally, it is necessary to move a patient under general anesthesia between the radiology department and the operating room. It is thus highly desirable that these two areas be situated close together.

It is not uncommon for neurosurgical patients to receive more than one anesthetic over a period of a few days (for angiography or CT scanning followed by anesthesia for craniotomy). Therefore, the anesthetic technique should ensure that there is minimal disturbance of the patient's general condition or neurologic state and that recovery is rapid, with minimal postoperative nausea or vomiting. Such attention is critical in pediatric patients since dehydration can occur much more rapidly than in adults.

Some other general problems commonly encountered in the diagnostic neuroradiology suite are (29):

1. The patient may be a poor anesthetic risk. In obtunded patients or in emergency situations, the medical history may be vague, and associated systemic or serious chronic disease states may not be recognized.
2. The x-ray suite often is dark and unfamiliar to anesthesiologists. This environment makes it difficult to observe the patient's color, respiratory pattern, and the flowmeters on the anesthesia machine.
3. Since the use of nonexplosive agents is almost universal today, hazards of explosion and electrocution have been removed, but there is radiation exposure for both patient and anesthesiologist.
4. Since certain diagnostic procedures are lengthy and may require repetition, fatigue and boredom can engender carelessness and loss of vigilance.
5. Preparation of the patient may be inadequate. Patients often come from hospital areas unfamiliar with usual anesthetic preparation and may not be premedicated or fasted. Procedures may be started without involvement of an anesthesiologist only to result in failure to obtain a complete study because the patient is not fully prepared.

6. Most radiologic areas are constructed without consideration for anesthesia requirements, resulting in a working environment that is not only unfamiliar to the anesthesiologist, but lacking in many vital requirements (oxygen, suction, intravenous administration equipment, etc.).
7. Maintenance of a clear airway can be difficult when access to the patient is poor and numerous postural changes are necessary for good diagnostic studies. Even the presence of an endotracheal tube does not provide complete assurance since tubes can kink, especially during CT scanning and PEG when the patient may be moved several times during the study.
8. Since most diagnostic procedures are considered to cause minimal physiologic changes, it is sometimes forgotten that the presence of a general anesthetic and sudden positional changes may precipitate cardiovascular instability.
9. Many patients are transported to the radiology department by messengers and then left unattended by medical personnel, perhaps resulting in increased patient apprehension.
10. X-ray rooms are usually not well ventilated and anesthetic gases may accumulate during long procedures if the proper devices for scavenging the environment are not available.
11. Radiologists and radiology technicians trying to complete a diagnostic study in haste may not realize the importance of communicating their plans to the anesthesiologist.

ANESTHETIC MANAGEMENT

Neuroradiologic procedures may be performed under local anesthesia with or without sedation or under general anesthesia. There is no consensus as to which method best fulfills anesthetic and radiologic requirements.

Local Anesthesia and Sedation

Local anesthesia provides a safe technique and if combined with appropriate sedation provides a calm, awake, and cooperative patient. By maintaining verbal contact with the patient, changes in levels of consciousness and physiologic responses to the study can easily be observed and evaluated. Sedation can be achieved with the following drugs used singly or in combination: benzodiazepines (diazepam), phenothiazines, butyrophenones (droperidol), and narcotics. Diazepam is a potent, relatively long-acting tranquilizer with minimal cardiovascular and respiratory depression and good amnesic properties (3). The narcotics can produce nausea and vomiting, respiratory depression, and cardiovascular instability; the phenothiazines are associated with hypotension that occasionally is prolonged and refractory to conservative therapy; the butyrophenones cause dysphoria and extrapyramidal effects. The combination of droperidol and fentanyl (neuroleptanalgesia) in careful administration can avoid most of these complications and is widely and safely used. The antiemetic action of droperidol may be useful during encephalography. Local anesthesia plus sedation, however, may not be the method of choice with young children, adults who are uncooperative or with mental disturbances, and in comatose or restless patients.

General Anesthesia

General anesthesia can safely provide many of the requirements needed for successful radiologic studies. It produces an immobile patient, which facilitates the production of clear and sharp x-ray films. It blunts reflex movements of the patient during injection of contrast media, and it avoids the restlessness and emotional stress that may be encountered during prolonged and sometimes painful investigations. The radiologist is provided more time and safety without concern for patient cooperation. The main disadvantages are those related to maintenance of the airway and of circulatory stability. Endotracheal intubation performed in children who may be moved during the procedure carries a risk of inducing croup and laryngeal edema postoperatively. Ketamine, an intravenous anesthetic agent, produces a state of "dissociative anesthesia-analgesia" and provides certain advantages over the more conventional inhalation-administered general anesthetics; there is a rapid and smooth induction, and the airway usually is well maintained during postural changes. Cardiovascular support is maintained due to release of catecholamines, and respiratory depression is rare and transient. Infants less than 6 months of age undergoing prolonged examinations must be carefully observed, however, since most cases of respiratory problems (apnea, periodic respiration) occur in this group. When ketamine was initially introduced, it seemed to offer a promising alternative to endotracheal intubation in children (4), but despite good airway maintenance, protection against gastric aspiration cannot be assured (5).

Certain side effects must be considered when ketamine is used in the patient with neurologic problems. It can markedly increase ICP in patients with reduced intracranial compliance from mass lesions or hydrocephalus. It probably should not be used when intracranial hypertension is suspected unless ventricular drainage has been established (6). Ketamine also has been shown to augment brain electrical activity to the point of inducing seizure discharges in experimental animals. It therefore could complicate the management of patients with seizure disorders (7). Marked individual variations can occur, such as delayed return to consciousness or a more prolonged effect that compromises poststudy neurologic examination.

ADVERSE REACTIONS TO CONTRAST MEDIA

Reactions to contrast media are not uncommon and vary from mild skin rashes to anaphylactic reactions. Common adverse effects of metrizamide include headache, nausea, vomiting, meningeal irritation as manifested by stiffness of the neck and Kernig and Brudzinski signs, and mild, acute psychoorganic reactions such as change of consciousness, anxiety, or panic (8). Rarely, localized spinal irritation may occur with spasm and stiffness in the lower extremities. Electroencephalographic (EEG) changes may be seen within 24 to 48 hours after instillation of metrizamide (9), even in patients with no history of epilepsy. Grand mal seizures have been reported (8,10). Phenothiazines may predispose the patient to metrizamide-induced seizures by lowering the seizure threshold (11) and should be avoided, as should enflurane and ketamine. Phenobarbital and benzodiazepines are the premedications of choice (12).

Marked responses to contrast materials include severe respiratory distress characterized by wheezing with bronchial and/or laryngeal spasm. In addition, this may be associated with giant urticaria, including swelling of the lips and eyelids. The other major response is one of cardiovascular collapse characterized by hypotension, tachycardia, dyspnea, confusion, cyanosis, and eventual loss of consciousness. The Committee on Contrast Media of the International Society of Radiology reported a 2.33% incidence of nonfatal reactions in over 27,000 vascular studies (13). Four fatalities occurred, including a patient undergoing cerebral angiography. Patients with a previous history of an untoward response had three times as many reactions as occurred in the general population. The mechanism for the reactions is unknown and predictive tests prior to the procedure usually are unreliable. Many radiologists prefer to schedule patients with a previous history of reactions when an anesthesiologist is in attendance so that vital signs can be carefully monitored. In addition, many radiologists prepare patients with steroids (150 mg of prednisone or its equivalent per day) starting 18 hours before and continuing 12 hours after injections of contrast media (14). In Zweiman's study, steroids were given only for patients in the "rush" and "anaphylactoid" categories; those in the "vasomotor" category received no steroids but were closely monitored. In 124 patients, only four mild reactions were seen (14). Other drugs commonly employed were antihistamines (diphenhydramine hydrochloride) either intravenously immediately or orally one hour prior to the procedure. In either case, it is common to use a test dose of contrast media either intravenously or intraarterially and to use small total quantities.

Treatment of adverse reactions depends primarily on their severity. Patients who develop skin rashes or mild vasomotor responses require minimal therapy such as intravenous fluids and/or the administration of an antihistamine (diphenhydramine, 50 mg). Severe anaphylactic reactions manifested by respiratory distress or severe cardiovascular collapse require immediate and aggressive treatment. Under these circumstances the main drugs used are epinephrine (0.25 mg subcutaneously) and steroids (hydrocortisone, 100 mg). The usual standard supportive measures must be available as in any situation requiring cardiopulmonary support. The special problems related to anaphylactic reaction after chymopapain are discussed in Chapter 9.

CEREBRAL ANGIOGRAPHY

Cerebral angiography is used to investigate cerebral vascular lesions such as aneurysm, arteriovenous malformation, arteriosclerotic cerebrovascular disease, brain tumor, head trauma, congenital cerebral anomalies, and cerebral infection (15).

Cerebral angiography can be performed by direct percutaneous puncture of the extracranial cerebral vasculature or via retrograde catheterization of the carotid, subclavian, brachial, or femoral arteries. Each method has its advantages and disadvantages. Local complications commonly occur related to the puncture site and include hematomas and peripheral neuropathies. Cerebral complications caused directly by angiography include dislodging of a thrombus or atherosclerotic plaque, air embolus, and subintimal injections leading to compression of branching vessels.

Carotid angiography is the most common procedure in these studies and involves the injection of contrast medium into the internal carotid artery in order to display this vessel in the neck and its major intracranial branches, the anterior and middle cerebral arteries. Only the circulation to the same side of the brain will be seen unless the opposite internal carotid artery is also compressed or if it is also involved in the occlusive process. Bilateral angiography is necessary when it is required to display the vasculature in both cerebral hemispheres as during the investigation of subarachnoid hemorrhage. These studies may reveal carotid artery disease or displacement of cerebral vessels and provide information concerning the localization and nature of space-occupying lesions. Abnormal tumor vessels, vascular spasm, aneurysms, and other vascular anomalies may also be detected.

The vertebral arteries and the circulation to the infratentorial structures and occipital lobes can be studied by vertebral angiography. One method allows for retrograde femoral catheterization, using the image intensifier as control to follow the tip of the catheter passing up the aorta, subclavian artery, and then manipulation of the tip into the origin of the vertebral artery.

Local analgesia can be used in selected and well-sedated patients undergoing unilateral carotid angiography. Diazepam can be given preoperatively and then neuroleptanalgesia can be used for induction (droperidol, 5 to 10 mg, and fentanyl, 0.1 mg intravenously 5 to 10 minutes prior to local infiltration of the neck). Additional doses of fentanyl, 0.025 to 0.05 mg, can be given during the procedure. Careful observation of the pulse and respiratory rates is necessary since both may become unduly slow from manipulation of the carotid vessels and the effects of fentanyl. Cessation of pressure in the neck may be necessary and the judicious use of naloxone, 0.2 to 0.4 mg intravenously should be given at the conclusion of the procedure.

In patients who are deeply comatose, an endotracheal tube will already have been inserted on admission to the hospital or in the intensive care unit. Such patients can be managed with local analgesia and controlled ventilation with oxygen.

General anesthesia is usually required for semicomatose patients who may move in response to painful stimulation or the injection of contrast material. It is also necessary for children, confused elderly patients, or those with subarachnoid hemorrhage (SAH). The common practice is to use an intravenous induction with thiopental, oxygenation, succinylcholine to facilitate endotracheal intubation, and then supplementation by either an inhalation technique (halothane, isoflurane, nitrous oxide/oxygen) if there are minimal signs of raised ICP or by intravenous agents thiopental and muscle relaxants if ICP is elevated. There is an increasing tendency to use nitrous oxide/oxygen narcotic relaxant techniques regardless of whether ICP is raised in preference to spontaneous ventilation with a volatile agent. Recovery from nitrous oxide/oxygen anesthesia is rapid, permitting early re-evaluation of neurologic status. It is claimed that mild hypocapnia (25 to 35 mm Hg) improves the quality of the angiographic films as well as producing a greater delineation of the nonautoregulatory tumor blood vessels (16). Overzealous hyperventilation could diffusely narrow cerebral vessels, however, thereby reducing cerebral circulation time, and give the false impression of diffuse vasospasm. Halothane anesthesia, by reducing arterial blood pressure, has occasionally made percutaneous vascular catheterization more difficult (17).

No matter what technique is used, continuous monitoring of blood pressure, pulse, and respiration is mandatory during and after injections of the contrast media until all systems are stable. Hypotension occurs, probably owing to baroreceptor discharge, but it is usually mild and transient. Note, however, that more severe falls in blood pressure can occur in patients with cerebrovascular disease and SAH. Commonly observed cardiac dysrhythmias include bradycardia, ventricular extrasystoles, nodal rhythms, and transient asystole in association with injection of contrast media.

Meglumine iothalamate (Conray) is now the most frequently used contrast material. As with previously used iodine-containing contrast media, adverse reactions, local and general, may occur. They are usually mild and transient and include psychosomatic responses (nausea, vomiting, headaches), arterial spasm, an intense burning sensation during injection, anaphylaxis (rare), and cardiovascular reactions involving thrombophlebitis or minor disturbances such as flushing or a feeling of warmth. Serious neurologic (convulsions, syncope, hemiparesis, aphasia, blindness) and hemodynamic (hypotension, bradycardia, and cardiac dysrhythmias) complications can occur.

COMPUTED TOMOGRAPHY (CT SCAN)

The introduction of computed tomography (CT) in the 1970s has provided a major advancement in the radiologic diagnosis of intracranial lesions. It involves taking tomographic films of horizontal brain sections (13 or 8 mm thick), each representing 15,600 numerical measurements of x-ray attenuation. By computerizing the data, tomographic slices of the head can be obtained in which the brain tissue, the ventricular system, and intracranial pathology can be clearly seen (18). In some patients with suspected neoplasms, an intravenous injection of contrast media is also given, which diffuses more readily into a vascular tumor than into normal brain tissue. The consequent increase in density is detectable by the scanner and furthers the diagnosis of an intracranial lesion.

Because the procedure is noninvasive (except for the injection of contrast material intravenously) and provides highly precise quantitative images unattainable with conventional x-ray systems, it has decreased the need for the more invasive studies of PEG, ventriculography, and angiography. Most centers report approximately a 25% decrease in carotid angiography and a 75% decrease in air-contrast studies.

The patient lies supine with his head inserted to the eyebrows into a radiologic chamber. The first commercial unit, the EMI scanner, required that the patient's head be placed in a rubber bag surrounded by water. The detection system was located on a scanning gantry in exact opposition to an x-ray tube. During the examination, the gantry rotates around the patient's head while a narrow collimated x-ray beam is transmitted through a thin section of the head. A complete rotation of the gantry takes approximately four and one-half minutes. New generations of scanners are now available that eliminate the need for the water-containing bag and have reduced the time of each rotation to approximately one minute.

The major radiologic requirement for a successful scan study is that the patient remain perfectly still during the examination. Anesthesia may be needed for cooperative patients who have movement disorders. Anesthesia frequently is necessary for patients who are confused, mentally incompetent, uncooperative, for restless patients with head trauma, and for many pediatric patients. Provision of anesthesia for outpatient CT scanning is becoming increasingly necessary as the noninvasive nature of the study has led to its early application in essentially well patients suspected to have intracranial lesions.

Recent statistics from major centers indicate that most adult studies can be performed in cooperative individuals without general anesthesia or anesthesia monitoring. Pediatric patients require a much higher incidence of general anesthesia, and this varies from one-third to one-half of all children undergoing CT scanning at major centers.

Since anesthesia problems that are present or liable to occur are discussed earlier in this chapter in the section on general considerations for neurodiagnostic procedures, only the major problems are presented here.

Attempts at sedation may fail and be especially dangerous when carbon dioxide retention occurs or the airway is obstructed. The head trauma patient who is restless or semicomatose with borderline or elevated ICP should be carefully monitored. If anesthesia is needed, close attention to technique and understanding of the underlying cerebrovascular pathophysiology are necessary. Scanning of posterior fossa lesions requires forward flexion of the head, and with a large mass located in a tense infratentorial compartment, compression of the brain stem can occur with such movement. It is essential that with the use of general anesthesia and muscle relaxants, excessive head and neck movements be avoided to decrease the incidence of this problem (2).

When anesthesia is indicated, either a thiopental nitrous oxide/oxygen relaxant technique with oral intubation can be employed or, after induction and intubation, an inhalation technique with halothane or isoflurane, nitrous oxide/oxygen can be maintained. With either technique, the aim is to provide a rapid postanesthetic recovery so that early assessment of neurologic status can be permitted. Care is taken to avoid kinking the endotracheal tube during positioning in the CT apparatus. Most CT scan rooms tend to be cold and well ventilated, and small infants have their head totally enveloped in the waterfilled bag, thus exposing a large proportion of body surface to heat loss via conduction. In children less than 12 months of age, the incidence of hypothermia (rectal temperature < 35°C) was 43% (19). Therefore, temperature monitoring is critical in this group of patients.

Previous studies have shown that the radiation exposure to the patient is similar to that of a conventional skull x-ray series, and much less than during a PEG or a carotid angiogram. Exposure values in the room are minimal, and anesthesia personnel might receive a skin dose of 1 to 2 mrad per hour. The use of a lead apron allows safe participation in a full daily schedule of cases.

Further caution is related to the use of contrast media. A large amount of hypertonic iodinated contrast media (usually metrizamide) is often given intravenously during the study to identify breakdown of the blood-brain barrier, as is seen in neoplasms and abscesses (10). This substance is a water-soluble agent that is absorbed from the subarachnoid space and need not be removed. Renal shutdown can occur if the patient is not well hydrated. Alternatively, fluid overload can precipitate pulmonary edema as well as unrecognized bladder distention in the recovery room.

In summary, CT has introduced a new dimension in neuroradiologic diagnostic studies. It is devoid of the risk of the more invasive procedures, and it is more rapid and highly accurate. The greatest risk for the patient undergoing CT might be the risk of general anesthesia, but an anesthesiologist who understands the principles of CT scanning and the pathophysiology of intracranial disease can minimize this risk.

PNEUMOENCEPHALOGRAPHY

Although PEG has greatly decreased in total number of cases since the use of CT scanning was introduced, it is still used from time to time in establishing a diagnosis. It still plays an important role in detecting small suprasellar mass lesions and small mass lesions in the cerebellopontine angle cistern region. There are still hospitals where CT scanning is not readily available, and complete PEG may still be carried out. Indications for PEG are hydrocephalus, cerebral atrophy, congenital intracranial anomalies, acoustic neuromas, sellar and suprasellar masses, brain-stem masses, intraventricular masses, parasagittal masses, and cerebral hemispheric masses. Ventriculography is usually employed when masses produce obstructive hydrocephalus (15). The necessary removal of cerebrospinal fluid

(CSF), injection of contrast gas, and subsequent maneuvering of the patient have resulted in morbidity and mortality sufficient to warn against casual use of the procedure. It should be applied cautiously, with great care at the outset to avoid undue risk to the patient. Principal contraindications to the performance of a PEG are the presence of increased ICP (over 15 mm Hg), the possible presence of a posterior fossa tumor, and children under 1 year of age.

The procedure involves the injection of air or oxygen into the lumbar subarachnoid space. The gas passes upward into the cranium if the patient is in the erect position. By appropriate positioning of the head, it enters the cisterna magna and the ventricular system of the brain. This outlines the size, shape, and symmetry of the ventricles. Some gas also passes over the cerebral hemispheres delineating brain sulci. Radiographs are taken with the patient in the erect, supine, and prone positions.

Premedication follows the usual criteria that one chooses for each patient. General anesthesia or local analgesia plus sedation may be used. The immobilization, prolonged duration, extreme positional changes, and airway management make general anesthesia a preferable technique over local methods, especially for children. Since this procedure is performed primarily on patients with normal ICP, practically all anesthetic agents have been used with excellent results. Many anesthesiologists prefer to avoid ketamine because the vasoconstriction may elevate ICP, but this is a relatively rare complication if the necessary precautions are taken. Nitrous oxide has also created considerable controversy because of its tendency to accumulate in gas-filled spaces but, once more, the complication rate is extremely variable. Many investigators have questioned the use of nitrous oxide during air encephalography since its high solubility in blood compared to nitrogen (30:1) will rapidly equilibrate into an air-filled ventricle, thereby adding to the intracranial volume on a relatively uncontrolled basis (20,21). Since air embolism is also a possibility as air is injected into the lumbar subarachnoid space, a number of investigators feel that nitrous oxide should not be used during air encephalography. When nitrous oxide replaces air as the contrast agent, there is no contraindication to using nitrous oxide as an anesthetic gas. Elwyn and associates (22) used nitrous oxide as the contrast gas in 475 pediatric patients anesthetized with nitrous oxide and halothane, and they found this method to be quite safe, with the advantage of more rapid excretion of nitrous oxide and reduction of postoperative headache as well as shorter hospitalization.

Air, oxygen, helium, and nitrous oxide have all been employed for intrathecal injection, and each may cause gas embolism if injected rapidly. Use of nitrous oxide for both anesthesia and contrast gas eliminates the danger of its diffusion into the ventricles, but nitrous oxide must be injected in larger quantities and more rapidly than air, thereby increasing the danger of gas embolism. Absorption of the bubbles is delayed by the presence of nitrous oxide in the blood, and the necessary rapid washout of the gas exposes the patient to cardiovascular collapse and cardiac arrest (23). The danger of air embolism during PEG in patients with ventriculoatrial shunts has been described by different investigators (24,25). Additional precautionary measures that have been advocated include use of a Doppler, a Swan-Ganz catheter, end-tidal carbon dioxide monitoring, and ligation of the shunt catheter prior to the study.

Cardiovascular changes during encephalography include hypertension, hypotension, bradycardia, and even cardiac arrest. When general anesthesia is used, management should be similar as for the patient anesthetized in the sitting position. Despite the potential cardiovascular depression associated with halothane anesthesia, it is still one of the most popular agents employed for this study. In one series of patients, blood pressure decreases of up to 25% were reported with 2% halothane in oxygen. This was accompanied by increases of 25% to 50% in cardiac output with the assumption of the sitting position (26). Because halothane anesthesia requires endotracheal intubation for safety in these circumstances and is associated with a slow recovery time, a number of alternative techniques have been employed. Ketamine rapidly induces general anesthesia, characterized by maintenance of both airway and circulatory stability. Its use probably should be limited to infants with open fontanelles where the risk of complications from endotracheal intubation is high, or in patients with ventriculostomies providing a means of CSF drainage for ICP control. The effects on the central nervous system (e.g., dysphoria, hallucinations) limit its usefulness among adults. Another technique is to use a combination of intravenous thiopental and lidocaine to achieve anesthesia (27). Anesthesia is induced with thiopental (125 to 350 mg) and oxygen, the trachea is topically anesthetized with lidocaine (40 mg) after succinylcholine is administered (1 mg/kg body weight), and maintenance of anesthesia is provided by an intravenous drip of thiopental and lidocaine (1.5 gm of thiopental and 0.2 gm of lidocaine in 500 ml of normal saline) using 100% oxygen and spontaneous respiration. Thiopental reduces ICP and provides amnesia, while lidocaine depresses the cough reflex and produces analgesia, slight sedation, and in low doses, cardiovascular-respiratory stimulation. The airway and spontaneous ventilation are maintained as evidence of neurologic function. Provided the dose of thiopental is carefully controlled and the study is not excessively long (more than two hours), a return to consciousness occurs within one to two hours after the study.

Anesthesia can also be maintained with either diazepam or neuroleptic agents. The use of fentanyl will reduce overall drug requirements and permit rapid recovery and may be antagonized at the end of the anesthetic. The use of muscle relaxants permits light planes of anesthesia without the attendant problems of coughing and vomiting. Controlled ventilation, by reducing arterial carbon dioxide tension, may counteract the increase of ICP caused by the anesthetic or contrast medium. Wolfson and associates (28) have used several combinations of drugs in attempts to reduce the severity of headache and nausea in patients undergoing PEG under local analgesia and sedation. At the same time, they tried to maintain consciousness, the ability of the patient to cooperate, and a patent airway. The authors concluded that the most satisfactory technique involved the use of diazepam as a tranquilizer and amnesic, combined with alphaprodine for headache, plus droperidol as an antinauseant (29).

In summary, the important features in preventing problems in PEG are to avoid rapid injection of contrast gas, to avoid nitrous oxide anesthesia, to avoid air for contrast gas, to avoid the procedure in the presence of high ICP, and to avoid adding to the risk by the use of complex safeguards (Swan-Ganz catheters). The replacement of PEG in a larger percentage of cases by CT scanning has markedly reduced the incidence of these complications. The report by Elwyn and associates (22) affirms that recognition of the hazards and careful technique overcome many theoretical disadvantages.

VENTRICULOGRAPHY AND MYELOGRAPHY

Ventriculography is considerably safer than PEG in patients with increased ICP caused by posterior fossa lesions or noncommunicating hydrocephalus. The procedure usually is performed under local anesthesia, even in children. General anesthesia may be required in very small children or in uncooperative patients. The ventricular system and the cisterna magna can be visualized following the injection of contrast media via a burr hole into one lateral ventricle. The patient remains in the supine position while the surgeon injects the local anesthetic, and in very small children an 18-gauge needle can be passed through an open coronal suture, or through a small drill hole in older children. After the injection of 25 to 30 cc of gas into the ventricles, films are taken in several positions. Headache during or following the procedure is the principal complication.

Myelography is accompanied by some discomfort during lumbar puncture and during final aspiration of the contrast material. There may be some manipulation of cauda equina nerve roots. Most patients tolerate myelography under local analgesia and moderate sedation. Uncooperative adults and small children will require a light general anesthetic in order to reduce the discomfort associated with the original lumbar puncture and permit the prolonged maneuvering, turning, and tilting that may be necessary for completion of the procedure. The primary problems involved are maintaining respiratory and cardiovascular stability during multiple position changes, close observation so that the endotracheal tube does not dislodge while the room is dark, and dislodgment of the spinal needle.

DIGITAL SUBTRACTION ANGIOGRAPHY

Digital subtraction angiography (DSA) involves computer processing of an x-ray image, often obtained at the time of angiography. In the most usual configuration, the information from an image intensifier is converted to digital form and introduced into a computer as an array of numbers varying according to the density of each point on the image. A computer stores these data and constructs the image according to a preset program. In DSA, the image just prior to the injection of a contrast agent is stored as a mask image, the image after the contrast injection is acquired and stored, and then the second image is subtracted from the first so that only the vessels containing contrast material are visualized on the reconstructed image.

Advantages over standard angiography include greater sensitivity of the image intensifier than standard x-ray film, ability to manipulate the contrast and definition electronically, and almost immediate availability of the image; also, long-term storage is less expensive on magnetic tape. In addition, because the sensitivity is so great, it is sometimes possible to obtain a satisfactory angiographic image after intravenous injection, so that arterial catheterization is not always necessary.

Disadvantages include poor definition of some intracranial structures when compared with standard angiography because of some artifact produced by bone. This is particularly apparent along the base of the skull, where vascular lesions are quite common. For extracranial carotid artery disease, however, DSA frequently is the only procedure required.

Anesthesia considerations for DSA are essentially the same as for angiography if intraarterial injection is performed, and frequently DSA is performed simultaneously with standard angiography. If intravenous contrast material is employed, the procedure has little discomfort associated with it, but the patient may require sedation to remain immobile throughout the study.

POSITRON EMISSION TOMOGRAPHY AND NUCLEAR MAGNETIC RESONANCE

These new techniques are being developed for both research and clinical medicine. Positron emission tomography (PET) is a technique that permits both the tomographic delineation of cerebral structures and the measurement of local tissue concentrations of injected radioactive tracers. The latter provides a means of implementing quantitative tracer kinetic techniques for the measurement of functional processes in the human brain. The first PET system was developed for human use in 1975 (30,31), and new generation devices are in present stages of development. Initial studies of brain pathology using this technique have focused on the major clinical diagnostic problems of neurologic disease. General areas of investigation include cerebrovascular disease, dementia, seizure disorders, degenerative diseases, and neoplasms. At present, PET techniques have been developed for the measurements of regional cerebral blood flow, cerebral blood volume, cerebral metabolic rate for glucose and oxygen, selective blood-brain barrier and cell membrane transport for glucose, and passive blood-brain barrier diffusion.

PET scanning is similar to radiologic computed tomography (CT) in that an array of detectors monitors radiation and reconstructs an image of a slice of tissue, based on the relative amount of radiation detected at each point on the array surrounding the head or body. In CT, however, the source of radiation is an x-ray tube, and the amount of radiation detected is a reflection of the radiodensity of the tissues through which it passes. In PET, the source of radiation is from injected radioisotopes that accumulate selectively in different tissues under various circumstances. Because the isotopes emit positrons in opposite directions simultaneously, the coincidental arrival at detectors opposite each other allow localization of the source of radioactivity within the area being scanned, so the computer reconstruction of the distribution of positron sources allows one to localize the source in specific tissues and calibrate its intensity. The derived picture resembles that of a CT scan in that it represents a slice through the brain or other body tissues, but the resolution is not as precise.

By selecting different isotopes as the source of positrons, it is possible to obtain different types of information from PET scanning. For instance, 2-dioxyglucose will accumulate in tissues in proportion to the amount of metabolic activity; areas of impaired metabolism or infarction can be readily identified.

Since most of the positron-emitting isotopes have short half-lives, it is necessary to have a local facility, such as a cyclotron, to manufacture the isotopes, which makes PET scanning prohibitively expensive for most institutions. In addition, the potential clinical usefulness of such information has not yet been demonstrated, so that PET scanning presently is considered more of a research effort than a clinical tool for general application.

Anesthesia considerations involve primarily the temporary immobilization of the patient during the period of scanning. The usual precautions for handling radioactive substances are employed, and a system for safe disposal of isotopes excreted through the lungs or kidneys must be incorporated into the system, although the short half-life of most of the isotopes minimizes this problem.

Nuclear magnetic resonance (NMR) is another revolutionary technique for medical diagnosis that may eventually replace CT scanning (32). Instead of using x-rays, this diagnostic device produces pictures that are based on the responses of atomic nuclei in a magnetic field. The images are similar to those produced by CT scanning but are sharper and show more distinctions without the use of x-rays, contrast media, or the problems of radioactivity. Although the major testing has been in experimental animals, five clinical facilities have begun using this diagnostic technique in humans. Again, the role of the anesthesiologist, if any, requires further elucidation.

Despite its apparent advantages, there are some problems with NMR imaging. It is large and must be kept in a place that protects it from extraneous radio signals and substances that contain magnetic iron. Any object with magnetic iron (e.g., a screwdriver) can become a flying missile when exposed to the device's magnetic force. NMR can be hazardous also to patients fitted with various devices; people with pacemakers, for example, could not be examined by NMR as it currently exists.

REFERENCES

1. Du Boulay G, Edmonds-Seal J, Bostick T: The effect of intermittent positive pressure ventilation upon the calibre of cerebral arteries in spasm following subarachnoid hemorrhage. Br J Radiol 1968;41:46–48.
2. Shapiro HM, Aidinis SJ: Neurosurgical anesthesia. Surg Clin North Am 1975;55:922–926.

3. Edwards JC, Flowertew GD: Diazepam and local analgesia for lumbar air encephalography. Br J Anaesth 1970;42:999–1003.

4. Corrsen G, Graves EH, Gomez S, et al.: Ketamine: Its place in anesthesia for neurosurgical diagnostic procedures. Anesth Analg (Cleve) 1969;48:181–188.

5. Penrose BH: Aspiration pneumonitis following ketamine induction for general anesthesia. Anesth Analg (Cleve) 1972;51:41–43.

6. Shapiro HM, Wyte SR, Harris AB: Ketamine anesthesia in patients with intracranial pathology. Br J Anaesth 1972;44:1200–1204.

7. Winters WD: Epilepsy or anesthesia with ketamine. Anesthesiology 1972;36:309–312.

8. Manus PM: Metrizamide: A review with emphasis on drug interactions. Am J Hosp Pharmacol 1980;37:510–13.

9. Kaada B: Transient EEG abnormalities following lumbar myelography with metrizamide. Acta Radiol (Kbh) (suppl) 1973;335–80.

10. Sackett JF, Strother CM, Quaglieri CE, et al.: Metrizamide-CSF contrast material. Radiology 1977;123:779–82.

11. Gonsette RE, Brucher JM: Potentiation of Amipaque-epileptogenic activity by neuroleptics. Neuroradiology 1977;14:27–30.

12. Pyles ST, Pashayan AG: Anesthesia and neuroradiology: Considerations regarding metrizamide. Anesthesiology 1983;58:590–591.

13. Shehadi WH: Adverse reactions to intravascularly administered contrast media; a comprehensive study based on a prospective survey. Am J Roentgenol Radium Ther Nucl Med 1975;124:145–152.

14. Zweiman B, Mishkin MM, Hildreth EA: An approach to the performance of contrast studies in contrast material-reactive persons. Ann Intern Med 1975;83:159–162.

15. Lin JP, Kricheff II: Central nervous system and spinal cord neuroradiologic diagnostic tools, in Cottrell JE, Turndorf H (eds.): Anesthesia and neurosurgery. St. Louis, CV Mosby, 1980;pp 119–137.

16. Dallas SH, Moxon CP: Controlled ventilation for cerebral angiography. Br J Anaesth 1969;41:597–602.

17. Lewis RN, Moore BA: Some aspects of general anesthesia for cerebral angiography. Br J Anaesth 1968;40:37–44.

18. Hounsfield GN: Computerized transverse axial scanning (tomography). I. Description of system. Br J Radiol 1973;46:1016–1022.

19. Aidinis SJ, Zimmerman RA, Shapiro HM, et al.: Anesthesia for brain computer tomography. Anesthesiology 1976;44:420–425.

20. Campkin TV, Turner JM: Blood pressure and cerebrospinal fluid pressure studies during lumbar air encephalography. Br J Anaesth 1972;44:849–853.

21. Saidman LJ, Eger EI, II: Change in cerebrospinal fluid pressure during penumoencephalography under nitrous oxide anesthesia. Anesthesiology 1965;26:67–72.

22. Elwyn RA, Ring WH, Loeser E, et al.: Nitrous oxide encephalography: 5-year experience with 475 pediatric patients. Anesth Analg (Cleve) 1976;55:402–408.

23. Collan R, Iivanainen M: Cardiac arrest caused by rapid elimination of N_2O from cerebral ventricle after encephalography. Can Anaesth Soc J 1969;16:519–524.

24. Paul W, Munson ES: Gas embolism during encephalography. Anesth Analg (Cleve) 1976;55:141–145.

25. Youngberg JA, Kaplan JA, Miller ED: Air embolism through a ventriculoatrial shunt during pneumoencephalography. Anesthesiology 1975;42:487–490.

26. Wilson RD, Overton MC, Waldron RL, et al.: Abrupt postural changes in patients undergoing air contrast studies. JAMA 1966;198:970–974.
27. Raudzens P, Cole AFD: Thiopentone/lidocaine anesthesia for pneumoencephalography. Can Anaesth Soc J 1974;21:1.
28. Wolfson B, Kielar CM, Shenoy NR, et al.: Analgesic "cocktails" for pneumoencephalography: Ketamine, diazepam, alphaprodine and droperidol. Anesth Analg (Cleve) 1973;52:779–783.
29. Wolfson B, Hetrick WD: Anesthesia for neuroradiologic procedures, in Cottrell JE, Turndorf H (eds.): Anesthesia and neurosurgery. St. Louis, CV Mosby, 1980, pp 138–148.
30. Phelps ME, Mazziotta JC, Huang SC: Study of cerebral function with positron computed tomography. J Cer Blood Flow Metabol 1982;2:113–162.
31. Ter-Pogossian MM, Phelps ME, Hoffman EJ, et al.: A positron emission transaxial tomograph for nuclear imaging (PETT). Radiology 1975;114:89–98.
32. Brownell GL, Budinger TF, Lauterbur PC, et al.: Positron tomography and nuclear magnetic resonance imaging. Science 1981;215:619–626.

PART II

Neurosurgical and Related Procedures

CHAPTER 6

The Management of Cerebrovascular Disease
George B. Jacobs and Elizabeth A.M. Frost

ISCHEMIC CEREBROVASCULAR DISEASE

Stroke caused by occlusion of intracranial or extracranial vessels is the third most frequent cause of death in the United States, and a common cause of partial or total disability. About 80% of all strokes are caused by arterial occlusive disease (1). Expanded neuroradiologic diagnostic capabilities and ready availability of the operating microscope have established neurovascular surgery as a separate specialty. Thus, increasing numbers of patients with intracranial arterial occlusive disease are candidates for surgical correction either by carotid reconstruction or extracranial-intracranial (EC-IC) revascularization procedures.

The extracranial blood supply of the brain consists of two carotid and two vertebral arteries. These vessels arise both directly and indirectly from the aortic arch. The common carotid arteries end in an arterial dilatation, the carotid bifurcation, which becomes the external and internal carotid systems (Fig. 6.1). The carotid sinus, which contains the baroreceptor mechanism, is located at the carotid bifurcation. Chemoreceptors, which are sensitive to oxygen changes, are present in the carotid and aortic bodies (2,3). The branches of the external carotid artery as they originate are: (a) superior thyroid, (b) ascending pharyngeal, (c) lingual, (d) external maxillary, (e) occipital, (f) internal maxillary, and (g) superficial temporal. The two arterial systems anastomose at the base of the brain to form the circle of Willis (Fig. 6.2).

The most common site of atherosclerotic stenosis is the carotid bifurcation. Plaques extend downward through the internal carotid system and upward through the external and internal carotid vessels (Fig. 6.3). These atherosclerotic plaques often are associated with small ulcerated irregularities on their luminal surfaces. Cerebral ischemia usually does not cause neurologic deficit until carotid artery stenosis is about 80% or, more commonly, as showers of small emboli, usually platelet aggregations, detach from ulcerated areas. The disease is bilateral in 50% of cases. In many patients, abnormalities of the circle of Willis—usually hypoplastic communicating vessels—are present. Thus the ability to augment contralateral flow is compromised and the margin of safety for cerebral perfusion

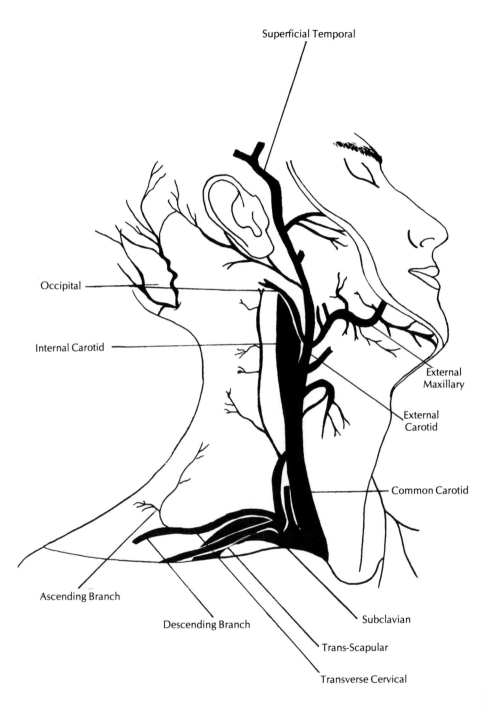

Figure 6.1 The carotid artery and its branches.

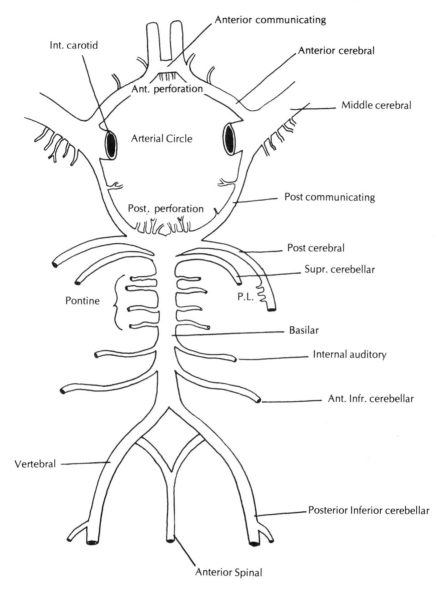

Figure 6.2 The circle of Willis.

reduced. Preoperative evaluation of patients with carotid artery disease should include a test of neck motion to ascertain that consciousness is maintained with lateral movement.

Surgery is indicated in patients who have a transient ischemic attack (TIA), characterized by deficits that persist for less than 24 hours and resolve completely,

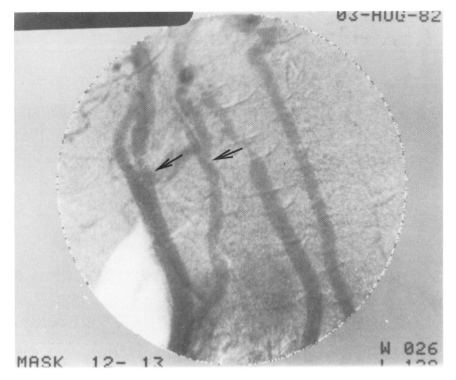
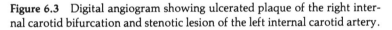

Figure 6.3 Digital angiogram showing ulcerated plaque of the right internal carotid bifurcation and stenotic lesion of the left internal carotid artery.

or in those who have sustained a reversible ischemic neurologic deficit (RIND), which implies that symptoms have persisted longer than 24 hours but resolved within one week. Surgery may also be scheduled for patients with a persistent older (six to eight weeks) ischemic neurologic deficit. Many patients with complete stroke have a history of a TIA. If untreated, approximately 30% to 40% of these patients will suffer a complete stroke within 3½ years of the first attack (4).

Initial criteria for extracranial carotid surgery traditionally have excluded patients with bilateral disease. With the development of more sophisticated surgical and anesthetic techniques, however, patients with bilateral disease can safely be offered surgical intervention.

Current surgical techniques undertaken in the treatment of ischemic cerebrovascular disease involve carotid endarterectomy with or without patch angioplasty and revascularization procedures using EC-IC microsurgical anastomosis. Procedures that have been used to increase intracranial blood flow include anastomosis of the superficial temporal to middle cerebral artery, the occipital artery to middle cerebral or posterior fossa vessels, or long vein grafts from the cervical carotid artery to branches of the intracranial carotid system.

Carotid Endarterectomy and Angioplasty

Complete neurologic and medical evaluation is essential for patients who are being considered for carotid surgery.

Neurologic Assessment

Preoperative preparation must include computed tomographic (CT) examination of the brain, electroencephalography, skull films, and conventional catheter four-vessel studies visualizing the extracranial and intracranial circulation and/or digital angiography (Figs. 6.4, 6.5). Experience with digital angiography suggests that this examination, with its lesser potential for complications, might replace conventional angiographic techniques in selected cases. Other noninvasive tests that have been developed include ophthalmodynamometry, assessment of flow reversal in the ophthalmic-facial collaterals with directional Doppler equipment, thermography, and oculoplethysmography (4). Quantitative assessment of regional cerebral blood flow (CBF) and metabolism is possible by monitoring the

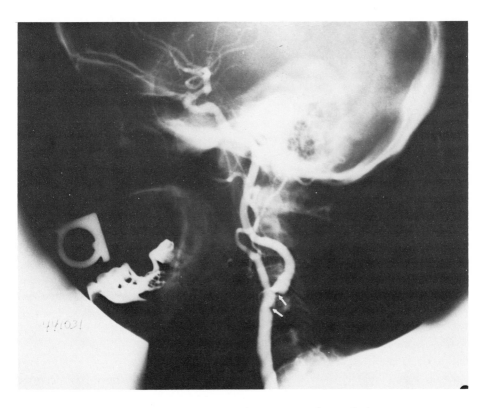

Figure 6.4 Carotid angiogram showing two ulcerated plaques.

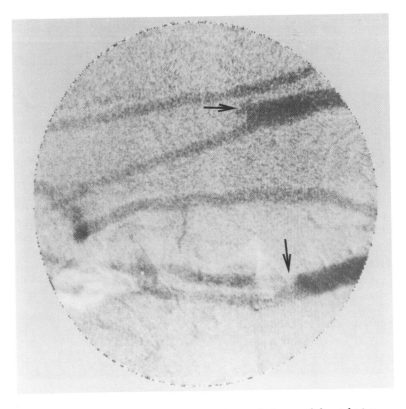

Figure 6.5 Digital angiogram showing ulcerated plaque of the right internal carotid artery (*bottom arrow*) and complete occlusion of the left internal carotid artery (*top arrow*).

washout of ¹³³Xenon from small areas of the brain. ¹³³Xe is administered by inhalation or intracarotid injection until saturation of the brain is achieved, at which time the isotope is in equilibrium with blood and brain and its washout rate will therefore be limited as a function of the blood flow rate. The blood flow rate is measured by external scintillation crystals, each of which looks at a small cylinder of brain tissue (5). Positron emission tomography (PET) provides even greater sophistication in diagnosis by measuring metabolic rates for carbon dioxide generation, ammonia turnover, oxygen consumption, and regional cerebral blood volume. Use of this technique is limited, however, as access to a cyclotron is required.

Medical Assessment

Because vascular disease rarely is restricted to the cerebral vessels, evaluation of multisystem disease preoperatively is usually essential. Most patients with cerebrovascular disease have systemic arterial hypertension. Not only is the hypertensive patient subjected to general anesthesia at increased risk of myocardial infarction, but he is particularly unstable during the anesthetic period, developing hypotension intraoperatively and further compromising ischemic areas of brain and hypertension postoperatively, which puts atheromatous cerebral vessels at risk of rupture. Arterial pressure should be brought under control preoperatively (6). All medications should be maintained up to and including the day of surgery. The only possible exception to this is the administration of clonidine, which has a very short half-life and is not yet available in parenteral form. Discontinuation results in severe rebound hypertension. Ideally, the drug should be stopped two weeks prior to surgery and the patient reestablished on another regimen. In the absence of ideal antihypertensive therapy, however, elective surgery need not subject patients to an added clinical risk provided that the diastolic pressure is stable and not greater than 110 mm Hg and that close monitoring and prompt therapy avoid hypotensive and hypertensive episodes perioperatively (7).

A history of previous myocardial infarction is obtained from 25% of patients and has been shown to correlate closely with postoperative cardiac complications irrespective of the time since or severity of the myocardial injury (8).

About 20% of patients have undergone previous major vascular surgery. Simultaneous scheduling of triple bypass coronary artery surgery with carotid endarterectomy is becoming common.

Approximately 85% of patients with cerebrovascular disease receive several drugs on a long term-basis (8). These include digitalis preparations, diuretics, antihypertensives, antiarrhythmics, anticoagulants, insulin, steroids, and antacid preparations. Hypertensive patients with generalized vascular disease who receive combinations of drugs constitute a very high-risk group, which can be identified by the criteria in the multifactorial risk index developed by Goldman et al. (9). This score affords a useful means for selecting patients suitable for anesthesia but does not indicate proper intraoperative or postoperative management.

The risk of complications from drug interactions rises in direct proportion to the number of drugs administered until approximately 10 medications are involved (10). There is then a sharp increase in complication rate, and when 20 drugs are involved, side effects occur in 45% of patients. These symptoms include delayed return to consciousness, prolonged neuromuscular block, and altered renal and cardiac function. As approximately 5 to 10 medications usually are given during general anesthesia (11), a potentially dangerous situation may quickly develop. It thus behooves the entire surgical team to prescribe additional drugs only after very careful consideration.

Diabetes mellitus is found in about 20% of patients with cerebrovascular disease (8) and usually requires insulin for control. Coincidental use of steroids in neurosurgical management to decrease cerebral edema may complicate the therapy and increase insulin needs. About 40% of patients have smoked one to two packs of cigarettes per day for more than 20 years. Consequently bronchitis, emphysema, chronic hypoxia, or even carcinoma are not infrequent complicating factors.

Hyperkalemia is a recognized danger in patients with central nervous system lesions with skeletal muscle paralysis. The phenomenon may occur in patients with both upper and lower motor neuron lesions. Elevated serum potassium levels are found in the venous blood from all paralyzed muscles for several weeks after injury, indicating that the source of the potassium is the abnormal muscle distal to the neural lesion (12). Subsequent administration of succinylcholine may increase serum potassium levels, causing cardiac arrhythmias or even arrest. Preoperative serum potassium levels must be known and be within normal limits. The patient should be pretreated with small doses of a nondepolarizing muscle relaxant, and succinylcholine should be avoided or used only in minimal amounts.

Surgical Technique

We favor a surgical approach under general anesthesia to allow meticulous dissection (13). With the patient in a supine position, the head is rotated to the side opposite the incision. The skin incision parallels the anterior border of the sternocleidomastoid muscle. The carotid artery is exposed through deep dissection. Occasionally, the descending hypoglossal branch must be sectioned from the hypoglossal nerve to permit more distal access to the internal carotid artery. This produces no demonstrable neurologic deficit. Care must be taken to avoid injury to the vagus nerve or the jugular vein.

An internal shunt introduced immediately following arteriotomy is used routinely in our practice (Fig. 6.6). Measurements of the internal carotid artery stump pressure are not reliable determinants of the safety of carotid cross-compression. Although a stump pressure of 55 to 60 mm Hg has been considered to be a safe indicator of adequate cerebral blood flow (14), these levels may be associated with definite regional flattening of electroencephalographic tracings (8). Although brisk retrograde bleeding from the arteriotomy after opening of the internal carotid artery clamp would suggest good cross-filling, this indicates only global pressure and cannot identify areas of regional insufficiency. It is reasonable to assume that if poor-risk patients require protection by shunting maneuvers, all patients should be so treated.

The use of shunting routinely has allowed us to perform a more adequate endarterectomy with careful attention to the internal lumen, with reduction of postoperative complications secondary to retained internal debris, and with the use of patch angioplasties to increase arterial diameter.

Stump pressures rise proportionately with systemic blood pressure (15). Increasing the systemic blood pressure therefore will increase collateral circulation from the opposite side, and thus increase pressure in the stump. Therefore, prior to cross-clamping, systemic blood pressure should be increased by 20 to 30 mm Hg.

Patch angioplasty commonly is performed using standard vascular techniques. Graft materials include double velour, dacron, Gore-Tex, and autogenous venous patches. Materials are chosen according to individual preference and to the length and size of the lesion. Compression of the suture line for five minutes usually is adequate to control hemorrhage, although occasionally reversal of heparinization may be necessary.

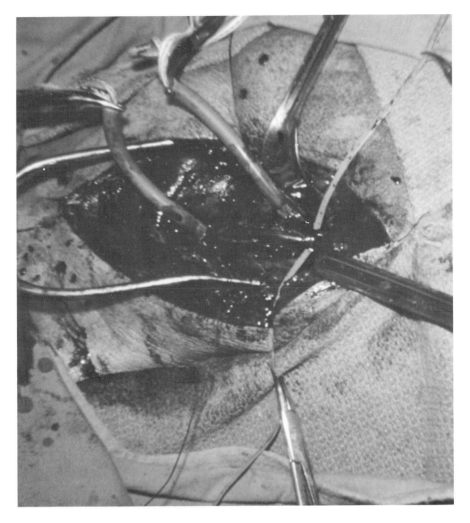

Figure 6.6   Shunt in place in the carotid arteriotomy.

Patients who are candidates for bilateral carotid endarterectomy should, in most cases, have the symptomatic side corrected first. If a marked differential exists in the degree of carotid stenosis, the site of the more significant stenosis is operated on first.

Staged bilateral carotid endarterectomy and angioplasty may be performed after a one-week interval if there is no evidence of neck swelling or incisional hematomas.

Emergency carotid surgery should be performed only in the early postoperative phase of endarterectomy if new thrombi have formed. This complication occurs rarely with proper anticoagulation therapy and attention to complete plaque removal.

Prophylactic antibiotics are recommended for 24 hours preoperatively, throughout the operation, and for 24 hours postoperatively to prevent infection carried in the open vascular system.

Postoperative complications of carotid artery surgery include emboli precipitated by the arterial dissection, a complication which can be reduced by gentle dissection and minimal palpation of the pathologic part of the carotid artery.

Rarely, hematomas may develop in subcutaneous tissues and occlude vascular structures or the airway. It is thus advisable to preserve easy access to the surgical site and keep emergency means of airway establishment, including tracheostomy equipment, immediately available. Should the patient develop hypertension, bradycardia, or any deterioration in neurologic status, immediate evaluation should be obtained to exclude intraarterial occlusion at the operative site.

Anesthetic Management

The major features of anesthetic management of patients presenting for carotid endarterectomy are listed in Table 6.1.

Undoubtedly, the most accurate assessment of adequate cerebral perfusion intraoperatively is obtained by maintaining voice and motor contact with the patient during a regional cervical plexus block technique. Such a technique causes anxiety and perhaps pain, which often results in tachycardia, hypertension, hypercarpnia (as the patient rebreathes under drapes), and increased myocardial and brain oxygen consumption. Moreover, neurologic damage may not occur immediately after carotid artery clamping and may even be delayed for up to 30 minutes, occurring at a time when attention may be directed elsewhere.

Table 6.1 Essential Requirements in Anesthetic Management of Patients Presenting for Carotid Endarterectomy

Time	Requirement
Preanesthetic assessment	Stabilize vascular condition
	Maintain medications
	Control diabetes
	Identify pulmonary pathology
Anesthetic management	Maintain adequate cerebral perfusion pressure
	Establish normocapnia
	Minimize drug additions
	Utilize agents to decrease cerebral oxygen requirements
Postanesthic care	Maintain normotension
	Ensure adequate respiratory exchange
	Trend record neurologic status

In the well-informed patient without systemic disease, a regional anesthetic technique is feasible. Otherwise, general endotracheal anesthetic management, and the control of ventilation which it affords, should be used (16). Continuous electro-encephalographic monitoring is used in some centers.

Adequate preoperative sedation may be achieved with a small oral dose of diazepam (5 mg) or lorazepam (0.5 mg) one hour prior to coming to the operating room. Atropine can be given intravenously before induction if necessary. Anesthesia is induced with small incremental doses of sodium pentothal (50 to 75 mg) to a total of approximately 250 mg. Although, ideally, arterial cannulation should be achieved prior to induction under nitrous oxide analgesia if necessary, if the patient is extremely apprehensive and if sufficient assistance is available, this maneuver may be postponed until after the patient has lost consciousness. If the patient does not have any muscle paresis, succinylcholine may be given to facilitate intubation. Following a stroke, however, and to avoid the cardiotoxic effects of sudden increase in serum K^+, nonpolarizing agents should be used.

Anesthesia may be maintained with 0.5% to 1% isoflurane, which has an inherent relaxant action and obviates the need for further administration of neuromuscular agents (17). Moreover, CBF and intracranial pressure do not increase from awake levels at 0.6 to 1.1 MAC (minimum alveolar concentration) when this agent is used (18). A dose-dependent decrease in the cerebral metabolic rate of oxygen utilization ($CMRO_2$) ensures further cerebral protection (19). Epileptic patterns cannot be evoked by increasing the depth of isoflurane anesthesia (20), in contradistinction to its isomer, enflurane.

CBF must be maintained. Early intraoperative stabilization of blood pressure frequently is difficult because of vascular disease and probably is best achieved by using low concentrations of a potent inhalation agent such as isoflurane supplemented with intravenous administration of lidocaine, 50 mg, shortly after induction of anesthesia. Judicious use of 0.02% phenylephrine hydrochloride solution is warranted. Toward the conclusion of the operative procedure and after removal of the plaque, blood pressure frequently rises. This response is attenuated by intravenous administration of hydralazine, 5 to 10 mg, and propranolol, 1 mg. We have also found that with prompt intraoperative treatment of developing hypertension, fewer cardiovascular problems are encountered in the recovery room. Clinical studies have also shown that an intravenous technique using sufentanil affords considerable cardiovascular stability (21).

Intraoperative surgical stimulation of the carotid sinus may occur, which causes bradycardia, hypotension, and a reduction in the flow gradient across the stenotic area. The reflex arc involves the ninth cranial nerve, the medulla, and the vagus nerve. The surgeon should be alerted immediately to any cardiovascular changes. The reflex may be blocked by infiltration of the carotid sinus with lidocaine or intravenous administration of 0.4% atropine. Occasionally, an elderly patient may have been maintained on sufficient doses of β-adrenergic blocking agents to prevent any tachycardic response from atropine. Such a situation is demonstrated in Figure 6.7. The heart rate trend shows remarkable stability over two and a half hours; however, there is wide variation in blood pressure. During

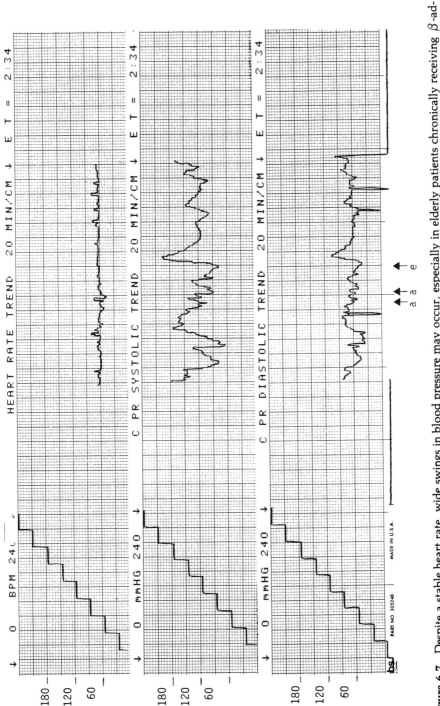

Figure 6.7 Despite a stable heart rate, wide swings in blood pressure may occur, especially in elderly patients chronically receiving β-adrenergic blocking agents (*a*, atropine; *e*, ephedrine).

traction on the carotid artery, the blood pressure fell and remained low despite 1.2 mg of atropine. Good response is obtained with ephedrine (5 mg). Isoproterenol (1 mg in 500 ml solution) may also be given by infusion.

Considerable controversy has continued over the merits of hypercapnia or hypocapnia during anesthesia for patients with cerebrovascular disease (22). Because CBF increases linearly with rising arterial carbon dioxide tension ($PaCO_2$), hypercapnia, by increasing collateral flow, might be beneficial. Ischemic areas of the brain probably are already maximally dilated and thus are no longer responsive to changing levels of carbon dioxide. Reduction in resistance in nonischemic areas may divert blood to normal areas of the brain by the so-called steal phenomenon. An increase in carbon dioxide usually causes a rise in systemic arterial pressure (which is beneficial) but increases the frequency of cardiac arrhythmias.

Hypercapnia by increasing cerebral volume decreases stump pressure and increases cerebral venous pressure, both of which decrease cerebral perfusion pressure. Hypocapnia, on the other hand, increases resistance in nonischemic areas of the brain, and thus blood may be shunted to ischemic regions. But this effect may jeopardize healthy brain and increase resistance in collateral vessels supplying ischemic areas. In addition, a shift of the oxygen dissociation curve to the left with respiratory alkalosis makes oxygen less available to the tissues. Therefore, if the awake patient is functioning normally, normocapnic values should be maintained intraoperatively.

Intraoperative monitoring should include electrocardiogram, arterial blood pressure and gases (from an arterial cannula), and temperature. The Cerebral Function Monitor (Critikon, Inc., Tampa, Florida), which is an electroencephalographic processor giving information essentially from a single pair of parietal electrodes, probably gives only a gross indication of activity. Continuous full electroencephalographic recording, especially during the period of carotid clamping, is preferable. Nevertheless, prevention of acute embolic complications, which are more common than ischemic problems, is not obtained.

Postoperatively, careful monitoring and trend recording in an intensive care unit setting for 24 hours is essential, with frequent evaluation of neurologic status to monitor for vessel obstruction or embolization that requires surgical reexploration.

Blood pressure should be maintained at slightly elevated levels to maintain flow. Reduced baroreflex function may cause both hypotensive and hypertensive episodes in the recovery phase. Hypotension reduces perfusion of both brain and heart, and hypertension increases the work and oxygen demand of the myocardium, with an end result of myocardial ischemia in both instances. Hypertension may also increase capillary hydrostatic pressure, especially in ischemic areas of the brain, leading to protein leak, edema, or hemorrhagic infarction.

Hypotension is treated by fluid replacement and infusion of 0.02% phenylephrine hydrochloride. Myocardial infarction, the most serious cause of postoperative morbidity in these patients, must be excluded. Hypertensive episodes, which occur more frequently, require prompt therapy when mean blood pressure rises more than 15% to 20% above baseline levels. Antihypotensive medications before operation should be restarted as soon as possible. Useful parenteral drugs include hydralazine 5 to 20 mg intravenously; diazoxide in a bolus injection of 50 mg, which may be repeated twice; labetalol, 0.5 mg/kg/hr; or sodium nitroprusside, 70 μ g/kg/hr. Addition of propranolol, 0.5 to 1 mg given slowly, augments the effects of hydralazine.

Particular attention should be paid to patients in whom bilateral carotid endarterectomy has been performed over the past 12 months, as damage to the carotid body may have resulted. This chemoreceptor reflexly induces an increase in ventilation in response to hypoxemia or acidosis. Although the medullary chemoreceptors contribute 87% of ventilation, the peripheral receptors in the carotid body are responsible for the remaining 13%. Patients should receive a high inspired oxygen concentration, and drugs that depress respiration should be used cautiously (23). If there is preexisting cardiac or pulmonary disease, deterioration in respiratory function should be anticipated postoperatively. Patients may complain of throat pain, which probably is related to retraction of the trachea or esophagus intraoperatively. Treatment consists of reassurance and topical anesthetic lozenges.

Extracranial to Intracranial Revascularization Procedures

The development of techniques of microvascular anastomosis have added a new dimension to the treatment of cerebrovascular insufficiency secondary to complete occlusions of the internal carotid or the middle cerebral system (24–29). Despite the small size of the anastomosis, a significant volume of blood can be delivered to the affected hemisphere through a normal vessel (4,26,30) (Fig. 6.8).

Surgical Technique

The technique has been described by Yaşargil, Krayenbuhl, and Jacobson (27), and Byer and associates (31). The patient is placed supine with the head rotated to the side opposite the surgical incision. The head is secured almost horizontally by a pin headrest. The site of the superficial temporal or, at times, occipital artery is determined by palpation, visualization, or Doppler ultrasonic identification. An incision is made over the superficial temporal artery, which is dissected in its entirety but kept intact until the anastomosis is performed. A small craniectomy is performed either through the same incision or through a separate incision about 6 cm above the external auditory canal. This dissection is carried out with loupe magnification. After opening the dura, the recipient artery, usually an angular branch of the middle cerebral artery, is selected and under microscopic magnification dissected free from the arachnoid membrane. Adequate dissection may require coagulation and section of perforating branches. Prior to arterial cross-clamping, heparain, 1500 units intravenously, is given. The superficial temporal artery is clamped, its distal connection sectioned, and a catheter placed within the lumen. The artery is irrigated with heparin-saline solution. A small terminal portion is dissected, and the donor artery opening is extended by a bias section to further increase the diameter. The artery is brought into the craniectomy

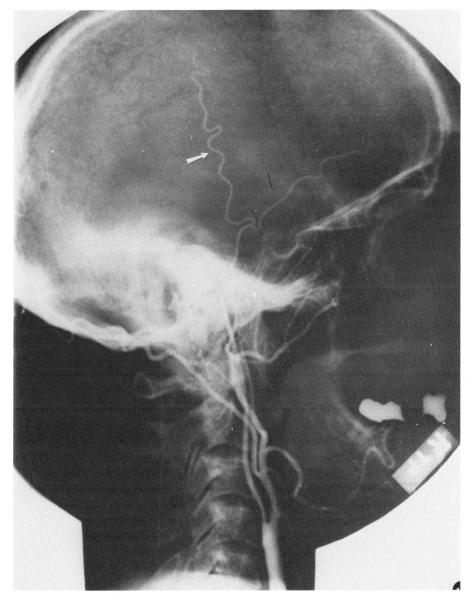

Figure 6.8 Complete occlusion of the right internal carotid artery. The superficial temporal artery (*arrow*) will be used for EC-IC bypass.

site through a subcutaneous tunnel if necessary, and an end-to-side anastomosis is completed using approximately 12 sutures of 10-0 size.

As soon as the occluding clips on the cortical vessel are removed, blood usually is seen flowing into the superficial temporal artery. After an intact suture line has been confirmed, the clamp on the superficial temporal artery is released. It is seldom necessary to reverse the mini heparin dose.

Occipital arteries can also be used as donor arteries. Posterior fossa revascularization procedures are performed utilizing the occipital artery as donor and branches of the vertebrobasilar system as recipient. Favorable results following anastomosis between the occipital artery and the posterior inferior cerebellar arteries have been reported (32–35). This procedure is much more complex than anterior circulation anastomosis because of the anatomy of the occipital artery and the lack of adequate instrumentation. Surgical complications involve a myriad of brain-stem syndromes and include cardiovascular and respiratory instability postoperatively and obtunded at depressed airway reflexes.

Complications of superficial temporal–middle cerebral artery anastomosis are usually transient and reversible. Aphasic difficulties following operations on the dominant hemisphere may occur but usually are reversible. Scalp necrosis and wound infection have been reported to occur in about 5% of cases (36).

Reports of long vein grafts from the cervical carotid artery to the intracranial circulation have not received wide acceptance (37–40). Although the initial blood volume delivered is much greater than that through an arterial anastomosis, the rate of postoperative occlusion is high. Direct anastomosis of the venous graft to the carotid artery carries a much higher incidence of surgical complications related to the necessity to perform an arteriotomy of the short internal carotid artery and interruption of the major collateral pathways to the involved hemisphere during the anastomosis.

Anesthetic Management

Many of the principles that apply to the anesthetic management of patients undergoing carotid endarterectomy are relevant to EC-IC bypass. Meticulous preoperative assessment of multisystem disease and polypharmacologic intake is essential.

The major intraoperative requirements of anesthetic care are listed in Table 6.2. Maintenance of normocapnic or slightly hypocapnic levels will decrease the deleterious effects of cerebral vasoconstriction in a compromised brain. Cerebral perfusion must be maintained. Following induction of anesthesia, a hypertensive response on intubation may be attenuated by intravenous and topical administration of lidocaine (41). Thereafter, in the absence of surgical stimulation, blood pressure tends to decrease and should be supported as necessary by a slow infusion of 0.02% phenylephrine hydrochloride. After removal of the arterial clamps, the blood pressure again tends to rise. Therapy at this time should include hydralazine, 5 to 15 mg, diazoxide, 50 mg, and propranolol if the pulse rate exceeds 80 to 90 beats per minute. Because the surgical technique involves clamping of a branch of the middle cerebral artery for approximately one hour, an agent such as a barbiturate, which may afford ischemic protection, might be preferable (42). This agent causes marked cerebral vasoconstriction, however, which might further decrease collateral flow to ischemic areas. Administration of low-dose inhalation agents, especially isoflurane, in combination with normocapnia

Table 6.2 Intraoperative Anesthetic Requirements for Patients Undergoing Extracranial-Intracranial Anastomosis

Requirement	Criteria or Means
Normocapnia	PaCO$_2$ 35 to 40 mm Hg
Maintain cerebral perfusion pressure	Phenylephrine HCl; Hydralazine
Decrease brain metabolic requirements	Isoflurane, barbiturates, narcotics
Monitoring and trend recording	Blood pressure
	Electrocardiogram
	Arterial gas tensions
	Input-output charting
	Temperature
Minimize brain bounce	Jet ventilation
	Low tidal volume
	Diuretics
	CSF withdrawal
Prompt return to consciousness	Light anesthetic technique

decreases cerebral metabolic rate of oxygen consumption while maintaining CBF to poorly perfused areas. The absence of the development of any new neurologic deficit immediately after operation in our series and the ability to perform accurate neurologic assessment because of prompt return to consciousness would indicate that this regimen is satisfactory (36). Routine monitoring in all patients should include arterial blood gas estimation and arterial pressure measurements, electrocardiogram, fluid balance, and temperature. Posterior circulation anastomoses are usually carried out in a sitting position, when all the precautions necessitated by this position must be observed (see Chapter 7).

Brain movement as a result of cardiac and respiratory action is problematic at high magnification. Initially the brain may appear swollen, and there is a temptation to increase ventilation to correct the situation; however, this state is most probably related to the cerebrovascular disease, and the area involved has lost reactivity to carbon dioxide. Thus, improved operative conditions are better achieved by use of a head-up position, less acute head turning, smaller tidal volumes with increased respiratory rate, drainage of cerebrospinal fluid after opening into the subarachnoid space, and judicious administration of small doses of furosemide (10 to 20 mg intravenously). A modification of jet ventilation will undoubtedly be most beneficial in these situations (43).

Low molecular weight dextran maintains flow through newly anastomosed vessels. It is usually infused at a rate of 50 to 100 ml/hr. In about 50% of cases, however, persistent oozing of blood develops. Dextran may also increase the tendency to hypertension. In both these situations, dextran therapy should be discontinued.

As EC-IC anastomosis involves only superficial cortical vessels, patients should be readily responsive and the trachea extubated on entry to the recovery room. Close observation of all vital signs for 48 to 72 hours, including careful, frequent neurologic assessment, is necessary. Patients with a previous history of myocardial infarction are at particular risk of cardiac complications after operation, and maintaining arterial pressure close to preoperative baseline values is essential (36). Early ambulation is possible and desirable to prevent embolic complications. Because little postoperative pain is experienced, narcotics with their depressant effects can usually be avoided.

SUBARACHNOID HEMORRHAGE

In the United States, the death rate from subarachnoid hemorrage is 16 per 100,000 population (44). The immediate mortality after rupture of an intracranial aneurysm is 43%. With conservative management, 35% of survivors will die following another bleed within one year, and 51% will be dead within five years (45). The mortality rate is greater after recurrent hemorrhage: 64% after the first rebleed and 96% after the second. Neurologic deficit occurs in 30% of survivors (46).

Cerebral arteries, like arteries elsewhere, are made up of several layers of tissues. The internal elastic membrane is thicker in cerebral arteries than in arteries in other parts of the body. With age, however, degenerative changes occur consisting of fenestration and folds (47,48). The medial layer, which consists of smooth muscle cells, is much thinner and contains less muscular and elastic tissue than other arteries. Defects and abnormalities of this layer, which thickens with age, frequently are found at arterial bifurcations. The adventitia in intracranial vessels is thinner than in other vessels (48). The defects in the muscular layer and in the internal elastic layer apparently predispose to the development of intracranial aneurysms (Figs. 6.9, 6.10).

Contrary to previous belief, it has been suggested that intracranial aneurysm is an acquired rather than a congenital disease. Evidence for this is based on the fact that aneurysms are rarely found at autopsy of infant brains, and on a clinical association between aneurysms and angiographically visible atheromas, which form on the internal elastic lamina (49).

Untreated systemic hypertension and smoking tend to predispose to aneurysmal dilations (49). There are two other infrequent causes for the formation of aneurysms. Mycotic aneurysms are caused by adhesion of septic emboli to an arterial wall with resultant necrosis. They occur as a complication of heart valve vegetations that develop in rheumatic fever. Most are broad-based and located in the middle cerebral system (48). Traumatic aneurysms develop as a result of direct trauma to an artery with injury to the wall.

Arteriovenous malformations consist of an abnormal arteriovenous communication containing both arteries and veins (50) (Fig. 6.11). Hemorrhage is usually from the venous end of the dilated arteriovenous malformation. Four types of abnormalities have been identified: (a) telangiectasia or capillary angiomas are composed of thin-walled capillaries without smooth muscle or elastic tissue; (b) varices are dilated venous channels such as occur in malformations of the great vein of Galen; (c) cavernous angiomas are formed of many thin-walled blood vessels

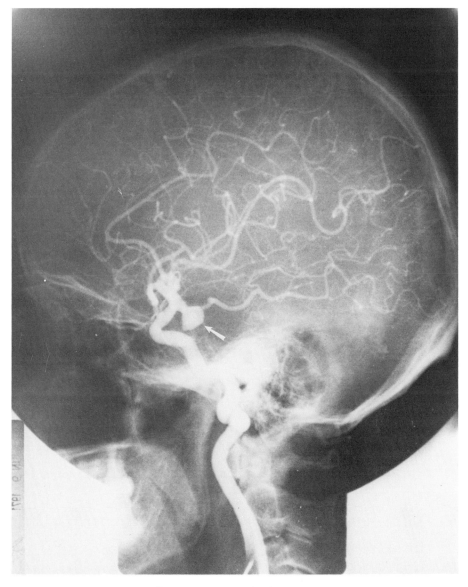

Figure 6.9 Posterior communicating artery aneurysm.

without separation by the supporting glial tissue; and (d) the classic arteriovenous malformation consists of large numbers of dilated, and sometimes arterialized veins, which usually are triangular and point toward the ventricle (48). Infrequently, arteriovenous malformations have an associated signal lesion in the scalp because of a common blood supply (50). Arteriovenous malformations usually share a common clinical triad consisting of severe, repetitive headaches, often in the same location, with episodes of neck stiffness and seizures.

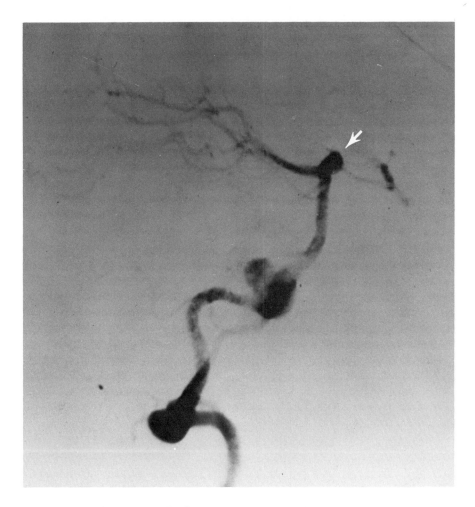

Figure 6.10 Basilar artery aneurysm, subtraction study.

Distinctly different from aneurysms, arteriovenous malformations may bleed repeatedly with complete recovery. They may also present as mass lesions. Intracerebral hematomas following rupture of an arteriovenous malformation are not uncommon and sometimes make surgical resection of the lesion much easier.

The aim of surgery for arteriovenous malformations is complete removal of the lesion, which is accomplished by block dissection. Wherever possible, the arterial supply must be obliterated prior to the venous return. Obliterating the venous return before the arterial side has been eliminated may lead to a rapid expansion of the malformation with hemorrhage and massive brain edema. Newer radiologic techniques for use in the surgically inaccessible arteriovenous malformations consist of embolization and obliteration of the malformation with plastic polymers. Complications of these indirect techniques include all the manifestations of cerebral ischemia.

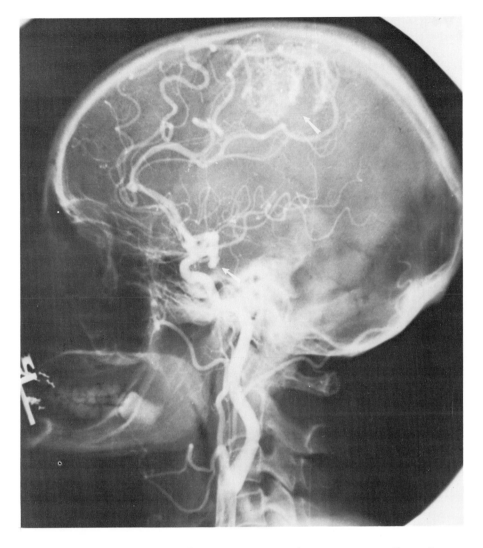

Figure 6.11   Internal carotid artery aneurysm and arteriovenous malformation.

Some arteriovenous malformations involve such large areas of the brain that they are not suitable for either surgical extirpation or embolization and obliteration techniques. Medical management of an arteriovenous malformation of this type is aimed at reducing blood pressure and the elimination of rapid increases in intracranial pressure secondary to Valsalva maneuvers. Prognosis, however, is grave.

Experimental obliteration of aneurysms through a percutaneous retrograde catheter technique is under way. The future may bring further refinements in the management of these lesions. If the experimental techniques prove successful, the treatment of intracranial aneurysms and arteriovenous malformations may eventually fall into the realm of interventional radiology.

Aneurysmectomy

Assessment and Preoperative Management

Twenty percent of patients presenting with subarachnoid hemorrhage have multiple aneurysms (48) (Fig. 6.12). Mirror aneurysms of the internal carotid system are most common, but other combinations of locations occur (44). The site of the bleeding aneurysm is best identified by CT studies, evidence of vasopasm in the immediate vicinity, and lobulation of the aneurysmal wall on angiographic studies.

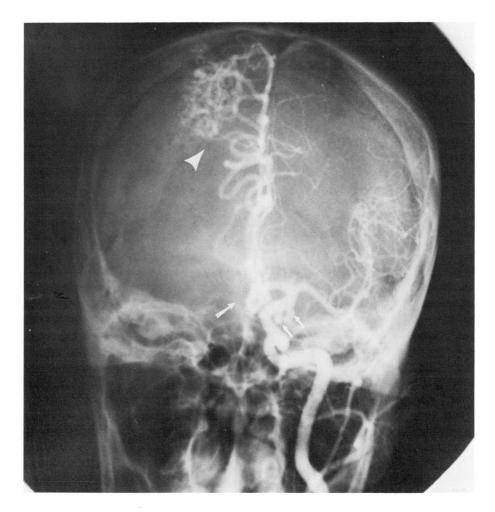

Figure 6.12   Anterior communicating artery aneurysm (*large arrow*), internal carotid artery aneurysm (*small arrow, left*), middle cerebral artery aneurysm (*small arrow, right*), and arteriovenous malformation (*arrowhead*).

Table 6.3 Grading System for Clinical Status and Outcome after Subarachnoid Hemorrhage

Grade	Pathology	Clinical Condition
I	Minimal bleed	Alert
		No neurologic deficits
		No signs of meningeal irritation
II	Mild bleed	Alert
		Minimal neurologic deficits
		(e.g., oculomotor palsy)
		Signs of meningeal irritation
III	Moderate bleed	Drowsy or confused
		Marked signs of meningeal irritation
		Major neurologic deficits
IV	Moderate to severe bleed	Stupor or coma
		Some purposeful movements
		Major neurologic deficits may or may not be present
V	Severe bleed	Coma
		Decerebrate movements
IV	Severe bleed	Moribund

Table 6.3 outlines a grading system adapted to clinical terminology to identify the severity of the disease and indicate prognosis (51). Patients in Botterell Grades I and II are much more likely to have a good surgical result than patients in Grades III through VI. Patients in Grade V and VI can be expected to succumb to their illness.

During childhood and adolescence, subarachnoid hemorrhage is rare and is more commonly due to arteriovenous malformations rather than to ruptured aneurysms (48). After the second decade, aneurysms predominate as the cause of intracranial hemorrhage. In 1.4% of patients with subarachnoid hemorrhage, arteriovenous malformations and aneurysms coexist (44). The frequency of locations of ruptured intracranial aneurysms is shown in Table 6.4 (44).

Table 6.4 Incidence of Aneurysms at Various Locations

Site	Incidence (%)
Internal carotid	38
Anterior cerebral system	36
Anterior communicating junction	30
Internal carotid at posterior communicating junction	25
Middle cerebral system	21
Vertebrobasilar system	5

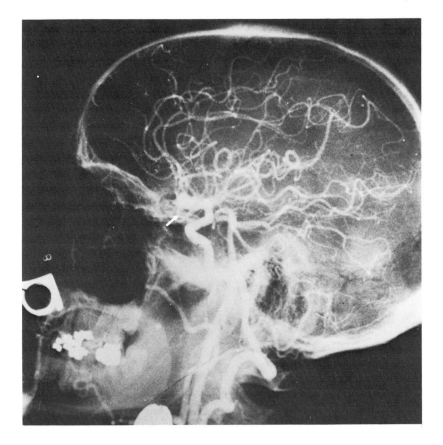

Figure 6.13   Carotid angiogram, lateral view, showing anterior communicating artery aneurysm giving rise to multiple branches.

With the exception of evacuation of intracerebral hematomas associated with rupture of a cerebral aneurysm, aneurysms are best operated semielectively, which allows scheduling of surgery without encountering brain edema or aggravating the vascular spasm caused by the initial subarachnoid hemorrhage.

Surgical Care

Medical management of subarachnoid hemorrhage, which usually is pursued for two to three weeks, may be considered an adjunct to surgical therapy. The goal is cerebral recovery with elimination of brain edema and arterial vasospasm, prevention of early rebleeding, and control of hypertension. Treatment involves bed rest, hypotensive therapy, antifibrinolytic therapy (including administration of epsilon aminocaproic acid), and control and management of increased intracranial pressure. Prevention of seizures by anticonvulsant medication is essential.

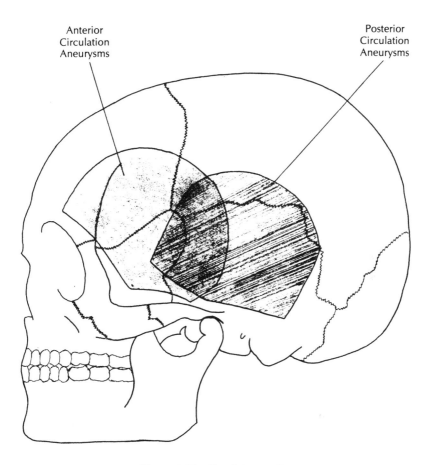

Figure 6.14   Craniotomy sites.

A careful bowel regimen must be maintained to prevent straining, and although administration of enemas may produce a vagovagal reflex, this is preferable to sudden increases in intraabdominal pressure and the resultant obstruction to cerebral venous return.

The timing of surgery affects the surgical result (52). Patients in Botterell Grades I and II are candidates for earlier operations than patients in Grades III through VI. The location of the aneurysm also influences timing of operation. Aneurysms of the internal carotid artery (see Fig. 6.11), which are approached without brain dissection, can be operated on earlier than aneurysms within the brain tissue itself, such as anterior communicating and middle cerebral artery aneurysms (Fig. 6.13). If multiple aneurysms exist, the defect that has bled most recently should be operated on first. If all the lesions can be exposed through the same craniotomy, multiple aneurysms can be operated on simultaneously.

Aneurysms located in the carotid, ipsilateral middle cerebral, and anterior

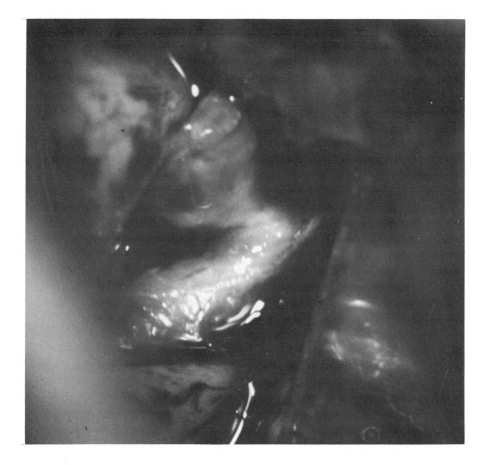

Figure 6.15 Internal carotid artery aneurysm exposed.

communicating arteries can be approached through a single frontotemporal craniotomy (52) (Fig. 6.14). Mirror aneurysms located in both carotid or posterior communicating arteries or in the contralateral middle cerebral arteries require separate exposures.

Three-point fixation of the head is essential for microsurgical exposures. A supine position with the head rotated about 20 to 30 degrees to the side opposite the surgical exposure is used for anterior approaches. Before the dura is incised, dexamethasone, furosemide, and mannitol may be administered intravenously to promote diuresis and decrease brain size. Additional drainage of spinal fluid is obtained through a catheter placed preoperatively, after anesthetic induction, in the lumbar subarachnoid space. Up to 100 ml of spinal fluid can be slowly drained by this technique at the time the dura is opened. While not always essential, the additional intracranial space obtained allows for gentler retraction and smaller operative approaches.

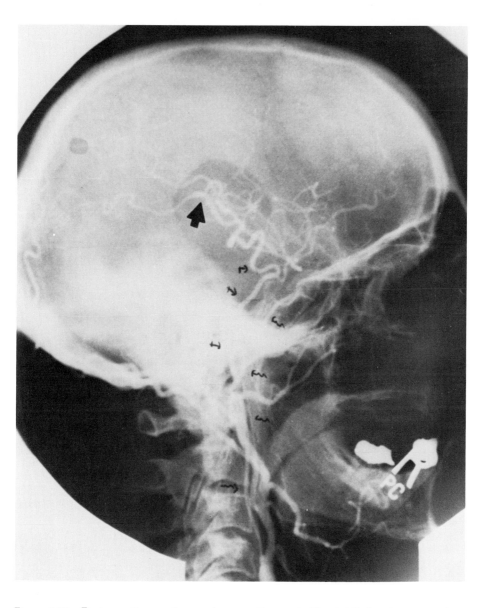

Figure 6.16 Postoperative angiogram (same patient as in Fig. 6.12) showing revascularized hemisphere. Arrow points to site of anastomosis.

Following elevation of an area of bone, the dura is opened and its edges secured to prevent epidural bleeding. Gentle retraction of the frontal lobe with loupe magnification is used until the optic nerve and carotid artery are visualized. A self-retaining retractor is placed and the operative microscope is brought into

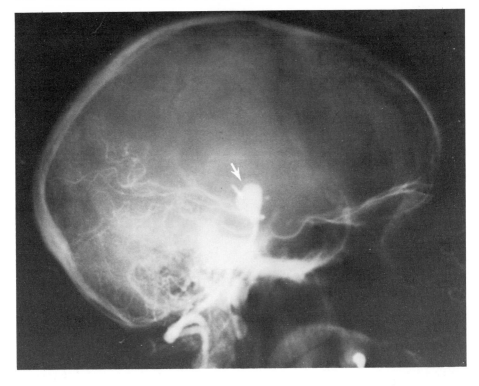

Figure 6.17 Basilar artery aneurysm.

the field. The remainder of the procedure is done under microscopic magnification. The subarachnoid (prechiasmatic) cisterns are opened and as much of the cerebrospinal fluid as possible evacuated.

The arachnoid around the carotid artery may then be dissected. The exposure allows visualization of anterior communicating, middle cerebral, and carotid artery aneurysms (Fig. 6.15). Aneurysms of the middle cerebral artery, high up in the Sylvian fissure, may be exposed without dissection of the carotid artery, but proximal control of the aneurysm whenever possible is preferred. Figure 6.16 is a postoperative angiogram showing a completed revascularization in a patient with multiple aneurysms of the anterior circulation.

Aneurysms of the basilar artery (Fig. 6.17) are reached through the subtemporal approach with a horizontal head position. The bone flap is located farther back, allowing for elevation and retraction of the temporal lobe. The anterior limb of the flap corresponds to the posterior limb of the incision to expose an aneurysm of the anterior circulation. Aneurysms of the vertebral arteries and their branches are approached through a suboccipital craniectomy with the patient in the sitting position.

A subtemporal transtentorial approach to the lower basilar artery and the vertebrobasilar junction is perfectly feasible. The suboccipital area may also be

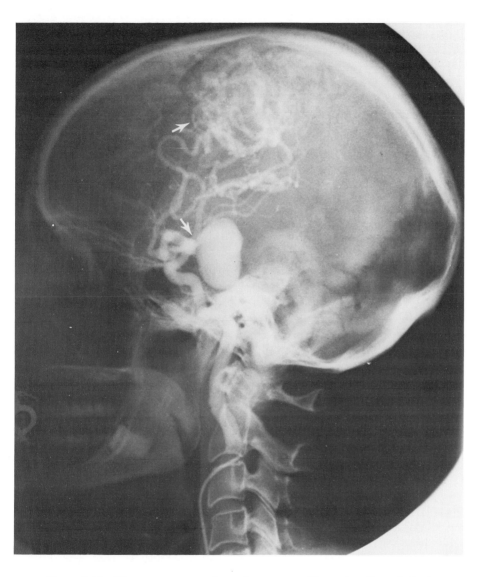

Figure 6.18   Giant aneurysm and arteriovenous malformation (lateral view).

approached in the lateral recumbent position (bench position). Skeletal fixation is again essential. Decision on the type of craniotomy employed in the exposure of an aneurysm of the posterior circulation depends on the location and projection of the aneurysm and, in some cases, the preference of the surgeon.

If the sitting position is employed, all precautions necessitated by the maneuver must be exercised (see chapter 7). Although carotid artery occlusion as the primary treatment of intracranial aneurysms has become an infrequently used

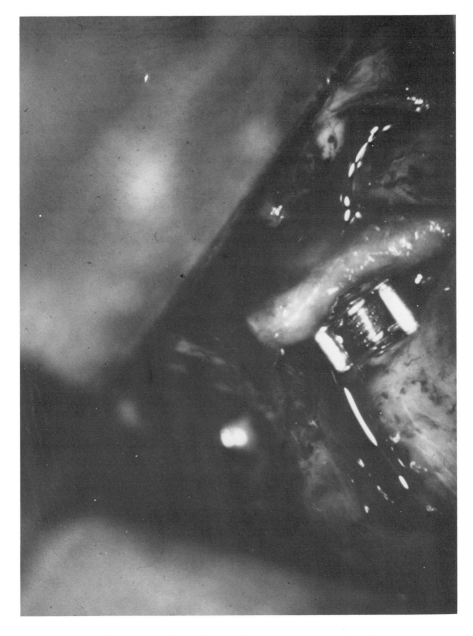

Figure 6.19 Internal carotid artery aneurysm clipped.

technique, indications for carotid ligation still exist. Among these may be included giant (Fig. 6.18) and inaccessible aneurysms of the internal carotid artery as well as anterior communicating artery aneurysms in the presence of unilateral circulation caused by hypoplasia or absence of one anterior cerebral artery. Because of the potential for a disastrous neurologic complication secondary to cerebral ischemia following carotid ligation, the procedure should be employed only if a contraindication exists to the intracranial approach and direct obliteration or wall reinforcement of the aneurysm. Gradual occlusion of the carotid artery allows for reversal of any induced cerebral ischemia (53,54). The aim of carotid ligation is to reduce arterial pressure in the aneurysm by decreasing the volume of blood in the immediate circulation.

Intracranial surgery of aneurysms aims to obliterate the dilation by occlusion of the neck of the sac with spring clips (Fig. 6.19) or ligatures, often in combination with bipolar coagulation. Some aneurysms, particularly those of the middle cerebral and the anterior communicating artery, may be part of the essential intracranial circulation through branches originating from the dome. Under these circumstances, obliteration of the aneurysm is potentially catastrophic because the necessary perforating blood vessels are eliminated. Wall reinforcement after a complete dissection of the aneurysm and its branches can be achieved by the use of plastic polymers and artificial wrapping material; however, the question of lasting cure persists with this maneuver.

Aneurysms of the carotid artery in the intracavernous portion may produce symptoms through enlargement or hemorrhage. The development of carotid-cavernous arteriovenous fistulas may occur as a complication of hemorrhage. Treatment includes carotid ligation, trapping procedures in which both the cervical and intracranial carotid arteries are occluded, embolization, and balloon occlusion techniques.

Giant aneurysms of the internal carotid and middle cerebral arteries occur and present as mass lesions rather than as acute intracranial hemorrhagic disasters. The use of EC-IC revascularization procedures prior to the trapping of some of these aneurysms is a definite consideration, although early clinical experience suggests that this staging mechanism may not prove quite as useful as hoped because the acute nature of the ischemia during surgery may be too extreme to be overcome by early blood flow shunting.

Anesthetic Management

Preoperative management of patients with subarachnoid hemorrhage includes bed rest and sedation. Thus predisposition to penumonic processes exists. Serial chest fims should be obtained and arterial blood gases and white cells measured immediately before surgery. Vigorous pulmonary function tests are obviously contraindicated, and all evaluations should be restricted to bedside estimations. epsilon aminocaproic acid (Amicar) is used as an antifibrinoloytic agent and has been reported to cause embolic phenomena and pulmonary embolization (55). We have also observed nonspecific electrocardiographic changes such as ST and T-wave abnormalities in the absence of other clinical cardiac signs. These findings may be associated with blood in the subarachnoid space or with the infusion of Amicar. In our patients, we have encountered no adverse cardiac effects of subsequent anesthetic administration.

For preoperative medication, oral sedation with relatively large doses of diazepam (10 mg) or lorazepam (2 mg) about one hour before surgery is adequate. Atropine is avoided, as it causes unpleasant dryness of the mouth, which may only increase the patient's anxiety. During induction, attempts should be made to preserve a stable transmural pressure across the aneurysm. Thiopental sodium causes cerebral vasoconstriction and modifies increases in intracranial pressure caused by laryngoscopy (56). Pretreatment with lidocaine, 1.5 mg/kg intravenously, has also been shown to be effective in reducing pressure increases (57). Liberal use should also be made of a topical lidocaine spray to attenuate the hypertensive response to intubation and to prevent bucking during insertion of the pinhead holder (41). Sodium nitroprusside has been used to control arterial pressure during laryngoscopy (58), but this drug causes a marked decrease in cerebrovascular resistance and consequent rise in intracranial pressure, and its use should be restricted until after the dural coverings have been opened (59). Hydralazine, which also increases intracranial pressure, should also be avoided before the dura is opened. The previous neurosurgical practice of scalp infiltration with epinephrine has been largely abandoned, as absorption of this agent after 10 to 20 minutes causes arterial hypertension (60). Controlled ventilation to maintain $PaCO_2$ values of 27 to 30 mm Hg is established almost immediately. Light inhalational anesthesia is preferable. Isoflurane concentrations, which provide adequate neurosurgical anesthesia (1 MAC), cause little or no depression of myocardial function, cardiac output, or tissue perfusion (61). CBF and intracranial pressure do not increase from awake levels at 0.6 to 1.1 MAC (18). Thereafter, a dose-dependent increase in flow occurs, which may be prevented by hyperventilation (62). Trend recording of blood pressure during an 8-hour period of surgery for clipping of a posterior cerebral aneurysm and arteriovenous malformation is shown in Fig. 6.20.

Insertion of the saw guide may also increase intracranial pressure, and care must be taken to establish adequate ventilation and early withdrawal of cerebrospinal fluid to ensure sufficient relaxation of the brain (56).

Necessary monitoring includes early establishment of direct arterial pressure recording, electrocardiogram, urinary output, temperature, and esophageal stethoscope. Although not generally available, monitoring of evoked potentials, cerebral metabolites, and mixed venous oxygen tension provides additional useful information.

Induction of systemic hypotension has long been advocated as an intraoperative neurosurgical adjunct to decrease surgical hemorrhage, permit a drier field, and facilitate microdissection prior to aneurysm clipping, arteriovenous malformation obliteration, vascular tumor resection, and during spine and cord surgery. As aneurysm sacs and necks become slacker and more pliable, application of occlusive clips is safer. Should rupture occur, hemorrhage is more easily controlled than under normotensive conditions.

Several techniques have been advocated and mostly abandoned, such as arteriotomy and extremity pooling with tourniquets, which both tend to result in cardiac failure; high spinal or epidural anesthesia to the first thoracic segment (a block which may cause profound, uncontrolled hypotension that is difficult to reverse); and intracardiac pacing to decrease effective cardiac output.

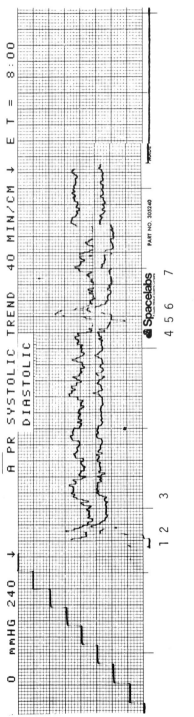

Figure 6.20   Blood pressure trend recording in aneurysm surgery.

Ganglionic blocking drugs that prevent sympathetic vasoconstriction and decrease peripheral resistance were introduced by Enderby in 1950 and included pentamethonium, hexamethonium, tetraethylammonium, pentolinium tartrate, and trimethaphan camsylate. Subsequently, several other drugs have been suggested as useful hypotensive agents. Sodium nitroprusside (SNP), a hydrated nitrosylpentacyanoferrate compound, was first described by Playfair in 1849. Administered intravenously, it acts directly on vascular smooth muscle to cause peripheral vasodilation. Diazoxide also is a rapid-acting smooth muscle relaxant of peripheral arterioles. As with SNP, cardiac output is maintained while cerebrovascular resistance and blood pressure are reduced. Inhalation anesthetic agents such as halothane and isoflurane cause vasodilation and, in sufficient concentration, decrease cardiac output. Nitroglycerin dilates capacitance vessels, which allows a rapidly reversible hypotensive effect. Finally, the calcium channel antagonists nifedipine and verapamil reduce blood pressure by altering the extracellular calcium flux.

Of all these means of producing a hypotensive state, only four are in common use. In order of preference, they are SNP, halogenated anesthetics, trimethaphan, and nitroglycerin.

SNP has an evanescent action because of its rapid conversion to thiocyanate. It is administered intravenously in a freshly prepared 0.01% solution which must be protected from light. Blood pressure fall is precipitous, within seconds, and the rate of infusion must be meticulously monitored. It does, however, afford precise control, and arterial pressure returns to normal values within one minute of discontinuing the infusion. Reduction in mean pressure to a level of 40 or 50 mm Hg has only negligible effect on cardiac output, but vascular resistance is significantly decreased (63). Vital organ blood flow remains near normal with maintenance of regional oxygen extraction.

Destruction of SNP may be along three pathways. It may be converted to thiocyanate by rhodonase, to cyanide by combination of the active radical with sulfhydryl groups, or it may combine with hemoglobin to form cyanmethemoglobin. Since 1 mg of SNP contains 0.44 mg of cyanide, toxic blood levels (i.e., 100 μg/dl) may occur if more than 1 ml/kg is given over two to three hours. Toxicity is recognized by development of metabolic acidosis, tachycardia, ventricular arrhythmias, hypotension, and hyperventilation. Treatment involves discontinuation of the infusion, administration of intravenous thiosulfate, sodium nitrite, hydroxycobalamine, sodium bicarbonate, and inhalation of amyl nitrite.

If SNP is started only when the surgeon begins to work in the immediate area of the aneurysm or arteriovenous malformation, the total dose rarely exceeds 10 to 15 mg and duration of administration is generally less than one hour. At this dosage range, the adverse effects of tachyphylaxis, cyanide toxicity, rebound hypertension, and platelet abnormalities are rarely encountered. Should arterial pressure rise more than 20 to 30 mm Hg above baseline on discontinuing SNP infusion, hydralazine in increments of 10 mg with small doses of propranolol, 1 mg, may be given. A rare complication of prolonged SNP administration is hypothyroidism, which may result from thiocyanate interference with thyroid iodide trapping mechanisms after prolonged administration (64).

Using postoperative angiographic studies of patients who developed a new deficit after surgery, we found that patients who received SNP showed less vasospasm than those in whom halothane had been used to produce controlled hypotension intraoperatively (65). We also found significantly fewer side effects that when trimethaphan was used. Use of SNP during pregnancy with apparently no untoward effects on the fetus has also been described (66).

The main advantage of simply increasing the percentage of the halogenated agent already being administered is that there is no need to add another potentially dangerous pharmocologic agent. Halothane and, to a smaller degree, isoflurane act as hypotensive agents at higher concentrations (above 2 MAC), increasing cerebral blood flow and intracranial pressure. Failure rate is low but the end point is variable. Tachyphylaxis is not seen, but relative overdose may delay emergence from anesthesia. Both agents exert a good cerebral protective effect but may increase intracranial pressure at higher concentrations, an effect offset by prior hyperventilation.

Trimethaphan is a ganglionic blocker with histamine-releasing properties. Administered as an intravenous infusion of 0.1% solution, it acts in about five minutes to lower the systolic blood pressure to around 70 to 80 mm Hg. It depends on the kidneys for excretion after destruction by serum cholinesterase. Potentiation of action by inhalation agents is marked.

Nitroglycerin has also been used successfully as a hypotensive agent in a dose of 0.5 to 1.5 μ.g/kg/min (67). This solution should be freshly prepared, must be protected from light, and has an expiration time of 8 hours. Hypotension is achieved within two minutes, but there may be considerable further downward drift. Recovery rate is also relatively slow (about 12 minutes). The total dose of nitroglycerin over a 45-minute period is about 3 mg (80 ml). Nitroglycerin has the same effect as SNP in increasing intracranial pressure but produces less pulmonary shunting. Rebound hypertension is extremely rare, as plasma renin is not increased and there is no danger of cyanide toxicity. Desired hypotensive levels may be difficult to maintain, however, since following discontinuation of administration considerable further downward drift of blood pressure may occur.

Because vasodilators act primarily by producing shifts in extracellular and intracellular calcium flux, current experimentation is directed toward developing calcium channel blockers as useful hypotensive agents. Verapamil, nifedipine, phentolamine, and labetalol have all been investigated in animal models. In a cat model, verapamil has been shown to decrease arterial pressure promptly while causing little change in intracranial pressure (68).

Intrapulmonary ventilation/perfusion inequalities increase during periods of hypotension, particularly if there is preexistent pulmonary disease (66). This probably is due to the ability of the hypotensive agent to overcome the normal compensatory pulmonary vasoconstriction that occurs in response to hypoxia. Reversal to previous values occurs promptly on discontinuing the hypotensive technique. Although there does not appear to be any correlation between the severity of the ventilation/perfusion abnormality that develops and neurologic outcome, patients who are more hypoxic for longer periods have an increased number of and more severe respiratory problems postoperatively.

Complications of induced hypotension are:

1. Decreased blood flow
   a. Cerebral thrombosis
   b. Myocardial infarction
   c. Renal failure
   d. Retinal artery thrombosis
2. Reactionary hemorrhage
3. Rebound hypertension
   a. Cerebral hemorrhage
   b. Cardiac failure
4. Persistent hypotension
5. Pressure necrosis
6. Hypothermia
7. Increased intracranial pressure
8. Respiratory distress syndrome
9. Delayed awakening

Although it may be seen that these complications of deliberate hypotension are formidable, they generally are potential hazards than can be avoided by careful monitoring and attention to detail. The safety of deliberate, controlled hypotension in patients without cerebrovascular disease has been documented. The overall mortality in a series of 27,930 cases was reported as 0.34% (0.25% were considered related to anesthesia or hypotension) (70). In another study of 9107 cases, deaths caused by anesthesia and hypotension were only 0.555% (71). Nonfatal complications are, of course, more common. In the first study, Hampton and Little reported 908 major and minor complications, an incidence of 3.3%. The more common nonfatal complications were reactionary hemorrhage, delayed awakening, blurred vision, oliguria, anuria, and persistent hypotension. The combined incidence of major and minor central nervous system complications was 1.3%. Cerebral thrombosis occurred in 0.014% and retinal arterial thrombosis in 0.01% (72).

Hypothermic techniques, which substantially increase anesthetic time, are no longer commonly used during vascular neurosurgery. They are associated with a much greater frequency of arrhythmias during and after surgery. Return to consciousness is also delayed.

Following aneurysm surgery, patients are less likely to exhibit cardiovascular instability than patients with generalized vascular disease. Intensive monitoring is still essential. A patient who was neurologically intact preoperatively and in whom no intraoperative catastrophe occurred should be awake, with the trachea extubated, on admission to the recovery room. Hypertension may develop and indicate vasospasm or clot formation. An associated bradycardia or deterioration in the level of consciousness requires prompt CT scanning to exclude an intracranial mass lesion. Currently postoperative care is aimed at maintaining a slightly increased arterial pressure, generally by increasing the blood volume. Because the arterial malformation is now clipped, it is no longer at risk of rupture. Thus all basic respiratory maneuvers may be carried out. Following frontotemporal procedures, edema formation frequently results in temporary closing of one eye or the other, hindering neurologic assessment. Again, trend recording of neurologic status is essential.

Aneurysms Associated with Pregnancy

Subarachnoid hemorrhage secondary to rupture of an aneurysm or arteriovenous malformation is reported to cause 12 to 24% of maternal deaths (73). Estimates of incidence range from 1/10,000 to 1/2,500 pregnancies (74).

If it becomes necessary to operate during pregnancy to secure the aneurysm, the anesthetic goals include maternal safety, avoidance of teratogenic drugs, fetal well being and uterine stability. If pregnancy continues to term, the anesthetic management requires provision of adequate pain control for safe vaginal or abdominal delivery without deterioration of the neurologic pathology.

Aneurysms tend to rupture during the thirtieth to fortieth gestational week and arteriovenous malformations during the second trimester or in the peripartum period. Increased blood volume and cardiac output may be contributing causes (75). The clinical picture may resemble that of severe toxemia with hypertension, proteinuria, headache, and coma (76).

Physiologic changes of importance to anesthetic management in these patients include a 20% reduction of functional residual capacity at term and 20% increased oxygen consumption, making the rapid development of hypoxia an ever-present hazard. Cardiac output increases by 30 to 40%. A relative anemia develops as plasma volume increases by 40% and red blood cell volume by 20%. Aortocaval compression may cause severe hypotension in the supine position and uterine displacement must be continued during anesthesia (73).

Inhalation anesthetic requirements are reduced during pregnancy as is the effective dose of succinylcholine. Dosage schedules should be adjusted downwards to avoid overdose. Osmotic diuretics cross the placenta and decrease fetal blood and extracellular volumes, which may cause severe fetal dehydration. Controversy exists over the safe use of induced hypotension (75,77). We have used a technique employing low-dose nitroprusside successfully (66). Long-term follow-up of the infants showed no neurologic abnormalities. Besides the usual monitors for intracranial surgery, an external Doppler fetal heart rate monitor and an external tocodynamometer to measure uterine tone are indicated.

The anesthetic management is similar to that for non-pregnant patients with the additional caveats for concern over rapidly developing hypoxia and the increased risk of regurgitation during intubation due to gastrointestinal changes (76) (increased gastric acid production and incompetence of the gastroesophageal sphincter). Caesarean section need only be performed if obstetrically indicated.

Postoperative monitoring of both the mother and the fetus should continue for at least 24 to 48 hours in an intensive-care setting.

If labor precedes intracranial intervention, therapy should be aimed at avoiding maternal straining and shortening the second stage of labor. This is best achieved by a skillfully placed segmental lumbar epidural or caudal anesthetic (73).

ACKNOWLEDGMENT

We gratefully acknowledge the contributions of: Digital angiography: Charles Herbstman, M.D., Holy Name Hospital, Teaneck, NJ   07666; and X-ray material: Leroy Kotzen, M.D., Hackensack Medical Center, Hackensack, NJ   07601.

REFERENCES

1.   Wylie EJ, Ehrenfeld WK: Extracranial occlusive cerebrovascular disease. Philadelphia, WB Saunders, 1970, pp 231.
2.   Mountcastle VB: Medical physiology, ed 13. St Louis, CV Mosby, 1974, vol 2, pp 1440–1441.
3.   Robertson JT, Auer NJ: Extracranial occlusive disease of the carotid artery, in Youmans JR: Neurological surgery, ed 2. Philadelphia, WB Saunders, 1982, pp 1562–1563.
4.   Fein JM: Contemporary techniques of cerebral revascularization, in Fein JM, Reichman OH (eds): Microvascular anastomoses for cerebral ischemia. New York, Springer Verlag, 1978, pp 161–177.
5.   Lassen NA, Ingvar DH, Skinhøj E: Brain function and blood flow. Sci Am 1978; 239:462–471.
6.   Foex P, Prys-Roberts C: Anaesthesia and the hypertensive patient. Br J Anaesth 1974;46:575–588.
7.   Goldman L, Caldera DL, Nussbaum SR, et al.: Multifactorial index of cardiac risk in noncardiac surgical procedures. N Engl J Med 1977;297:845–850.
8.   Frost EAM: Anaesthetic management of cerebrovascular disease. B J Anaesth 1981;53: 745–756.
9.   Goldman L, Southwick FS, Nussbaum SR, et al.: Cardiac risk factors and complications in noncardiac surgery. Medicine 1978;57:357–370.
10.   Cullen BF, Miller MG: Drug interactions and anesthesia, a review. Anesth Analg (Cleve) 1979;58:5413–5423.
11.   May FE, Steward RB, Bluff LE: Drug use in the hospital: Evaluation of determinants. Clin Pharmacol Therap 1974;16:834–845.
12.   Tobey RE, Jacobsen PM, Kahle CT: The serum potassium response to muscle relaxants in neural injury. Anesthesiology 1972;37:332–337.
13.   Pillone PR, Jacobs GB, Parikh S, et al.: Carotid endarterectomy utilizing the exclusion clamp. Int Surg 1975;60:2:105–108.
14.   Boysen G, Ladegaard-Pedersen HJ, Valentin N, et al.: Cerebral blood flow and internal carotid artery flow during carotid surgery. Stroke 1970;1:253–260.
15.   Geevarghese KP, Patel TC: Anesthesia and surgical treatment of cerebrovascular insufficiency. Int Anesthesiol Clin 1977;15:3:63–64.
16.   Sharbrough FW, Messick JM Jr, Sundt TM Jr: Correlation of continuous electro-

encephalograms with cerebral blood flow measurements during carotid endarterectomy. Stroke 1973;4:674-683

17. Homi J, Konchigeri HN, Eckenhoff JE, et al.: A new anesthetic agent—Forane[R]. Preliminary observations in man. Anesth Analg (Cleve) 1972;51:439-447.

18. Murphy FL Jr, Kennel EM, Johnston RE, et al.: The effects of enflurane, isoflurane and halothane on cerebral blood flow and metabolism in man, abstracted. Scientific papers, Annual Meeting, American Society of Anesthesiologists, 1974, pp 61-62.

19. Newberg LA, Michenfelder JD: Cerebral protection by isoflurane during hypoxemia or ischemia. Anesthesiology, 1983;59:1:29-35.

20. Eger EI, II, Stevens WC, Cromwell TH: The electroencephalogram in man anesthetized with Forane. Anesthesiology 1971;35:504-508.

21. McKay R: Short acting narcotics: Effects of intracranial tension and use in neurosurgery—Opioids in anesthesia, Cleveland Clinic Foundation, May 1983.

22. Geevarghese KP, Patel TC: Anesthesia and surgical treatment of cerebrovascular insufficiency. Int Anesthesiol Clin, 1977;15:3:59.

23. Lee JK, Hanowell S, Kim YD, et al.: Morphine induced respiratory depression following bilateral carotid endarterectomy. Anesth Analg (Cleve) 1981;60:64-65.

24. Donaghy RMP: Evaluation of extracranial-intracranial blood flow diversion, in Austin GM: Microneurosurgical anastomosis for cerebral ischemia. Springfield, Ill, Charles C Thomas, 1976, pp 256-275.

25. Donaghy RMP, Yaşargil MG: Microvascular surgery. St Louis, CV Mosby, 1967, pp 1-171.

26. Reichman OH: Extracranial to intracranial arterial anastomosis, in Youmans JR: Neurological surgery, ed 2. Philadelphia, WB Saunders Co, 1982, vol 3, pp 1585-1618.

27. Yaşargil MG, Krayenbuhl HA, Jacobson JH, II: Microneurosurgical arterial reconstruction. Surgery 1970;67:221-233.

28. Yaşargil MG, Yonekowa Y: Experiences with the STA-cortical MCA anastomosis in 46 cases, in Fein JM, Reichman OH (eds): Microvascular anastomoses for cerebral ischemia. New York, Springer Verlag, 1978, pp 272-277.

29. Yaşargil MG, Yonekowa Y: Results of microsurgical extra-intracranial arterial bypass in the treatment of cerebral ischemia. Neurosurgery 1977;1:22-24.

30. Fein JM: Microvascular surgery for stroke. Sci Am 1978;238:58-67.

31. Byer A, Moss CM, Hubbard HM, et al.: Experience with extracranial/intracranial bypass. J Med Soc NJ 1982;79:7:553-556.

32. Ausman JI, Nicoloft DN, Chou SN: Posterior fossa revascularization: Anastomosis of vertebral artery to PICA with interposed radial artery graft. Surg Neurol 1978;9:281-286.

33. Khodadad G: Atherosclerotic occlusive disease of the vertebral system in young adults and its surgical consideration. Acta Neurochir (Wien) 1978;45:147-154.

34. Khodadad G: Occipital artery-posterior inferior cerebellar artery anastomosis. Surg Neurol 1976;5:222-225.

35. Sundt TM, Jr, Piepgras DG: Occipital to posterior inferior cerebellar artery bypass surgery. J Neurosurg 1978;48:916-928.

36. Frost EAM, Arancibia CU, Kim Y, et al.: Anesthesia for cerebral revascularization. Meeting Proceed. 8th Annual Meeting Society of Neurosurgical Anesthesia and Neurologic Supportive Care, St Louis, Mo, 1980.

37. Lougheed WM, Marshall BM, Hunter M, et al.: Common carotid to intracranial internal carotid bypass venous graft. Technical note. J Neurosurg 1971;34:114-118.

38. Neblett CR: Large vessel vein grafts for cerebral ischemia. Presented at the Congress of Neurological Surgeons, Vancouver, Canada, Sept 25, 1974.

39. Tew JM, Jr: Reconstructive intracranial vascular surgery for prevention of stroke. Clin Neurosurg 1975;22:264–280.

40. Tew JM, Jr, Greiner AL, Berger TS, et al.: Intracranial vascular bypass: Can it prevent stroke? Mod Med 1977;45:58–61.

41. White PF, Schlobohm RM, Pitts LH, et al.: A randomized study of drugs for preventing increases in intracranial pressure during endotracheal suctioning. Anesthesiology 1982;57:242–244.

42. Smith AL, Hoff JT, Nielsen SL: Barbiturate protection in acute focal cerebral ischemia. Stroke 1974;5:1–7.

43. Kirby RB: High frequency positive pressure ventilation. Anesthesiology 1980;52: 109–110.

44. Sahs AP, Perret GE, Locksly HB, et al.: Intracranial aneurysms and subarachnoid hemorrhage. Philadelphia, JB Lippincott & Co, 1969, pp 1–296.

45. Nibbelink DW, Torner J, Henderson WG: Intracranial aneurysms and subarachnoid hemorrhage. Stroke 1977;8:202–218.

46. Adams CBT, Loach AB, O'Laoire SA: Intracranial aneurysms: Analysis of results of microneurosurgery. Br Med J 1976;2:607–609.

47. Baker AG: Structure of the small cerebral arteries and their changes with age. Am J Pathol 1937;13:453–460.

48. Smith RR: Pathophysiology and clinical evaluation of subarachnoid hemorrhage, in Youmans JR, Neurological surgery, ed 2. Philadelphia, WB Saunders 1982, vol 3, pp 1627–1644.

49. Bell BA, Symon L: Smoking and subarachnoid hemorrhage. Br Med J 1979;1:577–578.

50. McCormick WF: The pathology of vascular (arteriovenous) malformations. J Neurosurg 1966;24:808–816.

51. Botterell EH, Lougheed WM, Morley TP, et al.: Hypothermia in the surgical treatment of ruptured intracranial aneurysms. J Neurosurg 1958;15:14–18.

52. Jacobs GB, Rubin RC, Wille R: The treatment of intracranial aneurysms. J Neurosurg Nurs 1976;8:149–154.

53. Crutchfield WB: Instruments for use in the treatment of certain intracranial vascular lesions. J Neurosurg 1959;16:471–474.

54. Silverston B, White JC: A method for gradual occlusion of the internal carotid artery in the treatment of aneurysms, Proceedings, New England Cardiovascular Society 1952;9:24.

55. Sengupta RP, So SC, Villarejo-Ortega FJ: Use of epsilon aminocaproic acid in the preoperative management of ruptured intracranial aneurysms. J Neurosurg 1976;44: 479–484.

56. Shapiro HM, Wyte SR, Harris AB, et al.: Acute intraoperative intracranial hypertension in neurosurgical patients. Anesthesiology 1972;37:399–405.

57. Bedford RF, Winn HR, Tyson G, et al.: Lidocaine prevents increased ICP after endotracheal intubation, in Shulman K, Marmarou A, Miller JD, et al. (eds): Intracranial Pressure, ed IV. Berlin, Springer-Verlag, 1980, p 595.

58. Stoelting RK: Attenuation of blood pressure response to laryngoscopy and tracheal intubation with sodium nitroprusside. Anesth Analg (Cleve) 1979;58:116.

59. Turner JM, Powell D, Gibson RM: Intracranial pressure changes in neurosurgical patients during hypotension induced with sodium nitroprusside or trimethaphan. Br J Anaesth 1977;49:419–425.

60. Christensen KN, Jensen JK, Sogaard I: Blood pressure response to administration of local anaesthetics with noradrenaline during craniotomies. Acta Neurochir (Wien) 1980;51:157-160.

61. Stevens WC, Cromwell TH, Halsey MJ, et al.: The cardiovascular effects of a new inhalation anesthetic, Forane, in human volunteers at constant arterial carbon dioxide tension. Anesthesiology 1971;35:8-16.

62. Adams RW, Cucchiara RF, Gronvert GA, et al.: Isoflurane and cerebrospinal fluid pressure in neurosurgical patients. Anesthesiology 1981;54:97-99.

63. Tinker JM, Michenfelder JD: Sodium nitroprusside: Pharmacology, toxicology and therapeutics. Anesthesiology 1976;45:340-354.

64. Nurok DS, Glassock RJ, Solomon DH, et al.: Hypothyroidism following prolonged sodium nitroprusside therapy. Am J Med Sci 1964;248:129-138.

65. Frost EAM, Tabaddor K, Arancibia CU: Hypotensive drugs and outcome in aneurysm surgery. Anesthesiology 1979;51 (suppl 82):87.

66. Frost EAM: Anesthesia for elective intracranial procedures. Anesthesiol Rev 1980; 7:13-19.

67. Chestnut JS, Albin MS, Gonzalez-Abola E, et al.: Clinical evaluation of intravenous nitroglycerin for neurosurgery. J Neurosurg 1978;48:704-711.

68. Thiagarajah S, Orkin LR, Marmarou A, et al.: Intracranial pressure in the cat during verapamil induced hypotension. Proceedings 8th Meeting—Society of Neurosurgical Anesthesia, St. Louis, Mo, 1980.

69. Colley PS, Cheney FW: Sodium nitroprusside increases $\dot{Q}s/\dot{Q}t$ in dogs with regional atelectasis. Anesthesiology 1977;47:338-341.

70. Hampton LJ, Little DM Jr: Complications associated with the use of "controlled hypotension" in anesthesia. Arch Surg 1953;67:549-556.

71. Enderby GEH: A report on mortality and morbidity following 9,107 hypotensive anaesthetics. Br J Anaesth 1961;33:109-111.

72. Little DM: Induced hypotension during anesthesia and surgery. Anesthesiology 1955;16:320-332.

73. Rosen MA: Cerebrovascular lesions and tumors in the pregnant patient, in Handbook of Neuroanesthesia; Clinical and physiologic essentials. Boston, Little Brown, 1983, P. Newfield, JE Cottrell (eds): pp 226-244.

74. Miller HJ, Hinkley CM: Berry aneurysms in pregnancy; A ten year report. South Med J 1970;63:279-.

75. Robinson JL, Chir B, Hall CJ, et al.: Subarachnoid hemorrhage in pregnancy. J Neurosurg 1972;36:27-33.

76. Cannell TE, Botterell E: Subarachnoid hemorrhage and prognosis. Amer J Obstet Gynecol 1956;72:844-855.

77. Minielly R, Yuzpe AA, Drake CG: Subarachnoid hemorrhage secondary to ruptured cerebral aneurysm in pregnancy. Obstet Gynecol 1979;53:64-70.

CHAPTER 7

Posterior Cranial Fossa Surgery
Robert C. Rubin and
Elizabeth A.M. Frost

Although the skull is divided into an anterior, middle, and posterior cranial fossa, the anatomy and resulting pathology of the posterior fossa differ from that of the other compartments. The anterior and middle fossa contain the cerebral cortex and are separated from the posterior fossa by the tentorium. The cerebellum and brain stem are the main neural structures of the posterior fossa. These structures, which are vital for the control of respiration, blood pressure, and cardiac rate, are protected by the buttress of the temporal bone anteriorly and the occipital bone and extensive posterior cervical musculature posteriorly. Supratentorial pathologic processes therefore revolve around the cerebral cortex and its coverings, whereas the pathology of the posterior fossa involves the cerebellum, brain stem, and lower cranial nerves and their coverings.

POSTERIOR FOSSA ABNORMALITIES

Structures of the posterior fossa are affected by a unique set of pathologic conditions. Understanding this pathology, its presenting symptoms, and indications for surgery are essential to proper treatment.

Congenital Anomalies

Birth defects and congenital anomalies of posterior fossa structures usually present at birth or soon afterward (see Chapter 11). There are, however, several late effects of congenital anomalies that may require surgery. Both syringomyelia (syringobulbia) and the Arnold-Chiari (type 1) malformation may present symptomatically as headache, vertigo, cranial nerve palsies, ataxia, and hydrocephalus in adolescents or older patients. The surgery for this lesion consists of a suboccipital operative exposure and, in the case of the Arnold-Chiari malformation, often a decompression of bone afforded by a laminectomy at the level of the first and second vertebrae and free dissection around the tonsils. Constricting dural

155

and connective tissue bands may also require lysis. The procedure is performed with the patient in the semi-sitting position. The operating microscope is an essential adjunct. Respiratory failure, often of a sleep-induced apnea type, has frequently been noted postoperatively in these patients (1).

Tumors of the Posterior Fossa

Neurosurgical procedures for tumors arising in the posterior fossa involve essentially tumors that are intraaxial, that is, part of the brain substance itself, and those that are extraaxial, arising from the cranial nerves and coverings of the brain but extrinsic to the brain substance.

The majority of intraaxial tumors, which are of a primary neural origin, occur in children. In adults, tumors of diverse origin are hematogenously transported, often to areas of the cerebellum. Primary neoplasms of the posterior fossa neuraxis can be further subdivided into tumors affecting the cerebellum, tumors affecting the fourth ventricle, and tumors affecting the brain stem. The age of the patient and the location of the tumor often predict the pathology.

The surgical approaches to tumors of the cerebellar hemisphere are similar regardless of the pathology (2). Cerebellar astrocytomas, hemangioblastomas and, to a lesser extent, cerebellar sarcomas are found predominantly in the cerebellar hemispheres, as are metastatic tumors. These patients usually present with gait difficulty and signs of increased intracranial pressure caused by obstruction of the cerebrospinal fluid pathways, particularly those of the fourth ventricle and aqueduct. Symptoms are headache, nausea, vomiting, and progressive lethargy.

More commonly in children, increased intracranial pressure may cause papilledema and disturbances in vision such as enlargement of the blind spot without a change in visual acuity. Later, extraocular motor palsies may develop. The sixth nerve, which has a long intracranial course, is especially prone to traction pressures. Surgical intervention is aimed at relief of pressure caused by the mass lesion, establishment of a tissue diagnosis (particularly in some instances of metastatic lesions), and alleviation of focal neurologic signs occurring from the cerebellar deficit. In patients with extreme degrees of hydrocephalus, a ventriculoperitoneal shunt may be placed electively prior to definitive surgery.

Preoperative preparation includes administration of a steroid preparation, usually dexamethasone, 4 to 6 mg four times a day. Occasionally, external ventricular drainage may be established by inserting a ventricular catheter into the lateral ventricle. The tubing is led subcutaneously under the skin of the scalp and neck to minimize infection.

In most instances it is elected to position the patient in a modified sitting position, which affords good exposure to the suboccipital region, allows the head to be elevated and decreases venous pressure, and allows for gravitational removal of blood and cerebrospinal fluid.

Often, a small parasagittal right occipital skin incision and burr hole are made and extended down to the dura. If hydrocephalus exists and a shunt or ventricular drainage procedure has not been performed previously, cerebrospinal fluid can then be removed from the right lateral ventricle. The surgical approach is through a midline skin incision extending from the inion to the posterior cervical region. The suboccipital muscles are incised in the midline, exposing the occipital bone and the lamina of the first and second cervical vertebrae. During the course of this dissection, the operative field should be kept moist and under water and the patient monitored for infusion of air emboli, which is most likely to occur during the initial operative exposure when the rigid venous sinuses and channels are opened.

The lamina of the first cervical vertebra is often removed, particularly if there is evidence of significant tonsillar herniation. A burr hole is placed in the suboccipital region and enlarged to a craniectomy. If the bony removal is extended laterally to the level of the mastoid sinuses, opened mastoid emissary veins in this area may allow embolization of air. The bone edges should be meticulously waxed and the field kept moist and under water. Venous bleeding may be encountered from tears into the large dural sinuses, which may be a point of entry for bolus infusion of air.

When the tumor has been extirpated and adequate hemostasis obtained with bipolar coagulating current, the fourth ventricle may be visualized and an attempt made to ascertain that the cerebrospinal fluid pathways are open and that fluid egressing through the aqueduct is unobstructed in its course to the posterior fossa. It is often difficult to approximate the dural edges in the posterior fossa, and a dural substitute may be used. The anesthesiologist may be asked to increase the venous pressure by adding positive end-expiratory pressure or simulating a Valsalva maneuver to check for adequate hemostasis. The suboccipital bone is not replaced.

Intraaxial tumors involving the region of the fourth ventricle consist mainly of gliomas, ependymomas, medulloblastomas, and cerebellar sarcomas. Occasionally, congenitally arrested tumors such as dermoids may be found within the fourth ventricle. These tumors essentially occur in childhood. Rarely, metastatic tumors may proceed to the midline of the cerebellum and appear to be within the fourth ventricle. Lesions in and around the fourth ventricle usually present with signs of increased intracranial pressure. Lethargy and alterations in the level of consciousness are often present. Bradycardia and hypertension may also coexist. The operative procedure aims to extirpate the tumor, if possible, and relieve the ventricular obstruction. Tumors involving the floor of the fourth ventricle, such as ependymomas and occasionally medulloblastomas, are rarely amenable to total removal. Surgery is performed under magnified vision through a midline approach. Confirmation of ventricular patency can be established by the introduction of supravital dyes, such as indigocarmine, through a cannula in the lateral ventricle. Egress of contrast through the aqueduct can be visualized.

Brain-stem tumors usually are infiltrating astrocytomas of various grades of malignancy. They present more commonly in childhood but may be seen at any age. The hallmark of their presentation is a combination of cerebellar findings (ataxia), cranial nerve deficits (usually affecting the lower cranial nerves), and associated long-tract findings (spasticity of the limbs with extensor plantar reflexes). It is unusual for these patients to present with hydrocephalus. The history is usually insidious, extending over several months.

A diagnosis can generally be made radiographically by confirming enlargement of the brain stem with elevation of the floor of the fourth ventricle. These features were previously well seen on air studies and/or angiograms, but computed tomography (CT) has now become the definitive diagnostic tool. In the presence of these classic findings, the enthusiasm for surgical verification of the lesion is lessened. Occasionally other intraaxial lesions, such as granulomas, and other infectious processes, including abscesses, may present a similar picture when tissue verification is required.

Extraaxial tumors involving the posterior fossa consist mainly of meningiomas and acoustic neuromas involving cranial nerves, such as the fifth. Tumors involving the region of the pineal gland may be extraaxial and straddle both the posterior and middle fossas. Preoperatively these patients are usually not as acutely ill as are those with lesions of the fourth ventricule. They may have some degree of obstructive hydrocephalus, which should be pretreated with steroid administration and occasionally with osmotic diuretic agents.

Indications for surgery of extraaxial posterior fossa lesions consist of progressive specific neurologic abnormalities such as eighth nerve deficits (hearing loss and tinnitus) and seventh nerve and cerebellar deficits associated with acoustic nerve tumors. The proximity of the eighth nerve to the seventh and fifth nerves may result in ipsilateral facial palsy and numbness. Fifth nerve compression is much less common with acoustic nerve tumors. Large acoustic tumors may also cause compression of the ipsilateral cerebellum, with associated incoordination of the limbs on that side. Obstructive hydrocephalus with increased intracranial pressure may be another presenting symptom. Tumors involving the other cranial nerves cause symptoms unique to the nerve origin.

Acoustic nerve tumors are located in the cerebellopontine angle lateral to the cerebellum. The approach generally is with the patient in a sitting position, although a middle ear transmastoid approach is used successfully for very small tumors (3).

The goal of surgery is complete removal of the tumor with preservation if possible of the seventh nerve, although it is often markedly stretched over the tumor capsule and may not be salvageable. Stimulation of filaments of the seventh nerve is often performed, and the anesthesiologist is asked to observe the face for movements. Dissection of the tumor along the brain stem may result in changes in the respiratory pattern if the patient is breathing spontaneously. Although controversy has existed as to the benefits of controlled respiration, as opposed to allowing the patient spontaneous respiration and observing for changes in the vital signs, controlled respiration provides better oxygenation, and decreases intracranial pressure and prevents the gasp reflex of air embolism (4).

Microvascular Decompression

Dandy (5) and subsequently Jannetta (6) have shown that vascular compression of the nerve root entry zones of various cranial nerves may result in cranial nerve dysfunction syndromes. The best known of these is trigeminal neuralgia. Hemifacial spasm also is thought to represent compression of the seventh nerve at its root exit zone. Procedures have been designed to relieve this compression of the nerve root. In the case of the fifth nerve, this involves dissection of the vascular loop, usually a loop of the superior cerebellar artery or the anterior inferior cerebellar artery, although large venous branches have also been implicated. After the artery has been dissected from the nerve, a piece of muscle or other material is placed between the nerve and the artery, preventing further compression. Indications for the operation are dysfunction of the involved cranial nerve. In the case of the fifth nerve, this equates to trigeminal neuralgia unrelieved by analgesics or diphenylhydantoin.

Glossopharyngeal neuralgia has also been implicated in compression of the ninth nerve, and some instances of hypertension may be due to compression of the left tenth nerve (7). The procedure for decompression of the ninth nerve is similar to that for the fifth. The procedure, carried out usually in the sitting position, involves a small craniectomy with microscopic dissection of the appropriate cranial nerve from surrounding vascular compression.

Vascular Lesions

Multiple vascular lesions may occur in the posterior fossa and include arteriovenous malformations, aneurysms, and revascularization procedures involving the blood vessels of the posterior circulation (Chapter 4). Patients are usually operated on in a semi-sitting position, although for certain lesions the lateral decubitus position has been used.

Vein of Galen malformations are rare but difficult problems and are considered in Chapter 11.

Spontaneous cerebellar hemorrhages are similar in nature to those found in the deep nuclear structures of the thalamus and basal ganglia (8). They tend to occur in the dentate nucleus and present as a sudden onset of increased intracranial pressure and alteration of consciousness. CT scan now provides an excellent definitive diagnostic tool. Some alert patients would appear to be able to tolerate hemorrhages in the cerebellum and can be treated conservatively with careful observation. Patients presenting with signs of ventricular outflow obstruction and severe depression of their level of consciousness may require immediate evacuation of the hematoma. These patients may present with hypertension and severe impairment in respiratory ability. Intubation has often been performed in the emergency room and the patients are taken to the operating room in extremis. If their condition is stable, they may be positioned in a semi-sitting position after appropriate monitoring modalities have been instituted. In those patients whose preoperative condition is too poor to allow this, surgery may be performed in a lateral decubitus or prone position. Often the exposure required is minimal, involving a paramedian suboccipital incision and unilateral exposure of the appropriate cerebellar hemisphere. The hematoma can be evacuated through a small incision in the cerebellum, often without resection of the adjoining cerebellar tissues. These patients usually require respiratory support for several days if their initial state of consciousness has been impaired and their respiratory function is compromised.

Infectious Lesions

The preoperative condition of these patients is determined mainly by the prevalence of infection elsewhere in the body. The condition is controlled by antibiotics and the general status of the patient. These lesions may present with increased intracranial pressure and hydrocephalus. If the etiology is known, the patient should be treated with antibiotics prior to surgery. Abscesses of the posterior fossa, particularly those involving the cerebellum, were at one time quite common and were direct extensions of infections involving the mastoid sinuses. Subsequent to the antibiotic era, these lesions have become much less prevalent in the United States. Tuberculous and other parasitic lesions, however, may still be common in other parts of the world.

OPERATIVE APPROACHES

Approaches to the posterior fossa structures are unique and the basic techniques differ considerably from other intracranial neurosurgical procedures. Exposure is limited and the operative field small. Precise patient positioning and microscopic operative techniques are therefore imperative. Intraaxial lesions, that is, those involving the brain stem itself and the cerebellum, are in critical areas affecting primary vital control functions such as respiration and blood pressure, which must be monitored precisely. The need to visualize various structures in the posterior cranial fossa without the retraction of other neural structures has led to several operative approaches to the posterior fossa.

Posterior Suboccipital

The most common approach to the posterior fossa involves a direct approach through the occipital bone (2). This approach, with some modification, allows either a direct posterior approach or a more lateral approach to one or the other side of the cerebellum. It gives direct exposure to the cerebellum, the fourth ventricle, areas of the brain stem, and more laterally to the cerebellopontine angle and the cranial nerves. It also allows exposure to the vertebral artery and to the lower aspects of the basilar artery. Following induction of anesthesia, the patient's head is fixed in a skeletal head holder, the Mayfield design being most popular. The head and shoulders are gradually elevated into a sitting or semi-sitting position with the neck partially flexed and the legs elevated to improve venous return. This position affords decreased venous bleeding in the operative field as well as gravity removal of blood and cerebrospinal fluid. The venous structures are less distended and the operative exposure is improved. The semi-sitting position does, however, introduce additional hazards, which fall mainly to the anesthesiologist to prevent, diagnose, or treat. These hazards are outlined as follows:

I. Cardiovascular changes
   A. Hypotension
   B. Venous Pooling
   C. Cardiac arrhythmias
II. Air embolism
   A. Venous
   B. Arterial
      1. Patent foramen ovale
      2. Pulmonary shunts
III. Airway obstruction
IV. Pneumocephalus
V. Neurologic complications
VI. Macroglossia

In infants and in the aged, the sitting position may not be tolerated, and therefore either a prone position with the head flexed or a lateral decubitus position can be adopted (9,10). In both cases, the head should be elevated to improve venous drainage. The exposure from either of these positions is inferior to that of the sitting position and moreover introduces the distortion of rotation, particularly in the lateral decubitus position and in instances where elevation of the cerebellum is useful to gain exposure to the fourth ventricle.

Transentorial

The subtemporal transtentorial approach to the posterior fossa involves placing the patient in a lateral decubitus position with the head elevated about 15°. A temporal scalp and bone flap is removed to expose the temporal lobe of the brain, which is retracted superiorly and the tentorium exposed and incised. This approach has the advantage of affording easy access to lesions that may be above and below the tentorium, such as certain meningiomas involving the tentorium and clivus. It also gives excellent exposure to the anterior aspect of the brain stem, including the basilar artery, and has been used as an approach to tumors of the cerebellopontine angle, affording good visualization of the fifth, seventh, and eighth cranial nerves.

This approach involves techniques similar to those employed in other supratentorial neurosurgical procedures. The use of spinal drainage and/or hyperosmolar agents, such as furosemide and mannitol, are necessary to ensure adequate retraction of the temporal lobe. In those instances where large neoplasms of the posterior fossa exist, spinal drainage is contraindicated because of the risk of herniation.

Although exposure to the anterosuperior aspects of the posterior fossa is excellent by this approach, it does not provide access to the more caudal structures such as the fourth ventricle and posterior aspects of the cerebellum. It also provides a unilateral rather than a bilateral exposure to the posterior fossa. It has the additional drawback of often requiring resection of venous structures draining the temporal lobe and, particularly if the dominant side is operated, is often followed by a disturbance in speech function. The fourth cranial nerve impinges on the edge of the tentorium and may be damaged in this approach. The third nerve, although less vulnerable and more easily visualized, is also at risk.

Transmastoid

The transmastoid approach to the middle fossa involves an incision through the mastoid antrum. It has been used primarily to drain abscesses of the cerebellum that also involve the mastoid or to remove tumors of the acoustic nerve that extend into the internal acoustic meatus (11,12). This approach does not gain exposure of the posterior fossa primarily but is used to complete the extirpation of lesions in the mastoid and middle-ear region that may have extended into the posterior fossa. The seventh and eighth nerves are at risk of damage in this approach, but there should be no risk to the brain stem. The patient is generally operated in the lateral decubitus position.

Anterior Approaches

The transoral or transclival approach to the posterior fossa has been used occasionally for very select applications involving exposure of the anterior brain stem and basilar arteries (13) or other extradural compression lesions at the level of the first cervical vertebra. It may require preplacement of a tracheostomy tube or a specially designed airway. The approach is through the oropharynx. The risk of postoperative infection if the dura is violated is high. The procedure is performed with the patient in a supine position.

Supracerebellar

The supracerebellar approach to tumors of the pineal region and structures at the junction of the middle and posterior fossas is essentially through a suboccipital craniectomy with the patient positioned semi-sitting (14). An incision is made in the midline over the posterior occipital and suboccipital region and, with the muscles incised and retracted laterally, the suboccipital bone is removed. The exposure is extended with bone removed over the transverse sinus, which allows superior retraction of the tentorium and inferior retraction of the cerebellum. The pineal region is then approached through the space between the cerebellum and tentorium. Bone excision is more extensive than with some other neurosurgical approaches to the posterior fossa, and the risk of air embolism is higher. The bridging veins between the cerebellum and tentorium must be sectioned.

CLINICAL CHARACTERISTICS OF LESIONS IN THE POSTERIOR FOSSA

Mass lesions of the posterior fossa often obstruct the cerebrospinal fluid pathways, and patients may present with signs and symptoms of increased intracranial pressure such as nausea, vomiting, dehydration, hypertension, and bradycardia. Patients with marked signs of elevated intracranial pressure (with hydrocephalus) often benefit from a cerebrospinal fluid diversionary procedure such as a ventriculoperitoneal shunt, which reduces intracranial pressure, stabilizes the vital signs, and affords a smoother intraoperative and postoperative course. Patients with intracerebellar hemorrhages and alterations in their level of consciousness require appropriate modifications of both surgical and anesthetic techniques. They often are in the older age group and may not tolerate the sitting position. Intracerebellar hemorrhages usually require only a limited operative exposure, and the lateral decubitus or prone position is adequate.

Patients with severe trigeminal neuralgia may also be in a hypovolemic state owing to inability to eat and drink. Adequate hydration prior to anesthetic and surgical intervention is essential.

ANESTHETIC CONSIDERATIONS

Meticulous monitoring of cardiovascular, respiratory, and brain function are required for posterior cranial fossa procedures. These stringent requirements arise from the often precarious preoperative condition of these patients, use of the sitting position, and the surgical trauma that may be imposed on brain-stem structures by operating in close proximity to them. Each of these factors imposes stresses on the cardiovascular system and may cause modifications in its function that require prompt responses on the part of the anesthesiologist or neurosurgeon. As in any neurosurgical procedure, there are standard or routine measures of physiologic function that must be monitored. Additionally, special precautions appropriate to posterior fossa neurosurgery must be taken in accordance with the surgical position adopted. These particularly include measures to monitor for the presence of air embolism.

General Monitoring

Routine measurements include those of blood pressure, preferably with an intra-arterial and continuously recording device, as well as electrocardiogram, temperature probe, esophageal stethoscope, measurements of urinary output, arterial blood gases, and end-tidal carbon dioxide tension.

Evoked Potentials

Much thought has been given to the direct monitoring of neuropathways in an attempt to guide the surgeon in operative procedures in and around the brain stem (15) (see Chapter 4). This is particularly relevant to tumors and other masses involving the brain stem itself and to lesions such as acoustic neuromas, which may impinge on the brain stem and require meticulous dissection from it. Procedures involving tumors of the floor of the fourth ventricle such as ependymomas and medulloblastomas may tempt the surgeon to radical resection with potential extirpation of vital structures lying on or in the floor of the fourth ventricle. Somatosensory and brain-stem evoked potentials, which measure the function of neuropathways traversing these areas, have been proposed as methods to guide against excessive zeal in these areas. It was hoped that early and reversible changes might alert the surgeon to critical areas. These techniques certainly have shown some promise, but they are cumbersome and may in fact only serve to alert the surgeon after the structures have been rendered functionally impaired. There are further difficulties in that the evoked potentials measured may not traverse the pathways in or adjacent to the operative field, and may be affected by anesthetic agents and temperature. Such is the case in certain spinal procedures where the evoked potential may measure posterior column function and not ventral or ventrolateral cord function, which is the area affected by surgery (16).

At present this area is under extensive investigation and shows promise for more accurate diagnosis in the future.

Intracranial Pressure Monitoring

Technical measurement of intracranial pressure has been simplified with the advent of solid state recording devices such as the Ladd system, which involves the introduction of a small fiberoptic pressure-sensitive monitor into the epidural space. The dura is left intact, reducing the potential for infection. Intraoperative measurement of intracranial pressure is of only limited application, however, as cerebrospinal fluid is drained during most posterior fossa procedures, and this results in a negative pressure. In most patients with mass lesions, when the initial intracranial pressure is elevated, attempts are made to reduce the pressure before the dura is opened. In these situations, measurement of pressure may be valuable. On a practical basis, however, the intracranial pressure is lowered with ventricular drainage or osmotic agents such as furosemide or mannitol and by hyperventilation. This again results in zero or negative intracranial pressure when the dura is opened, and further monitoring of this pressure is of limited value. Rarely, unexpected rises in intracranial pressure may signal the presence of subdural or intracranial hemorrhage not visible in the direct operative field. It may also warn of airway obstruction, which raises intracranial pressure by increasing cerebral blood flow. Because most of these procedures are performed with skeletal fixation maintaining the head in a rigid position, the possibility of the pin fixation causing epidural hemorrhages must be kept in mind. At present, however, it is not the uniform practice of most active neurosurgical services to record intraoperative intracranial pressure during posterior fossa surgery.

Venous Air Embolism – Monitoring and Pathophysiology

The sitting position used in posterior fossa neurosurgery increases the pressure gradient between the operative field and the right atrium. A sump effect is generated between open venous structures and the right heart, and air may be entrained in the venous system. Because air usually is embolized as a slow infusion rather than a bolus, early detection of small amounts of air in the vascular system allows prompt therapy to be instituted and prevents cardiovascular decompensation.

Much debate has ensued as to the most sensitive monitor of air embolism (17,18). It has been clearly demonstrated, however, that the classic methods of monitoring—such as esophageal or precordial stethoscope, electrocardiogram, arterial blood pressure, or central venous pressure—do not detect air within the vascular system before physiologic deterioration is well established. Precordial monitoring by Doppler ultrasound has previously been reported as the most sensitive method to detect air (19–21), and a recent study quantitatively defined this sensitivity (22) (Fig. 7.1). Venous air embolism was usually detected by the use of a precordial Doppler ultrasound monitor at an infusion rate as low as 0.015 ml/kg/min and consistently at a rate of 0.021 ml/kg/min. The first physiologic change, a gasp that is a reflex response initiated by alveolar stimulation, occurred at 0.36 ml/kg/min (4). End-tidal carbon dioxide tension decreased and central venous pressure began to increase at 0.4 ml/kg/min. Heart rate increased at 0.42 ml/kg/min. Electrocardiographic changes (peaking of the P wave) were observed at 0.6 ml/kg/min and blood pressure began to decrease at 0.69 ml/kg/min. Changes in heart sounds detectable through an esophageal stethoscope were not heard until the air infusion rate reached 1.7 ml/kg/min and cardiopulmonary decompensation was well established. Thus Doppler ultrasound is approximately 40 times more sensitive than the next most commonly advocated monitor, the capnograph. Advantages of the capnograph include a visual tracing and an audible alarm. Although the Doppler monitor may be "too sensitive" in that it detects clinically unimportant amounts of air, the operating team should be aware of even these small amounts since they could lead abruptly to a bolus infusion, especially if the patient is breathing spontaneously and the gasp reflex occurs.

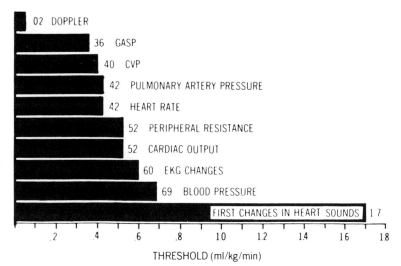

Figure 7.1 Thresholds at which the first changes occur on infusion of increasing volumes of air into the jugular vein. Air embolism is detected by Doppler monitoring before the earliest physiological change takes place (*CVP*, central venous pressure; *EKG*, electrocardiogram). (From Gildenberg PL, et al.: The efficacy of Doppler monitoring for the detection of venous air embolism. J Neurosurg 1981;54:75–78. Reprinted by permission.)

A survey of these changes in various physiologic parameters indicates that at lower rates of infusion, the blood pressure drops moderately and the heart rate increases (4). The central venous pressure shows a progressive increase, whereas the pulmonary artery pressure increases quite early to a plateau. This initial rise in pulmonary artery pressure appears to be due to constriction of the pulmonary vasculature since it occurs with amounts of air too small to cause widespread mechanical obstruction. A later plateau may occur and represent the opening of shunts within the lung, a concept consistent with the changes in arterial blood gases. The decrease in peripheral resistance is initially compensated by an increase in the aortic blood flow to maintain the blood pressure at an only slightly lowered level despite the progressive decrease in peripheral resistance. At succeedingly higher infusion rates, however, the cardiac output reaches a maximum, after which the blood pressure drops significantly.

Thus three different phases of physiologic effects of venous air embolism are seen. The initial changes take place at threshold infusions between 0.4 and 0.6 ml/kg/min. An increase in cardiac output compensates for the decrease in peripheral resistance, and blood pressure is only moderately depressed. Second, between 1.2 and 1.8 ml/kg/min, compensation begins to fail and the blood pressure decreases further. This corresponds to the infusion rate at which the ST-segment changes are first seen on the electrocardiogram. If the air entry is blocked within three minutes, survival is still likely. In the third phase, however, decompensation occurs at an infusion rate greater than 1.8 ml/kg/min, when blood pressure falls precipitously. Profound shock is usually evident after three minutes and, at least in the experimental setting, survival is rare (4).

These observations suggest that the physiologic response to slow infusion of air is initiated via a reflex in the lung. A sympatholytic effect with deteriorating peripheral resistance and increased intrapulmonary vascular resistance, at first compensated for by increased cardiac output, progresses to shock when compensation is exceeded. With slow infusion, the pulmonary-mediated sympatholytic reflexes appear to be the dominant factor. Slow infusion directly into the pulmonary artery demonstrates that cardiovascular collapse can occur even with no air in the heart on the first pass.

Use of the electrocautery in conjunction with Doppler monitoring causes a distressing noise. It can be avoided by use of a detector that incorporates interference sensing and rejection circuits to silence the audio detector during electrocautery (such as the Roche Embosonde air emboli detector manufactured by Roche Medical Electronics, Inc., Cranbury, New Jersey). The monitor then is silenced temporarily during use of the cautery (as is the practice, of course, with the electrocardiographic monitor).

As air in the pulmonary vascular system is absorbed only slowly, ventilation/perfusion abnormalities and pulmonary complications may occur postoperatively. Although it has been suggested that pulmonary edema occurs only following aspiration of massive amounts of air (> 140 ml), other authors have demonstrated perfusion defects and interstitial edema in cases in which only 1 to 1.5 ml of air could be aspirated (23). In this respect, a lung scan with technetium MAA is a more sensitive indicator than chest roentgenograms (24).

Although some workers have suggested that the Swan-Ganz catheter is superior in retrieving air, subsequent studies of a multiple-orifice atrial catheter showed greater access to the venous circulation (24). Nevertheless, should right atrial pressure exceed pulmonary capillary wedge pressure, as may happen in the seated position, the risk exists of paradoxical air embolism through a probe-patent foramen ovale. Monitoring with the Swan-Ganz catheter would afford advance warning of the development of this potentially dangerous situation (25). As increases in pulmonary artery pressure tend to occur prior to changes in arterial blood pressure and cardiac output, the return of pulmonary artery pressure toward normal values following an embolic episode can also be used as a guide to the appropriate time for resumption of surgery (26).

The mass spectrometer may also be a useful if not as yet universally available tool in early detection of venous air embolism. Nitrogen in an air bubble is quickly released into the alveoli, particularly following denitrogenation (FIO_21). From the area under the resultant curve, the volume of air embolized can be calculated. If nitrous oxide is employed, the diffusion of nitrogen would be much slower, that is, nitrous oxide would diffuse from the alveolus across the capillary into the air mass. On the other hand, if a 50:50 air/oxygen mixture is inhaled, diffusion would be from the air bubble in the capillary (80% nitrogen) into the alveolus (40% nitrogen).

Air in both the venous and arterial system may also be detected by use of transesophageal Doppler detection (27). Use of the esophageal Doppler sensor avoids the likelihood of dislodgement from the skin. The efficacy is unaffected by chest shape or form. It can detect air bubbles as small as 0.05 to 0.2 cc, making it as sensitive as the more conventional chest Doppler. An analog record may be obtained to record the pressure and time course of infused air.

An even more elaborate means of detecting air is by transesophageal echocardiography (28). For venous injection of air, the threshold dose detected by bolus was 0.02 ml/kg. When given by infusion, air could be detected by both contrast echocardiogram and Doppler sound change at 0.05 ml/kg/min. The threshold dose for air injected to the left ventricle is as low as 0.001 ml/kg with contrast echocardiography. The device has also been used to detect paradoxical arterial air embolism caused by intracardiac or pulmonary shunts.

Early monitoring devices suppose that air is infused slowly. Rarely, if a major sinus is entered or torn, a bolus of air may be sucked in, causing cardiovascular collapse owing primarily to an air lock in the right side of the heart. The physiologic mechanisms observed differ in that the gasp reflex is not seen, nor is peaking of the P-wave (4) seen. The increase in pulmonary artery pressure that characterizes a slow infusion does not occur. Instead, pulmonary artery pressure decreases, suggesting that an air lock has occurred proximal to the pulmonary artery. Autopsy findings have confirmed that air from a bolus is found in the right side of the heart, but air from a slow infusion is found more consistently in the lungs.

ANESTHETIC MANAGEMENT OF POSTERIOR FOSSA SURGERY

Premedication should be minimal to avoid depression of the respiratory center and the possibility of postural hypotension as the patient is moved into a sitting position. Atropine, preferably given intravenously immediately prior to induction, is useful to prevent bradycardia and maintain an adequate cardiac output.

A standard intubation sequence of thiopental, 2 to 3 mg/kg, lidocaine 1 to 1.5 mg/kg, and succinylcholine, 1 mg/kg, may be used over a five-minute period. Large or too rapidly administered doses can cause hypotension. Anesthesia can then be maintained with 1% to 2% isoflurane in a 50:50 mixture of oxygen and air. Because there is a risk of air embolism early on in the case with insertion of the pin head holder, nitrous oxide, which increases the size of entrained air bubbles, should be avoided. Use of an intravenous technique may prove difficult as excessive doses of narcotics may be required to ensure anesthesia in the absence of nitrous oxide, and recovery may be delayed. The best technique probably combines isoflurane (1%) with incremental doses of fentanyl (50 mg) every 30 to 60 minutes as vital signs dictate.

If the patient is to be operated on in the sitting position, an arterial cannula should be placed prior to position change to enable accurate monitoring of blood pressure. After rapid infusion of 100 ml of fluid to acutely increase the intravascular volume, the upright position is attained slowly, alternately raising the back and head and increasing the height of the legs. Correct position is achieved with flexion of the thighs and elevation of the knees to the level of the heart.

If the patient is to be operated on in a prone position, he should be anesthetized in his bed, all monitors established, and then turned onto the table. Great care must be taken to ensure that all pressure points are adequately padded and his eyes are closed and protected from undue pressure and the risk of retinal thrombosis.

After any position change, lung ventilation must be rechecked as the tip of the endotracheal tube migrates toward the carina and right main-stem bronchus with neck flexion. Conversely, with extension and lateral rotation of the neck, the endotracheal tube moves up and there is a risk of accidental extubation, especially in children who have short tracheas.

Armored types of anode tubes have been advocated as a means of preventing airway obstruction; however, several problems have been associated with their use. If these tubes are resterilized, parts of the rubber often become brittle and weaken, making the balloon either difficult to inflate or unevenly distensible. Moreover, the balloon, which is often of the high-pressure type, may overlap the open distal end and cause obstruction during position change. Finally, passage of an armored tube is technically more difficult, requires a stylet (which is rarely sterile), and may cause damage to the tracheal mucosa from small protruding broken pieces in the wire. For all these reasons, a disposable soft plastic tube with a flexible adaptor is preferable. The Oxford tube, with its molded-in pharyngeal cuff, is also useful.

Controversy has existed over the use of controlled ventilation in operations done in the sitting position. It has been suggested that spontaneous respiration should be maintained, as a change in the pattern of respiration is an important indicator of excessive manipulation of the brain stem. Controlled ventilation, however, allows the anesthesiologist to adjust and monitor the gas flow rate, the tidal volume, the inspiratory pressure, and the end-tidal carbon dioxide tension and $PaCO_2$. With controlled ventilation the gasp reflex of air embolism either does not occur or is greatly attenuated. In a spontaneously ventilating patient, on the other hand, the sudden negative pressure generated by a vigorous gasp will convert a slow rate of embolization into a catastrophic event. Finally, it has been demonstrated that the Doppler ultrasound is a much more sensitive indicator than respiration of deleterious surgical stimulation (19).

At the end of the procedure, care should be taken to ensure that the patient does not buck while still secured by the pin head holder. To prevent undue movement, lidocaine, 1 mg/kg, should be given intravenously during skin closure.

COMPLICATIONS OF POSTERIOR FOSSA SURGERY

Intraoperative complications of posterior fossa surgery are related mainly to airway and anesthetic management and to blood loss during the surgical procedure.

Cardiovascular Problems

The change of position from supine, in which the patient is initially anesthetized, to sitting results in rapid redistribution of fluids and a change in cardiac filling pressure and cerebral perfusion pressure. While postural hypotension occurs in about 30% of patients, the drop in blood pressure is usually short-lasting and of relatively small degree (20 to 30 mm Hg) (19). To maintain the patient as close to normotensive levels as possible the lower extremities should be completely wrapped to prevent venous pooling. Anesthesia should be maintained in as light a plane as possible with minimal hyperventilation. Infusion of fluid immediately prior to slow position change will usually suffice to prevent significant problems. In 2% of patients, use of a vasopressor such as ephedrine sulfate (12.5 mg intravenously) or phenylephrine is necessary. Transient hypertension not requiring therapy has been reported in 10% of patients (19).

Cardiac arrhythmias frequently occur during surgical manipulation around the brain stem. The most frequent abnormalities are bradycardia and ST-wave depression (Figs. 7.2, 7.3); however, multifocal ventricular bigeminy proceeding to ventricular tachycardia and even cardiac arrest may be a later development (Figs. 7.4, 7.5). Although many of these abnormalities may be treated successfully by pharmacologic means (atropine or propranolol), such therapy probably is ill advised, as cardiac arrhythmias represent an extremely valuable warning of deleterious surgical stimulation (Fig. 7.6). To prevent postoperative respiratory catastrophes, the better part of valor is to desist from further dissection. Occasionally, during dissection around the area of the brain stem, as for example prior to isolation and occlusion of a posterior inferior cerebellar artery aneurysm, hypertension may be problematic. The surgeon must be immediately alerted to this change. Sodium nitroprusside may be required to control the blood pressure. All the precautions necessitated by the technique of controlled hypotension must be adopted (Chapter 6).

Continuous monitoring of the electrocardiographic tracing is an essential part of postoperative care. Development of bradycardia and hypertension in the recovery room may herald the onset of brain-stem compression owing to hematoma formation. Immediate neurosurgical consultation and CT scan are indicated. In the absence of mass lesions, hypertension (increase in mean arterial pressure of more than 30%) and tachycardia may be treated with small doses of hydralazine (5 to 10 mg) and propranolol (1 mg), repeated at one-hour intervals.

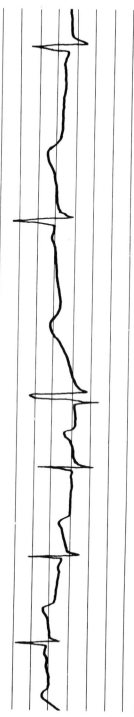

Figure 7.2   The first cardiac arrhythmia caused by brain-stem stimulation is usually sinus bradycardia.

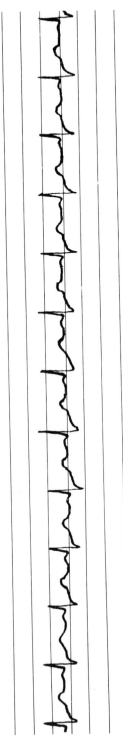
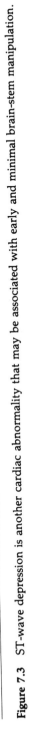

Figure 7.3   ST-wave depression is another cardiac abnormality that may be associated with early and minimal brain-stem manipulation.

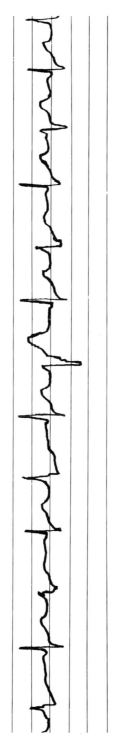
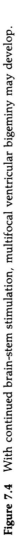

Figure 7.4 With continued brain-stem stimulation, multifocal ventricular bigeminy may develop.

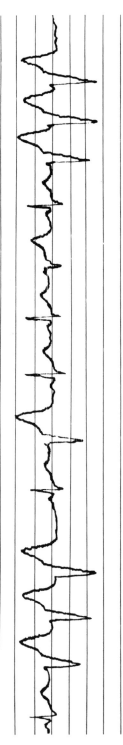

Figure 7.5 The most severe cardiac arrhythmia associated with dissection around the brain stem is ventricular tachycardia, which may proceed to cardiac arrest.

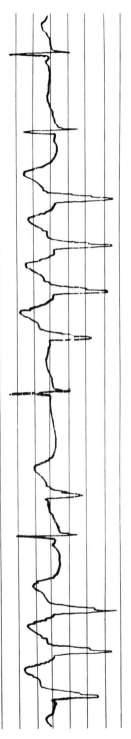

Figure 7.6 Ventricular tachycardia occurring during manipulation of the brain stem may be successfully treated with intravenous propranolol, 1 mg. It should be noted that this maneuver removes a warning sign that the surgeon is working in dangerous proximity to the respiratory center.

Intracranial Hypertension

Increase in intracranial pressure may occur during the operative procedure but is more likely to be present at the start of surgery as a result of the underlying pathology. It is noted most frequently prior to opening the dura and removing the responsible mass lesion. Often posterior fossa pathology creates increased intracranial pressure by obstructing cerebrospinal fluid outflow pathways and producing hydrocephalus. This situation can be alleviated by initially venting the ventricular system or by performing a ventriculoperitoneal shunt at some time prior to the definitive posterior fossa surgical procedure.

Usually measures to reduce intracranial pressure, particularly prior to the opening of the dura, consist of hyperventilation to lower the $PaCO_2$ and decrease the vascular volume of the intracranial contents and the use of hypertonic solutions such as mannitol. Diuretics such as furosemide are also valuable. Pharmacologic therapy is preferable to additional operative manipulation aimed at removal of cerebrospinal fluid, as there is no danger of further damage to the cortex or hemorrhage, which may occur as a catheter is passed. Spinal subarachnoid catheter drainage is contraindicated in posterior fossa lesions as it may cause tonsillar herniation.

Secondary causes of intracranial pressure increases are airway obstruction or intracranial hemorrhage. Respiratory difficulties may occur during positioning if the head is flexed, causing the endotracheal tube to migrate into the right mainstem bronchus (29). Other causes of airway obstruction, particularly if armored endotracheal tubes are used, include collapse of the tube inside the inflated cuff, obstruction caused by folding of the inner wall around the connector, double layering of the cuff preventing deflation, or nitrous oxide infiltration of the tube wall intraoperatively (30). Diagnosis is made by careful attention to inspiratory pressures and to frequent blood gas analyses. Intracranial hemorrhage can occur, particularly in the sitting position, as a result of bleeding from veins that bridge from the cerebral cortex and the cerebellum to venous sinuses. With rapid decompression of the intracranial contents from drainage of cerebrospinal fluid and/or opening of obstructed cerebrospinal pathways, the contents of the brain may remain tethered by venous structures extending between brain cortex and venous sinuses. These veins may tear, resulting in subdural bleeding. Subdural hematomas over the cortex are usually not discernible during the operative procedure, but may be detected on the postoperative CT scan. They may eventually become symptomatic and present as a focal mass lesion over the cerebral cortex or cerebellum.

Hemorrhage can also occur directly from the operative site or from associated feeding arteries or draining veins. It may be particularly pronounced in cases of arteriovenous malformations or aneurysms. Replacement of lost blood and maintenance of systemic blood pressure are essential. If copious bleeding is expected it may be elected to perform part of the procedure under controlled hypotensive techniques. The need for such management should be taken under consideration when the operative position is selected. It has been shown that internal carotid flow is reduced an average of 14% in the anesthetized patient in the sitting position (31). Pressure transducers should be positioned at the level of the base of the brain to reflect cerebral blood pressure more accurately.

Epidural bleeding may occur with introduction of the skeletal fixation pin head holders and usually is not symptomatic under general anesthesia, but is identified in the postoperative period when the patient fails to regain consciousness appropriately or develops hemiparesis or unequal pupils.

Venous Air Embolism

A widely recognized complication of surgery performed in the sitting position is venous air embolism (32). Subatmospheric pressures develop in the cerebral venous system and these channels (dural sinuses or diploic veins), when cut, are held open by bone or by muscle contraction, which allows air to enter the vascular system, usually as a slow infusion rather than as a large bolus. It is only after several minutes that a potentially fatal chain of events is initiated. The earlier the embolism is detected (preferably before physiologic changes occur), the greater the possibility of avoiding serious consequences. The reported incidence of venous air embolism has varied according to the method of detection and type of surgery but is probably about 25% (19). A higher incidence (up to 80–90%) is detected if nitrous oxide is part of the anesthetic technique. Theoretical calculations allow a maximum increase in gas volume of 34 times if venous blood is in equilibrium with nitrous oxide concentrations of 70% because of the differential solubility of the analgesic gas (33).

Therapy of venous air embolism includes flooding the operative field with saline or application of bone wax to prevent further infusion, discontinuation of nitrous oxide, use of positive end expiratory pressure (which temporarily increases central venous pressure and may identify the open venous site), application of bilateral jugular pressure, and aspiration of air through a previously placed right atrial catheter (32–34). These measures usually suffice to stop the infusion of air. It is rarely necessary to put the patient into a head-down position, which carries a severe risk of wound contamination. Placing the patient in a left lateral position offers no protection if significant air embolism has already occurred as air is already distributed to both lungs. The use of the G-suit is not an adequate preventive measure against air embolism, as the initial increase in jugular venous pressure it induces is soon dissipated to the upper extremities and highly distensible splanchnic system (35). If the site of air entry cannot be identified, surgery should be concluded as quickly as possible and the patient returned to the supine position.

Right atrial catheterization has been advocated as a prerequisite for all procedures performed in a sitting position (19). Routine use of an atrial catheter, especially during posterior fossa craniectomies for nerve decompression, has been questioned recently. In 220 patients operated in the sitting position, intracardiac air was detected in 22%, although in no case could it be aspirated through the central venous catheter (36). Morbidity associated with the use of the catheter in this series included four episodes of pneumothorax and one of hemothorax produced by the insertion of catheters by a subclavian route when the preferred peripheral introduction could not be achieved. Transient and recurrent arrhythmias necessitating repositioning of the catheter were observed in 30%, and phlebitis occurred in 10% (Figs. 7.7, 7.8). Furthermore, the authors reported that not infrequently patients described the placement of the catheter as a frightening and painful experience. Other serious complications of central venous catheterization include hydrothorax, pericardial tamponade, vena cava obstruction, knotted or broken catheters, and cardiac arrest (37). In a subsequent study of 34 patients undergoing posterior fossa craniectomy in the sitting position for nerve decompression, the right atrial catheter was omitted (36). Although air was detected by Doppler ultrasound in 35% of cases, with prompt routine therapy no postoperative neurologic deficits occurred. The authors concluded that right atrial catheterization was not justified in this particular surgical circumstance, as it offered no advantage and subjected the patients to unnecessary risks. This attitude probably is reasonable when one considers the many other surgical procedures in which negative-pressure venous channels are opened without apparent incident (tonsillectomy, head and neck surgery, pelvic surgery in the Trendelenburg position). Other surgical situations may dictate different measures, however. If surgery involves arteriovenous malformations or dissection of tumors contiguous with large venous sinuses when a bolus of air may be entrained, use of a right atrial catheter is strongly recommended.

Pneumocephalus

Hyperventilation and use of diuretics decrease brain size, and in a head-up position, air is trapped in the frontal areas as the cerebral hemispheres settle into the lower cranial vault. Diffusion of nitrous oxide into intracranial air pockets increases the size of the gas space because of its high solubility compared to that of nitrogen. As long as the dura is open and the gas is allowed to exit freely, complications are unlikely. But if nitrous oxide administration is continued after meningeal closure, combined with reexpansion of the brain owing to increased

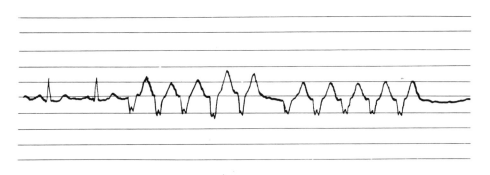

Figure 7.7 Placement of a central venous catheter through an internal jugular vein may cause sudden ventricular tachycardia and even cardiac arrest.

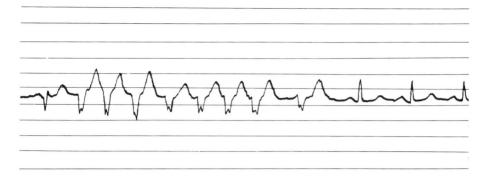

Figure 7.8 Repositioning of the tip of a central venous catheter allows rapid reestablishment of regular sinus rhythm.

$PaCO_2$ and rehydration during the postoperative period, tension pneumocephalus may develop (38,39). Moreover, if the patient is hypothermic on admission to the recovery room, the gas pocket may expand even further as the temperature returns to normal. Characteristically, this syndrome is suspected because of delayed return to consciousness and neurologic deterioration postoperatively. Diagnosis is confirmed by CT scan. Aids to decrease problematic intracranial gas postoperatively include flushing the subdural space with saline to displace as much gas as possible and introduction of ventriculostomy drains, which should be left open during dural closure. Small rubber drains through which fluid is irrigated may be placed at the upper and lower levels of the dural incision until dural flaps are approximated.

Baseline levels for intracranial pressure are reestablished within 10 minutes of discontinuing the use of nitrous oxide (40). Therefore, nitrous oxide should probably be discontinued at least 15 minutes before the dura is closed, although it has been suggested that if anesthesia is maintained with nitrous oxide, an intraoperative pneumocephalus would be more quickly reabsorbed (41). A situation has been described in which, despite discontinuation of nitrous oxide one and one-half hours prior to the dural closure, considerable difficulty with intracranial gas was encountered postoperatively (41). If possible, hyperventilation should be decreased to allow brain expansion as the dura is closed; however, ventilation must be controlled again when bone and muscle are manipulated to prevent the gasp response of air embolism. All attempts (such as warming parenteral and irrigation fluid and surface heating) should be taken to maintain normothermia.

As the effects of pneumocephalus may be obscured by prolonged anesthetic effect, skull radiographs or CT scans can be performed early in the postoperative period. Frequently in these procedures, neurosurgical technique includes a ventriculostomy cannula for drainage, and this route may serve as a convenient means to measure intracranial pressure. As air is absorbed only very slowly from the intracranial compartments, nitrous oxide should probably be avoided if surgical reexploration becomes necessary during the following one or two weeks. Indeed, it probably is advisable to avoid the use of nitrous oxide in all patients operated on in the sitting position. On the one hand, the analgesic capability of the gas decreases the required concentration of the more potent and depressant inhalation agents, and thus is the principal component of a balanced technique. But, on the other hand, the potential to cause or increase tension pneumocephalus and the size of air emboli exists. Reasonably, nitrous oxide probably will be replaced in future years by administration of air.

Respiratory Complications

Respiratory changes in the sitting position include a decrease in ventilation of the upper lobes and increase in ventilation/perfusion abnormalities. While these changes are usually transient and reverse as soon as the patient is returned to the supine position, preexistent lung disease may aggravate the condition and cause postoperative respiratory complications. The importance of intraoperative monitoring of arterial blood gases and appropriate adaptation of inspired gas concentrations and pressures cannot be overemphasized.

Pulmonary edema and frank adult respiratory distress syndrome (ARDS) have been reported after air embolism in young, otherwise healthy individuals (42,43). Lung scans with technetium MAA can detect small perfusion defects, while initial chest roentgenograms usually remain unchanged from films obtained before the air embolism. Although one study suggested that the extent of the perfusion defects were proportional to the volumes of air aspirated (44), in another case, in which ARDS developed, only small amounts of air were returned from a pulmonary catheter (43).

The mechanism of pulmonary edema induced by air embolism is probably one of pulmonary hypertension from mechanical obstruction of the precapillary arterioles and vasoconstriction of precapillary and postcapillary vessels forcing fluid into the alveoli. Moreover, if systemic hypotension occurs, whether caused by air embolism or position change, effective cerebral perfusion pressure may drop below 50 mm Hg and evoke a centrineurogenic reflex and postcapillary vasconstriction. Inhalation of 100% oxygen for a relatively long time may also contribute to local and central neurogenic edema formation (45). For this reason, it is recommended that inspired oxygen be reduced and air (50%) be added. Repeated episodes of pulmonary hypertension, as occurs during multiple episodes of air embolism, may damage pulmonary vascular endothelium. Protein aggregates may form at the gas-liquid interface and increase pulmonary capillary blockage into the postoperative period (43).

The perfusion defects thus caused can be readily confused with pulmonary thromboembolism. Nevertheless, the lesions resolve without the use of heparin therapy, which can be particularly hazardous in the neurosurgical patient.

Therapy combines assisted ventilation with supplemental oxygen and positive airway pressure as necessary diuretics, and antibiotics if a pneumonic infiltrate becomes superimposed.

Neurologic Complications

Midcervical quadriplegia after operations with the patient in the sitting position has been recognized (46). The precise etiology is unclear (47). It has been suggested that acute flexion of the cervical spine with the patient in the sitting position, particularly in a patient with narrowed cervical canal secondary to cervical spondylosis, provides either direct compression of the spinal cord or compression of its vascular supply. Angiographic and autopsy findings in patients who have developed infarctions in the vertebrobasilar artery distribution following neck manipulations have indicated that injury to the intima of the vertebral artery at the atlantoaxial joint forms a nidus for thrombus formation that may propagate or embolize to other vessels in the system and result in brain-stem infarction (48).

A further suggestion is that in the sitting position, intraspinal arterial blood pressure may be lower than normal, and with the additional reduction in cardiac output and stroke volume that may occur during anesthesia in the sitting position, the cerebral and spinal cord blood flow may be impaired (49).

Levy, Dohm, and Hardy (50) recently reported five cases of central cord syndrome occurring several days following decompressive cervical laminectomy, with the patients developing midcervical quadriplegia during operations in the sitting position. They postulated that episodes of hypotension and/or abnormal positioning of the neck may have initiated this phenomenon. Their patients developed typical central cord syndromes characterized by upper limb weakness greater than lower limb weakness with long tract findings in the lower extremities. Weakness was greater distally than proximally. Recovery was slow and incomplete (50). It is of interest that reports of central cord syndromes are usually associated with hyperextension rather than hyperflexion injuries (51).

Careful attention to positioning preoperatively will prevent both damage to peripheral nerves and macroglossia, which is due to protrusion of the tongue through the teeth or against a hard airway. Should these complications occur, therapy is nonspecific and involves reassurance, physical therapy, consultation, and documentation.

Cranial nerve dysfunction may result from direct operative intervention in and around the cranial nerves, particularly in those tumors involving the eighth nerve when the seventh nerve may be functionally or anatomically interrupted. In those patients, the cornea must be protected from abrasion caused by inability of the eyelid to close. Dust and foreign material must be prevented from entering the eye.

Lower cranial nerve dysfunction may cause vocal cord paralysis, swallowing difficulty, and airway obstruction, resulting in respiratory stridor, retained secretions, and risk of aspiration. Prior to extubation, laryngoscopy will confirm the presence of adequate protective laryngeal function. Should the reflexes be diminished, tracheal extubation should be postponed until there is complete return of consciousness, and the patient should be maintained in a lateral and slightly head-up position. Pharyngeal and tracheal edema may develop during prolonged intubation in a flexed position. Symptoms are usually transient, responding to racemic epinephrine and high-humidity inhalation. Rarely, tracheostomy may be required to provide an adequate airway.

Posterior fossa surgery, particularly that involving the brain stem and cerebellum, may result in various combinations of abnormal eye findings, particularly skew deviation, dysconjugate vision, and other extraocular motor dysfunction syndromes. These often resolve postoperatively if the primary offending lesion has been removed without permanent damage to nuclear structures or to the cranial nerves themselves. The most common late neurologic complication of posterior fossa surgery is the development of hydrocephalus. This occurs more commonly if wide and bilateral exposure of the posterior fossa contents is accomplished, such as after removal of tumors in and around the fourth ventricle (ependymomas, medulloblastomas, or cerebellar astrocytomas).

Adhesive arachnoiditis often results, obliterating the cerebrospinal fluid pathways over the posterior fossa. Swelling of the cerebellum may compress the fourth ventricle and lead to transient inability to absorb cerebrospinal fluid produced in the ventricular system, which then egresses through the cerebral aqueduct into the fourth ventricle. Often this is self limiting, and as the edema resolves the pathways may reopen. If not, hydrocephalus may be manifested by headache, nausea and vomiting, lethargy, and relative bradykinesis. Symptoms may be resolved by ventricular drainage, but if the situation persists, a ventriculoperitoneal shunt may be required.

Hydrocephalus is less common after unilateral procedures in the posterior fossa, such as microvascular decompression of the fifth nerve or the removal of acoustic tumors.

Infection

Posterior fossa surgery carries the usual risk of sepsis. Infections in this area that result in wound dehiscence and/or are associated with cerebrospinal fluid leaks may be particularly difficult to control. The presence of persistent cerebrospinal fluid leaks may indicate continued elevation of intracranial pressure and the presence of hydrocephalus. Treatment is ventricular drainage, usually of a permanent kind such as a ventriculoperitoneal shunt. This usually allows secondary closure of the wound, if needed, and eliminates formation of a pseudomeningocele, which occurs in the posterior fossa if intracranial pressure remains elevated.

REFERENCES

1. Raimondi MS: Respiratory hazards in surgery of Arnold-Chiari malformation. J Neurosurg 1962;19:675–678.
2. Kempke LG: Operative neurosurgery. New York, Springer-Verlag, 1970, vol 2, pp 1–80.
3. Rand RW: Microneurosurgery, ed 2. St. Louis, CV Mosby, 1978, chapter 13.
4. Adornato DC, Gildenberg PL, Ferrario CM, et al.: Pathophysiology of intravenous air embolism in dogs. Anesthesiology 1978;49:120–127.
5. Dandy WE: Concerning the cause of trigeminal neuralgia. Am J Surg 1934;24:447–455.
6. Jannetta P: Microsurgical approach to trigeminal nerve in tic douloureux, Progress in neurological surgery, Basel, Karger, 1976, vol 7, pp 180–198.
7. Laha RK, Jannetta PJ: Glossopharyngeal neuralgia. J Neurosurg 1977;47:316–320.
8. Ojemann RG, Mahr JP: Hypertensive brain hemorrhage. Clin Neurosurg 1976; 23:220–224.
9. Matson D: Neurosurgery of infancy and childhood. Springfield, Ill, Charles C Thomas, 1969.
10. Shillito J, Matson D: An atlas of pediatric neurosurgical operations. Philadelphia, WB Saunders, 1982.
11. House WF: Surgical exposure of the internal auditory canal and its contents through the middle cranial fossa. Laryngoscope 1961;71:1363–1385.
12. House WF: Monograph II. Acoustic neuromas. Arch Otolaryngol 1968;88:576–715.
13. Stevenson GC, Stoney RJ, Perkins RK, et al.: A transcervical transclival approach to the ventral surface of the brain stem for removal of a clivus chordoma. J Neurosurg 1966;24:544–551.
14. Stein BM: The infratentorial supracerebellar approach to pineal lesions. J Neurosurg 1971;35:197–202.
15. Greenberg RP, Ducker TB: Evoked potentials in the clinical neurosciences. J Neurosurg 1982;56:1–18.
16. Grundy BL: Intraoperative monitoring of sensory-evoked potentials. Anesthesiology 1983;58:72–87.
17. Breckner VL, Bethune RWM: Recent advances in monitoring pulmonary air embolism. Anesth Analg (Cleve) 1971;50:255–261.
18. Munson ES, Paul WL, Perry JC, et al.: Early detection of venous air embolism using a Swan-Ganz catheter. Anesthesiology 1975;42:223–226.
19. Albin MS, Babinski M, Maroon JC, et al.: Anesthetic management of posterior fossa surgery in the sitting position. Acta Anaesthesiol Scand 1976;20:117–128.
20. Edmonds-Seal J, Prys-Roberts C, Adams AP: Air embolism. A comparison of various methods of detection. Anaesthesia 1971;26:202–208.
21. English JB, Westenskow D, Hodges MR, et al.: Comparison of venous air embolism monitoring methods in supine dogs. Anesthesiology 1978;48:425–429.
22. Gildenberg PL, O'Brien RP, Britt WJ, et al.: The efficacy of Doppler monitoring for the detection of venous air embolism. J Neurosurg 1981;54:75–78.
23. Pattion WJ: End-tidal carbon dioxide levels in the early detection of air embolism. Anesthesia and Intensive Care 1975;3:58–59.
24. Buckland RW, Manner JM: Venous air embolism during surgery. Anaesthesia 1976; 31:633–643.

25. Perkins-Pearson NAK, Marshall WK, Bedford RF: Atrial pressures in the seated position. Anesthesiology 1982;57:493–497.
26. Marshall BM: Air embolism in neurosurgical anesthesia: Its diagnosis and treatment. Can Anaesth Soc J 1965;12:255–261.
27. Martin RW, Colley PS: Evaluation of transesophageal Doppler detection of air embolism in dogs. Anesthesiology 1983;58:117–123.
28. Furuya H, Suzuki T, Okumura F, et al.: Detection of air embolism by transesophageal echocardiography. Anesthesiology 1983;58:124–129.
29. Conrardy PA, Goodman LR, Lainge F, et al.: Alteration of endotracheal tube position. Flexion and extension of the neck. Crit Care Med 1976;4:7–12.
30. Ohn KC, Wu WH: Another complication of armored endotracheal tubes. Anesth Analg (Cleve) 1980;59:215–216.
31. Tindall GT, Craddock A, Greenfield JC: Effects of the sitting position on blood flow in the internal carotid artery of man during general anesthesia. J Neurosurg 1967;26: 383–389.
32. Michenfelder JD: Multiple episodes of air emboli: Report of a case. Anesth Analg (Cleve) 1968;47:355–356.
33. Munson ES: Effect of nitrous oxide on the pulmonary circulation during venous air embolism. Anesth Analg (Cleve) 1971;50:785–793.
34. Stallworth JM, Martin JB, Postlethwait RW: Aspiration of the heart in air embolism. JAMA 1950;143:1250–1251.
35. Cuypers J, Matakas F, Potolicchio SJ: Effects of central venous pressure on brain tissue pressure and brain volume. J Neurosurg 1976;45:89–94.
36. Appelbaum RI, Duncalf D, Phillips PL: Is central venous catheterization necessary for neurosurgical procedures in the sitting position? Abstract American Associations Neurological Surgeons annual meeting NY, 1980, p 142.
37. Schapira M, Stern WZ, Frost E: Complications and pitfalls of subclavian vein cannulation. Conn Med 1977;41:140–143.
38. Grundy GL, Spetzler RF: Subdural pneumocephalus resulting from drainage of cerebrospinal fluid during craniotomy. Anesthesiology 1980;52:269–271.
39. Kitahata L, Katz JD: Tension pneumocephalus after posterior fossa craniotomy, a complication of the sitting position. Anesthesiology 1976;44:448–450.
40. Saidman LJ, Eger EL, II: Changes in cerebrospinal fluid pressure during pneumoencephalography under nitrous oxide anesthesia. Anesthesiology 1965;26:67–72.
41. Friedman GA, Norfleet EA, Bedford RF: Discontinuance of nitrous oxide does not prevent tension pneumocephalus. Anesth Analg (Cleve) 1981;60:57–58.
42. Still JA, Lederman DS, Reim WH: Pulmonary edema following air embolism. Anesthesiology 1974;10:194–196.
43. Perschau RA, Munson ES, Chapin JC: Pulmonary interstitial edema after multiple venous air emboli. Anesthesiology 1983;45:364–368.
44. Carroll RG, Albin MS, Maroon J, et al.: Intraoperative pulmonary air embolism. Follow up of 8 documented cases. Crit Care Med 4:2 97, 1976.47.
45. Moss G: The role of central nervous system in shock: The centroneurogenic etiology of respiratory distress syndrome. Crit Care Med 1974;2:181–185.
46. Hitselburger WE, House WF: A warning regarding the sitting position for acoustic tumor surgery. Arch Otolaryngol 1980;106:69.
47. Wilder BL: Hypothesis: Etiology of midsurgical quadriplegia after operation with the patient in the sitting position. Neurosurgery 1982;6:530–531.

48. Sherman DG, Hart RG, Easton JD: Abrupt change in head position and cerebral infarction. Stroke 1981;12:1,2–6.

49. Michenfelder JD, Gronert GA, Rheder K: Neuroanesthesia. Anesthesiology 1969; 30:65–100.

50. Levy WJ, Dohm DF, Hardy RW: Central cord syndrome as a delayed postoperative complication of decompressive laminectomy. Neurosurgery 1982;11:491–495.

51. Schneider RC, Cherry G, Pantek H: Syndromes of acute central cervical cord injury with special reference to the mechanisms involved in hyperextension injuries of the cervical spine. J Neurosurg 1954;11:546–577.

CHAPTER 8

Hypophysectomy
Carlos U. Arancibia and
Elizabeth A.M. Frost

The term *pituitary* can be traced to the ancient concept of "pituita." Hippocrates (460–370 BC) related the brain to intelligence, dreams and ideas, and postulated that it was a cooling device by means of the secretion of phlegm, or pituita, into the nose (1). The first accurate description of pituitary anatomy is contained in the seventh book of the *Fabrica* by Andreas Vesalius (1514–1564), Professor of Anatomy at Padua. The end of the nineteenth century was witness to significant advances in understanding of the physiology of the gland. Rudolf Magnus (1873–1927), Professor of Pharmacology at Utrecht, demonstrated the antidiuretic action of glandular extracts. Pierre Marie, while working at the Salpêtrière, described acromegaly in 1886. A year later, Minkowski associated the syndrome with the pituitary and considered it to be caused by glandular insufficiency, an interpretation that persisted for 20 years (2). Histologic identification of the cells into chromophobe, basophil, and eosinophil were made depending on their staining properties by Flesch, Dostojewsky, and Schonemann (3). In 1888, Sir Byron Bramwell, a surgeon at the Royal Infirmary in Edinburgh, published a book on brain tumors that contains a description of the effects of pituitary tumors on the hypothalamus (1).

The first recorded surgical approach to the sella turcica through a lateral subtemporal craniotomy is credited to Caton and Paul, who reported a case of acromegaly surgically treated on February 2, 1893 (4). Victor Horsley (5), who had described a frontal approach to the pituitary in 1889, had recommended surgery, but Paul did not consider it feasible to attack the tumor directly and simply removed the right temporal bone without opening the dura to relieve intracranial hypertension. The patient died three months later before definitive removal of the tumor could be undertaken. Over the next few years, Horsley emphasized that surgery was indicated primarily to relieve pressure and avert blindness. He described 10 cases operated by the temporal approach with two deaths (5). Krause described a frontal approach that he used to remove a bullet and later demonstrated on a cadaver at a meeting of the Berlin Medical Association in 1900. Several clinical cases followed (3). The results were generally poor, however, and in his writings in 1908 Cushing paid scant attention to surgical approaches to the pituitary (6).

The emphasis switched to a nasal approach. In 1907, Schloffer described the transnasal approach with splitting of the nose in the midline (7). The technique was enthusiastically adopted and underwent many modifications. Three years later Hirsch introduced the endonasal transseptal approach (8) and published a report of two successful cases in the *Journal of the American Medical Association* (9). Harvey Cushing for many years used a similar method, the sublabial transseptal approach, but later on he preferred the transfrontal craniotomy because "in increasing numbers, both in children and adults, suprasellar tumors giving secondary hypophysial symptoms are being recognized, and if the sella is not enlarged, an approach from above is necessitated" (10).

Several technical advances after the Second World War led to renewed interest in the transsphenoidal route. The leaders of this renewal were Carl Axel Hamberger, an otolaryngologist from Sweden, Jules Hardy, a neurosurgeon from Canada, and G. Guiot of France (11,12).

The first case of pituitary adenoma treated by irradiation was reported in 1909 (13). Although other isolated case reports occurred, the first large series was not described until 1926 (14). This form of therapy received mixed reviews. Indications, timing and duration of treatment were controversial.

PATHOPHYSIOLOGY

Anesthetic considerations in hypophysectomy include management of patients with hypophyseal-hypothalamic dysfunction and intracranial hypertension. The presenting signs and symptoms of any endocrine abnormality may dictate considerable modification of the anesthetic technique. Thus the anesthesiologist should be aware of normal function of this axis and the effects of the major disease processes.

In the normal adult the pituitary gland weighs about 0.6 gm. After repeated pregnancies the weight may double. The gland, which is divided into an anterior part and a posterior lobe, rests in the sella turcica and is bounded superiorly by a lamina of dura mater. Above the diaphragm is the optic chiasma. The diaphragm sella is perforated by the pituitary stalk that connects the gland to the hypothalamus. The stalk contains neurosecretory fibers that go from the supraoptic and paraventricular nuclei of the hypothalamus to the posterior hypophysis and the very complex hypothalamic-hypophyseal system of portal vessels that connect to the anterior hypophysis. Lateral to each side of the gland is the internal carotid artery and the third, fourth, and sixth cranial nerves, contained in the cavernous sinuses.

Hormones secreted from the pituitary are shown in Table 8.1. The anterior hypophysis produces at least seven hormones that structurally can be classified in three groups. Normal blood levels are listed in Table 8.2. The glycoprotein hormones, with molecular weight of about 30,000, comprise the first group. These are thyroid-stimulating hormone (TSH), follicle-stimulating hormone (FSH), and luteinizing hormone (LH). It appears that these hormones have two subunits,

Table 8.1 Hormones of the Pituitary

Site Molecular Weight	Hormone
Anterior pituitary	
30,000	Thyroid-stimulating hormone (TSH)
	Follicle-stimulating hormone (FSH)
	Luteinizing hormone (LH)
20,000	Growth hormone (GH)
	Prolactin (PRL)
4,000	Adrenocorticotrophic hormone (ACTH)
	Melanocyte-stimulating hormone (MSH)
Posterior pituitary	Antidiuretic hormone
	Oxytocin

alpha and beta. The beta subunit determines biologic specificity. The second group, polypeptide hormones with molecular weight around 20,000 include the growth hormone (GH) and prolactin (PRL). Finally, the other two hormones, which are smaller (molecular weight around 4000), are adrenocorticotrophic hormone (ACTH) and melanocyte-stimulating hormone (MSH).

The traditional concept of three types of cells in the anterior hypophysis has been challenged, and it now appears that there are at least five, each of which is specific for one hormone. The release of each hormone is under the influence of releasing or inhibiting factors from the hypothalamus. These substances are secreted into the portal system of the pituitary stalk in response to acetylcholine-, serotonin-, dopamine- or norepinephrine-mediated receptor stimulation.

It is unknown if these hypothalamic factors act on the synthesis of the hormones or only on their release (15). The function of the anterior hypophysis depends on neural, hormonal, and chemical factors. Release of TSH, ACTH, LH,

Table 8.2 Blood Levels of the Pituitary Hormones

Hormone	Level (nl)
Cortisol (morning level)	4.9 µg/dl (7–18 µg/dl)
Tetraiodothyronine (T_4)	6.1 µg/dl (4–11 µg/dl)
Tri-iodothyronine (T_3 uptake)	25.2% (25%–36%)
Follicle-stimulating hormone (FSH)	7.4 mIU/ml (1–15 mIU/ml)
Thyroid-stimulating hormone (TSH)	3.5 µU/ml (10 µU/ml)
Luteinizing hormone (LH)	3.1 mIU/ml (1–15 mIU/ml)
Prolactin (PRL)	12.7 ng/ml (1–20 ng/ml)
Estradiol	16 pg/ml (0.8–2.4 pg/ml)
Growth hormone (GH)	2–5 ng/ml

Note: nl = normal range.

and FSH is governed primarily by the level of hormone in their target glands. The control of GH excretion is complicated and includes chemical, neural, and hypothalamic factors. The level of prolactin is dependent on neural reflexes. An inhibitory hypothalamic factor, tentatively identified as the neurotransmitter dopamine, is associated with PRL. Control of MSH production by the hypophysis has still not been completely clarified. The hormones of the anterior hypophysis profoundly influence normal growth, maturation, reproduction, and metabolism. Furthermore, endorphins have also been isolated from human hypophyseal tissue.

The function of the posterior hypophysis is completely different. Two hormones, the antidiuretic hormone (ADH) and oxytocin, are produced in the hypothalamic nuclei and transported through the axons of the stalk to the posterior hypophysis, where they are stored until their release. That the posterior hypophysis is essentially a reservoir is evident since it can be removed without discernible effects; however, if the neurons in the stalk are damaged high enough to produce degeneration in the hypothalamus, there will be symptoms of glandular dysfunction.

ADH acts on the distal tubule of the kidney, modifying the reabsorption of water in order to maintain normal levels of plasma osmolarity. The osmolar receptors of the hypothalamus are the principal factors in determining the level of the hormone. Also, ADH produces contraction of smooth muscles in arterioles and gastrointestinal tract. Oxytocin stimulates uterine contraction and secretion of milk by contracting the myoepithelial cells of the breast (16).

Tumors of the pituitary may be classified as secretory or nonsecretory. Endocrine abnormalities caused by excessive levels of hormones usually make the diagnosis obvious before undue enlargement of the gland has occurred. Nevertheless, nonfunctioning tumors may extend to cause considerable perisellar tissue invasion and intracranial hypertension before surgery is contemplated. The most common secretory tumors produce ACTH, PRL, and GH.

ACTH Release

Pituitary basophilic cells are stimulated by hypothalamic corticotrophic releasing factor to release ACTH. The system is mediated by serotonin and acetylcholine and inhibited by norepinephrine-sensitive receptors. Normal resting levels of ACTH are 0.1 to 1 mU/ml. ACTH causes adrenal secretion of cortisol at a rate of about 16 mg/day. The diurnal variation of serum cortisol levels is between 25 and 10 μ g/100 ml at 4 to 8 AM and 4 to 8 PM, respectively. Half-life is 60 to 90 minutes. Urinary cortisol levels range from 75 to 378μg/24 hr in males and 36 to 297μg/24 hr in females.

Cushing's disease, which refers to primary pituitary ACTH excess from a discrete basophilic adenoma, is characterized by truncal obesity, supraclavicular and posterior cervical fat pads, abdominal striae, moon facies, hirsutism, coagulopathies, osteoporosis, hyperaldosteronism, hypokalemic alkalosis, high serum glucose levels, and hypertension.

Cushing's syndrome is due to hypothalamic, pituitary, adrenal, or exogenous causes of cortisol excretion such as cortisol excretion from oat cell carcinoma of the lung or adrenal adenomas.

Cushing's disease is confirmed by elevated morning and evening serum cortisol levels with absent diurnal variation, elevated urinary 17-hydroxycorticoid levels (>12 mg/24 hr), increased plasma ACTH levels, and urinary free cortisol levels of > 500 μg/24 hr. Plasma ACTH radioimmunoassary confirms the origin of the cortisol production. Dexamethasone administration may be palliative in cases of pituitary adenomas but not for adrenal adenomas or carcinoma. Radiologic evidence of sella erosion may be seen in only about 20% of cases (17).

Prolactin Secretion

PRL is produced in response to breast stimulation. Diurnal variations are 1 to 25 ng/ml. Dopamine-mediated receptors in the hypothalamus control secretion. The hormone is inhibited by a self-feedback mechanism. PRL may be elevated by anesthesia, surgery, endogenous opiates, estrogens, thyrotropin-releasing hormone, cimetidine administration, reserpine, α-methyldopa and stress. L-Dopa, norepinephrine, and bromocriptine all reduce PRL secretion. Excess secretion causes infertility and galactorrhea.

Although accurate radioimmunoassay methods are available for all hormones, these tests are especially important in allowing detection of PRL-secreting tumors prior to radiologic or anatomic evidence of enlargement of the gland (18). Most laboratories have a normal upper limit of 20 ng/ml. Kleinberg, Noel, and Frantz (19) have shown that with serum levels over 300 ng/ml, all patients had a tumor, and when the level was over 100 ng/ml, 57% had a pituitary tumor. If galactorrhea is also present, levels of > 50 ng/ml are significant. The diagnosis of a PRL-secreting tumor is confirmed if the serum level falls to less than 7 ng/ml in response to L-Dopa administration. The finding of high hyperprolactinemia is indication for further studies, which should include a detailed review of medication, polytomograms of the sella, visual field testing, and endocrinologic testing. Especially important are the thyroid studies, since there are some cases of hyperprolactinemia with enlarged sella caused by primary hypothyroidism (20).

Growth Hormone

GH is released from acidophilic pituitary cells by hypothalamic stimulus and hypoglycemia. Release is inhibited by hyperglycemia.

GH-secreting microadenomas cause the clinical syndrome of acromegaly. Soft-tissue proliferation is followed by bony enlargement and degenerative joint disease. Hepatomegaly, cardiomegaly, and dyspnea may all be apparent. Cardiomyopathy, which histologically comprises interstitial fibrosis and lymphomononuclear infiltrative myocarditis, is not uncommon.

Because of the disproportionate size of the jaw and tongue and other soft tissues, airway management is often difficult. Vocal cord paralysis may be caused by stretching the recurrent laryngeal nerve as the larynx or thyroid enlarges.

GH levels > 10 ng/ml and lack of suppression of GH in response to glucose infusion confirm the diagnosis of acromegaly.

Nonsecretory Pituitary Tumors

Autopsy studies have shown that asymptomatic adenomas are present in 25% of all pituitary glands (21). The most common clinically apparent type of tumor in this group is chromophobe adenoma, which comprises 15% of all primary intracranial neoplasms. Craniopharyngiomas, which account for 4% of all intracranial neoplasms and 30% of pituitary tumors, are also nonsecretory. Although they occur more commonly in young adults, persons of any age may be affected (22). Meningioma and, rarely, aneurysms may also present as sellar or suprasellar masses.

As those tumors usually are larger than secretory ones, presenting factors generally are related to panhypopituitarism with neurologic symptoms such as headache or visual field defects. Destruction of the sella turcica is generally seen on roentgenogram, and compression of the optic chiasma occurs. Pressure beneath the third ventricle by upward extension may give rise to internal hydrocephalus. Endocrine disturbance usually is evidenced by hypopituitarism. Although these tumors may grow to considerable size, signs of generally raised intracranial pressure are absent, probably because the lesions are so slow growing.

Pituitary Apoplexy

Between 5% and 10% of patients with pituitary tumors first present with the life-threatening constellation of symptoms termed *pituitary apoplexy*. Conditions predisposing to this situation are listed in Table 8.3. The syndrome, characterized

Table 8.3 Conditions Predisposing to Pituitary Apoplexy

Normal Pituitary	*Abnormal Pituitary*
Trauma	Radiation therapy
Mechanical ventilation	Drug therapy
Septic shock	Estrogen
Open-heart surgery	Bromocriptine
Increased intracranial pressure	Chlorpromazine
Meningoencephalitis	Anticoagulation
Sphenoid sinusitis	Diabetic ketoacidosis
Subarachnoid hemorrhage	Sepsis
Diabetes mellitus	Trauma
Thrombocytopenia	Hypertension
Pregnancy	

by the sudden onset of severe headache, visual impairment, diplopia, alteration of consciousness, and autonomic dysfunction, is caused by sudden enlargement of the gland or tumor, usually because of hemorrhagic necrosis (23). Mortality is about 45%. Treatment, which should be immediate, includes correction of secondary adrenal insufficiency with corticosteroids and transsphenoidal decompression.

PREOPERATIVE ASSESSMENT

Patients with Endocrine Abnormalities

Preoperative assessment of endocrine function should include estimation of the pituitary adrenal response to stress, which can be made following intravenous injection of insulin. Normally a decrease in blood glucose concentration of at least 50% occurs, and a plasma cortisol level increase to at least $20\mu g/100$ ml occurs. A reduced rise in plasma cortisol in response to insulin-induced hypoglycemia indicates impaired ACTH release and underscores the need for preoperative and intraoperative replacement therapy. Carpal tunnel syndrome is a rare complication of pituitary dysfunction, especially in acromegaly. Thus, an Allen's test may indicate inadequate ulnar arterial blood flow. Under these circumstances, an arterial cannula should be inserted to the posterior tibial or dorsalis pedis arteries.

If endocrine tests indicate the need for replacement therapy, this is best started with cortisone, L-thyroxine, and testosterone some two weeks before surgery. Additional dexamethasone (4 mg every 4 hrs) should be given starting 24 hours prior to operation.

As patients with panhypopituitarism are susceptible to water intoxication and hypoglycemia, the type and amount of intravenous fluid therapy must be carefully charted. Rarely, diabetes insipidus may become apparent with cortisol replacement as this hormone is necessary to allow the kidneys to secrete a water load. A hypersensitivity to central-nervous-system-depressant drugs has also been shown and should be considered prior to ordering preoperative medication. Occasionally, hypercalcemia from hyperparathyroidism may indicate multiple type endocrine hyperfunction.

Patients with Anatomic Abnormalities

The acromegalic patient with a large tongue and epiglottis must be carefully assessed for airway management. Problems with intubation of the trachea are not unusual. If subglottic stenosis and edema develop intraoperatively, early extubation may not be possible.

Patients with Metastatic Disease

These patients usually have neither endocrine nor anatomic abnormalities. Surgery is directed to control or modify some aspects related to their advanced cancer. In these patients anemia, hypovolemia, and pulmonary involvement (metastasis, pleural effusion, etc.) are the rule rather than the exception. They pose a significantly higher risk as well as a series of added problems to the anesthetic management.

Radiation pneumonitis may make it difficult to maintain adequate oxygenation intraoperatively. Pleural effusions due to metastatic disease may be conveniently drained after induction of anesthesia and before the neurosurgical approach is started. Bony metastases of the temporomandibular joint may make opening of the mouth difficult. These patients frequently are in great pain and any movements must be accomplished very slowly. Movement from the bed to the table should be performed carefully to avoid causing pathologic fractures.

Irrespective of the reason for hypophysectomy, the goal of preoperative preparation is to restore physiologic parameters as close to normal as possible with adequate control of adrenal and thyroid function, diabetes mellitus, and diabetes insipidus. Patients must be warned that they will have to breathe orally postoperatively because of nasal packing.

SURGICAL APPROACH

Presently there are three approaches to the hypophysis: stereotactic, transsphenoidal, and frontal craniotomy.

Stereotactic hypophysectomy has not achieved great popularity since its introduction 30 years ago. The intrasellar implant of yttrium-90 is better than previously used radioactive material, but is far from ideal. Proton beam irradiation has also been used to ablate the pituitary, although it is a technique not widely available. The transsphenoidal technique is indicated in cases of disease limited to the sella in those patients in whom the sphenoid sinus is adequately visualized. Hardy has proposed that selected degrees of suprasellar or parasellar extension may be amenable to transsphenoidal surgery (24). The operation involves incisions through the nasal septum and vomer to the sphenoid or through an incision in the upper jaw (Figs. 8.1 and 8.2). There are some clear advantages to this approach when properly indicated, including easy access to lesions without having to transverse normal glandular tissue and avoidance of brain retraction. It would appear that it is a less traumatic procedure for patients who are elderly or debilitated (e.g., patients with metastic cancer of the prostate or breast). Also, the cosmetic results are far superior when compared to a frontal craniotomy.

Some disadvantages must be considered. The leak of cerebrospinal fluid and possibly of meningitis or other intracranial infection are uncommon but potentially very serious problems. The possibility of damage to the carotid artery, visual damage, or injury to the hypothalamus are further considerations. More specifically related to this technical approach are nasal septum damage (abscess, hematoma, perforation), alterations of nasal function, numbness of the upper incisors, and fracture of the hard palate.

The intracranial approach is a frontal craniotomy with retraction and eleva-tion of the frontal lobe. A decision on which approach to use depends on the nature of the lesion and its degree of extension in the suprasellar area.

ANESTHETIC MANAGEMENT

From an anesthetic point of view, management of the frontal craniotomy does not differ from that of other craniotomies. The specific problems posed by the pituitary pathology are common to all surgical approaches. The transsphenoidal approach to the hypophysis is more commonly done through a sublabial transseptal technique as a combined procedure involving otolaryngologists and neurosurgeons. The rhinologist performs the approach to the sella and the closure, including patching of any leak of cerebrospinal fluid. The neurosurgeon performs the intrasellar dissection. The surgeons operate from the right side of the patient, using fluoroscopy and the microscope. This arrangement places the anesthesiologists and all related equipment on the left side of the patient. The pa-tient is usually positioned in a semi-sitting position, and thus all precautions regarding air embolism should be taken.

When the patient is brought to the induction room, he/she is placed on an operating room table with a split mattress. Standard monitoring includes con-tinuous electrocardiogram, blood pressure cuff, nerve stimulator on the left arm,

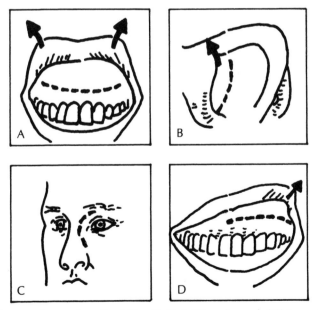

Figure 8.1 Approaches to the sella: (A) sublabial; (B) endonasal; (C) transethmoidal; (D) sublabial, transantral. (Modified from Kenan 1980.)

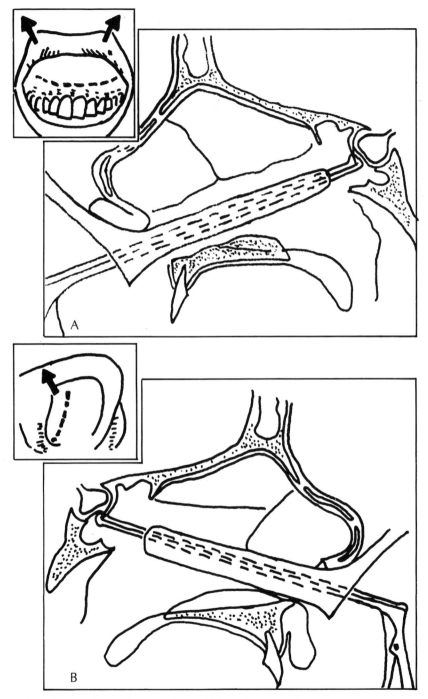

Figure 8.2 Approaches to the sella: (*A*) sublabial, transseptal; (*B*) endonasal, transseptal. (Modified from Kenan 1980.)

and precordial stethoscope. An arterial cannula is inserted percutaneously in the left radial artery or foot. After induction of anesthesia the patient's bladder is catheterized and a rectal temperature probe is inserted for continuous temperature monitoring. A spinal drainage system, which may also be used to measure spinal subarachnoid pressure, is inserted in the lumbar area and maintained closed using sterile technique.

After routine induction, the trachea is sprayed with 4 ml of 1.5% lidocaine. A flexible endotracheal tube is inserted. Except for cases of acromegaly where a difficult intubation is anticipated, we prefer the use of pancuronium bromide as a muscle relaxant for intubation as well as maintenance of muscle relaxation if necessary during the procedure. The endotracheal tube is secured to the left angle of the mouth. An oral airway is not used so normal nasolabial relations are better maintained. Packing of the pharyngeal area prevents aspiration of blood into the stomach or around the endotracheal tube. Maintenance of anesthesia is accomplished with enflurane or isoflurane in oxygen/nitrous oxide. Vasoconstriction may be achieved by the use of epinephrine or cocaine (the latter drug has a longer effect and causes fewer cardiac arrhythmias). The submucosa of the turbinates, septum, and floor of the nose may be injected with a solution of 0.5% lidocaine with epinephrine 1:200,000. After injection the nose is packed with gauze soaked in 0.5% neo-Synephrine (25,26). The average amount employed is 12 ml of solution.

The use of a solution with epinephrine and the packing with neo-Synephrine are sources of potential problems. Limitation of the amount injected usually avoids the problem of drug-related arrhythmias. In this respect, the use of enflurane or isoflurane over halothane is preferable. Another problem is elevation of blood pressure. A moderate increase, in the range of 25 to 30 mm Hg of systolic pressure, not accompanied by alterations of rhythm save for moderate increase in heart rate, is not uncommon after 20 to 30 minutes. The rise is usually controlled by simply increasing the concentration of inhaled anesthetic agent for 10 to 15 minutes. This reaction is different in etiology, management, and outcome from that seen occasionally after intravascular injection of epinephrine-containing solution, in which there is a sudden and severe increase of blood pressure that may reach 220 to 250 mm Hg systolic, associated initially with marked tachycardia and frequent premature ventricular contractions. If not controlled, it is followed by bradycardia that is frequently of nodal origin. This is a most serious occurrence. Rarely, blood pressure can be controlled by using a solution of sodium nitroprusside. Narcotic relaxant techniques would be advantageous in that it would decrease the incidence of arrhythmias, but the procedure lasts an average of slightly more than two hours. Doses of $10 \mu g/kg$ of fentanyl with a 70:30 mixture of nitrous oxide/oxygen would produce a patient who is awake at the end of the operation. At this dosage level of the narcotic there may be significant problems in the control of blood pressure, especially in those cases where it is necessary to discontinue the use of nitrous oxide intraoperatively. It is possible to solve the problem partially by increasing the dose of fentanyl. The minimum dosages required for adequate control of the cardiovascular system is the range of 25 to 30 μg/kg. The use of these amounts of narcotics usually necessitates mechanical ventilation postoperatively.

Reversal of narcotics with antagonist may cause excitement with increases in pulse rate and blood pressure that can be dangerous. The risk of renarcotization is ever present. This last aspect is particularly troublesome in patients after transsphenoidal surgery, since normal breathing is altered by the packing of the nose. After control of initial cardiovascular changes, the maintenance of anesthesia is simple but requires careful attention to every detail. We employ mechanical ventilation, adjusting the PaCO$_2$ to around 32 mm Hg, and monitor with a capnograph and frequent arterial blood gas determinations. On occasion, additional brain relaxation is required. The use of osmotic diuretics in these patients can create significant problems of water and electrolyte balance. Draining of moderate amounts of cerebrospinal fluid through the spinal drainage may be beneficial. When it is necessary to use mannitol, extra care should be exerted in the accurate measurement of urinary output, fluid replacement, blood glucose concentration, and osmolalities. Blood glucose should be measured at hourly intervals with the aim to maintain it at normal or slightly elevated levels by judicious use of replacement solutions supplemented when necessary by small amounts of short-acting insulin.

Blood loss may be deceptive during this procedure because of its constant and insidious nature. Continuous suctioning through the speculum ensures that the field is always dry, and thus estimation of hemorrhage is difficult unless constant watch is made of the suction bottles. A one- to two-unit blood replacement will be required in about 2% of cases.

Frequently toward the end of the dissection 2 to 5 ml of air is injected into the subarachnoid catheter in an attempt to identify the sella turcica on the fluoroscope and confirm complete removal of the tumor. Unless nitrous oxide is discontinued 10 to 15 minutes prior to air injection, intracranial pressure will increase by about 100% because of the fast rate of diffusion of this gas into the air. Although nitrous oxide or oxygen may be injected into the subarachnoid space instead of air, increase in intracranial pressure may still occur if air is sucked in through the open sphenoid. Therefore, nitrous oxide should probably not be used again for the duration of the surgical procedure, and certainly not until the sella has been irrigated and the opening sealed with muscle or cement substances (27).

Urinary output monitoring is most important, as diabetes insipidus may develop intraoperatively, although it is much more likely to occur some 12 hours later. Should urine excretion exceed one liter per hour, initial fluid restriction is recommended. If decreased output is not evidenced within 30 minutes, 5 units of pitressin tannate may be given subcutaneously. Careful electrocardiographic monitoring is essential as coronary vasoconstriction may cause ST- and T-wave changes. Should the surgery be extended, dexamethasone, 4 mg, should be given every four hours, which by itself may cause increased urinary output. As surgery is performed in a slightly head-up position, the potential for air embolism exists. Doppler monitoring should be used. Pathophysiology and therapy of air embolism are covered in Chapter 7.

At the end of surgery the patient should be responsive. The trachea should be decannulated only after careful suctioning of the mouth and pharynx under direct vision. An oral airway may facilitate breathing as the nose is usually packed. Occasionally, soft red rubber nasopharyngeal airways are used with Vaseline gauze packing around them. If these tubes are too long they may irritate the pharyngeal area and be poorly tolerated. Local application of lidocaine may be beneficial.

POSTOPERATIVE CARE

After hypophysectomy, patients should be responsive on arrival in the recovery room. Hormonal supportive therapy must be continued (hydrocortisone, 50 mg q.i.d.; L-thyroxine, 0.1 mg b.d. initially, decreasing by 50% as oral intake recommences).

While patients undergoing craniotomy routinely receive large doses of corticoids for the first five days and then are tapered quickly to their oral maintenance doses, lower doses are used during hypophysectomy. Usually by the third postoperative day the maintenance dose has been achieved. Systemic antibiotics generally are given prophylactically until the nasal packing is removed on the third day.

Potential complications associated with transsphenoidal surgery include intraoperative and postoperative bleeding, cerebrospinal fluid leak, meningitis, blindness, temporary or permanent diplopia, nasal septum perforation, or dehiscence of the suture line of the hard palate.

The most serious complication of pituitary ablation is diabetes insipidus, which is usually self-limiting over 1 to 3 days and occurs in about 10% to 20% of patients (28). Diagnosis is based on findings of polyuria (2 to 15 liters/24 hr), hypernatremia, and decreased urine osmolality (50 to 100 mOsm/kg) and specific gravity (1.001 to 1.005). Urine to serum osmolality ratio is less than one, indicating negative water balance.

Severe cases or undiagnosed situations may lead to muscle irritability, seizures, and coma.

As estimation of the amount of dehydration may be obtained from the formula:

$$\text{Actual body water} = \frac{\text{Decreased serum Na}^+}{\text{Actual serum Na}^+} \times \frac{\text{Normal total body water}}{(60\% \text{ of wt. in kg})}$$

The therapy of diabetes insipidus includes replacement of urine losses with hypotonic solution on an equal volume basis, addition of K^+, subcutaneous injection of pitressin tannate or nasal insufflation of DDAVP (1-desamino-8 arginine vasopressin) (this latter maneuver, which is quickly effective, may be hampered by the presence of postsurgical nasal packing). Preoperative prophylactic therapy with pitressin is not indicated, as diabetes insipidus occurs only in a small minority of patients. In addition, such preoperative management would deny the anesthesiologist the useful intraoperative sign of urinary output. Replacement therapy with sugar-containing solutions should be carefully monitored, as hyperglycemia alone causes diuresis. In addition, in acromegalics and in some patients with Cushing's disease, body water is in excess and postoperative diuresis may resemble diabetes insipidus.

Cerebrospinal fluid leak is another infrequent complication that may occur hours but usually days after surgery. This happens if the packing becomes dislodged. Meningitis may result. Therapy includes antibiotic administration and surgical reexploration.

Respiration must be carefully monitored. Because the nares generally are packed, the patient is dependent on oral breathing. Although pain is usually not severe, the patient requires constant reassurance in the recovery room that all is well. Coughing and deep breathing must be encouraged. A chest film should be carefully checked to ascertain that no blood clots have resulted in small areas of collapse. Hospital discharge is usually possible in five to seven days.

REFERENCES

1. Lawrence C, McHenry LC: Garrison's history of neurology. Springfield, Ill, Charles C Thomas, 1969.
2. Minkowski O. Uber einen Fall von Akromegalie. Berl Klin Wochenschr 1887;24:371–374.
3. Walker AE: A history of neurological surgery. New York, Hafner, 1967, pp 152–157.
4. Caton R, Paul FT: Notes of a case of acromegaly treated by operation. Br Med J 1893;2:1421–1423.
5. Horsley V: On the technique of operations on the central nervous system. Br Med J 1906;2:411–423.
6. Cushing HW: Surgery of the head, in Keen WW (ed): Surgery, its principles and practices. Philadelphia, WB Saunders, vol 3, 1908, pp 17–276.
7. Schloffer H: Erfolgreiche Operation eines Hypophysentumors auf Nasalem Wege. Wein Klin Wochenschr 1907;20:621–624.
8. Hirsch O: Demonstration eines nach einer neuen Methode operierten Hypophysentumors. Verh Dtsch Ges Chir 1910;39:51–56.
9. Hirsch O: Endonasal method of removal of hypophyseal tumors. JAMA 1910;55:772–774.
10. Cushing H: Disorders of the pituitary gland. Retrospective and prophetic. JAMA 1921;76:1721–1726.
11. Kenan PD: The rhinologist and the management of pituitary disease. The Laryngoscope 1979;89 (suppl 14):1–26.
12. Kenan PD: Surgical approaches for pituitary tumors. Clin Obstet Gynecol 1980;23:413–423.
13. Gramegna A: Un cas d'acromégalie traité par radiothérapie. Rev Neurol (Paris) 1909;17:15–17.
14. Heinismann JI, Czerny LI: Die Rontgen Therapie der Hypophysentumoren. Strahlentherapie 1926;24:331–335.
15. Reichlin S: The control of anterior pituitary secretion, in Wyngaarden JB, Smith LH (eds): Cecil textbook of medicine, ed 16. Philadelphia, WB Saunders, 1982, pp 1164–1198.

16. Ryan WG: Endocrine disorders: A pathophysiologic approach. Chicago, Year Book, 1975.

17. Abboud CF, Laws ER: Clinical endocrinological approach to hypothalamic-pituitary disease. J Neurosurg 1979; 51:271–291.

18. Kramer RS: Prolactin-producing pituitary tumors: Surgical therapy. Clin Obstet Gynecol 1980;23:425–440.

19. Kleinberg DL, Noel GL, Frantz AG: Galactorrhea: A study of 235 cases including 48 with pituitary tumors. N Engl J Med 1977;296:589–592.

20. Quigley MM, Haney AF: Evaluation of hyperprolactinemia: Clinical profiles. Clin Obstet Gynecol 1980;23:337–348.

21. Costello RT: Subclinical adenoma of the pituitary gland. Am J Pathol 1936;12:205–215.

22. Love JG, Marshall TM: Craniopharyngiomas. Surg Gynecol Obstet 1950;90:591–601.

23. Rovit RL, Fein JM: Pituitary apoplexy, a review and reappraisal. J Neurosurg 1972;37:280–288.

24. Hardy J: Transsphenoidal hypophysectomy. J Neurosurg 1971;34:582–594.

25. Katz RL, Bigger JT, Jr: Cardiac arrhythmia during anesthesia and operation. Anesthesiology 1970;33:193–213.

26. Reisner LS, Lippman M: Ventricular arrhythmias after epinephrine injection in enflurane and in halothane anesthesia. Anesth Analg (Cleve) 1975;54:468–470.

27. Frost E: Nitrous oxide and intraoperative tension pneumocephalus. Anesthesiology 1983;58:197.

28. Shucart WA, Jackson I: Management of diabetes insipidus in neurosurgical patients. J Neurosurg 1976;44:65–71.

CHAPTER 9

Surgery of the Spine
Robert F. Bedford

Although frequently performed on otherwise healthy patients, spinal surgery may in some instances pose considerable problems for the anesthesiologist. Thus, an understanding of some of the general principles of the most commonly performed procedures is highly desirable.

POSITIONING

An important aspect of spinal operations is that, of necessity, they must be performed in the prone, seated, or lateral decubitus position. Less frequently, anterior cervical spine surgery is done in the supine position. Thus, in addition to the usual considerations given to neuroanesthetic care, patient positioning becomes critically important.

The prone position affords access to the dorsal aspect of the entire spine, but presents several problems. Blood wells up within the surgical field, rendering meticulous dissection near nerve roots more difficult. Malpositioning of the head, neck, and upper extremities may result in neurovascular injury, abrasion of the corneas, central retinal thrombosis, cerebrovascular ischemia from twisting the neck and skin breakdown at pressure points such as the elbows, cheeks, and forehead. Finally, chest wall and abdominal compression in the prone position decreases respiratory compliance and increases pressure in veins about the neuraxis. The last of these problems usually is alleviated by raising the patient's torso either on a frame or cylindrical sandbags placed from the shoulders to the iliac crests (Figs. 9.1, 9.2) so that unrestricted movement of the abdomen and anterior chest is possible. This allows maximal respiratory excursion with minimal airway pressures and minimizes venous compression and subsequent intraoperative venous blood loss.

Because of the problems associated with the prone position, some centers prefer the lateral decubitus or lateral sitting position (1). This position has the advantage of minimizing thoracoabdominal compression, permits free egress of blood and cerebrospinal fluid (CSF) from the incision, and allows maximal flexion of the thoracolumbar spine. Careful positioning is still mandatory, however, primarily because the dependent axillary artery and/or brachial plexus may be

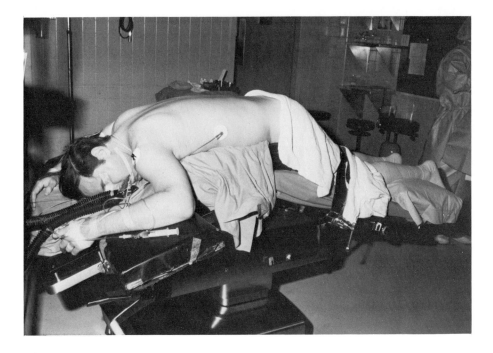

Figure 9.1 Patient placed in prone position for lumbar laminectomy with cylindrical sand-bags supporting the lateral thorax and pelvis so that free respiratory excursion is permitted and intraabdominal pressure is minimized. Note the ace bandages wrapped about the legs to prevent venous stasis. The eyes are taped closed to reduce the risk of corneal abrasion.

compressed unless a soft protective roll is placed under the axilla. Although the lateral decubitus position causes less respiratory and cardiovascular compromise, it probably is used less frequently than the prone position because of surgical considerations. First, the patient cannot be stabilized as readily as in the prone position, and second, the spine cannot be maintained aligned in the midline, thus rendering surgical orientation and tissue dissection more difficult.

Still another alternative to the prone position is the crouch, or "Mohammedan praying," position. Although moderately difficult to achieve in a flaccid, anesthetized patient, this position does allow free movement of the abdomen and minimizes spinal venous pressure. Potential problems related to this position, however, include acute flexion of the hips and knees, which may result in neurovascular compression.

The seated position is often used for cervical spine operations because it allows maximal flexion of the spine and access to compressed nerve roots. It also permits gravity drainage of blood and CSF, allows access to the patient's face and airway, and causes relatively minimal compromise of respiratory excursion (Fig. 9.3). Disadvantages, however, include the risks of venous air embolism (2) and

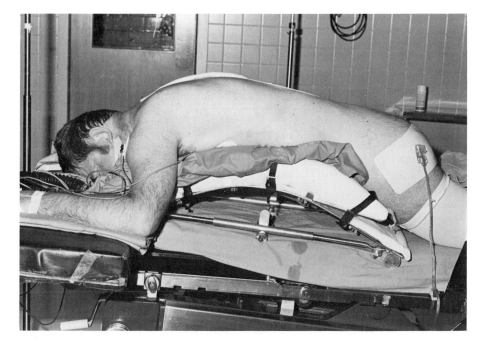

Figure 9.2 Patient supported on a frame for thoracic laminectomy. Extra padding is applied to the arm boards to avoid pressure-point injury.

hemodynamic instability (3). More hazards of positioning such as sciatic nerve stretch if the knees are not slightly flexed, ulnar nerve compression if the elbows are not protected from the edge of the operating table, and brachial plexus compression by the clavicles if the arms are not supported (4) may be encountered.

Patients placed in either the prone or seated position are subject to venous stasis in the lower extremities. Our routine clinical practice is to wrap the legs with ace bandages to promote venous return to the central circulation, whereas some centers prefer to use a G-suit (5). Generally adequate hydration with rapid infusion of balanced salt solution (approximately 10 ml/kg) and slow movement will assure a stable blood pressure during pronation. Some patients, particularly the elderly, may not tolerate pronation without vasopressor support, such as 10 to 15 mg of ephedrine given intravenously.

Occasionally, the supine position is used for thoracic and cervical spinal surgery, usually if fusion of the vertebral bodies is to be performed after removal of an intervertebral disk or tumor mass. The anterior cervical approach confronts the anesthesiologist with the problems of potential tracheal displacement and acute airway obstruction, puncture of the endotracheal tube cuff, or possible carotid artery compression with resultant baroreceptor stimulation from overzealous surgical retraction. The transthoracic approach to the dorsal spine entails all the considerations given to a formal thoracotomy, including documen-

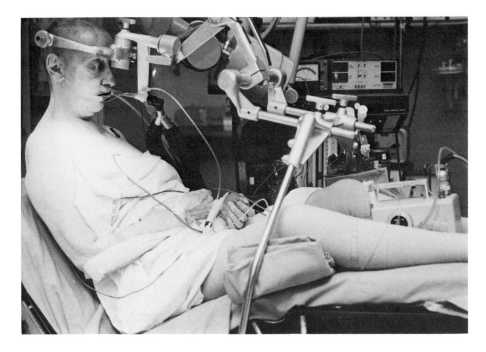

Figure 9.3 The seated position for cervical laminectomy. The neck is anteroflexed, but there is still space between the chin and the chest. The knees are bent and padded to avoid nerve injury, and the arms are supported away from the edge of the table. Note precordial Doppler in place for air embolism detection.

tation of arterial blood gas tensions to ensure adequacy of ventilation and oxygenation, continuous electrocardiographic (ECG) monitoring for arrhythmias caused by irritation of the myocardium by packs and retractors, and consideration of one-lung anesthesia via a double-lumen endobronchial tube in order to facilitate surgical exposure by collapsing the lung on the side of the incision.

REGIONAL ANESTHESIA

Although the vast majority of neurosurgical procedures require general anesthesia, relatively brief lumbar spinal procedures, such as uncomplicated laminectomy and disk excision, can be performed easily using either epidural (6) or single-dose subarachnoid technique (7). These patients have all undergone myelography prior to surgery and are acquainted with lumbar puncture. Since the patient's usual fear of "seeing the operation" is not a problem, those who have had a satisfactory experience with myelography are often surprisingly willing to have regional anesthesia for their laminectomy. Some clinicians feel that regional techniques should not be used for fear that residual neurologic symptoms may be blamed on the anesthetic, but we believe that this is a nonissue. In our practice, we use either 20 ml of epidural anesthetic solution (0.5% bupivacaine, 2% mepivacaine, or 1.5% lidocaine) or 10 mg of subarachnoid tetracaine dissolved in CSF to make an isobaric solution. Negligible spread of anesthetic is required since the operative site coincides with the level of injection. I usually perform subarachnoid blocks with the patient in the lateral decubitus position since low CSF pressure after myelography owing to leakage of CSF through the dural puncture often makes it difficult to obtain CSF when lumbar puncture is performed in the prone position. After injection of tetracaine at a high lumber (L2-3 or L3-4) interspace, the patient is placed in the prone position and the sensory level evaluated by pinprick. The level can be moved cephalad by asking the patient to cough or "clear the throat" if the operative site is not analgesic within a few minutes of injection.

After myelography many patients complain of post-lumbar puncture headaches. Since these occur when the patient is upright, the seated position is rarely useful for performing epidural or spinal anesthesia. On the other hand, no one complains of post-lumbar-puncture headache after a laminectomy, presumably because there is enough postoperative tissue reaction to seal any dural CSF leak that might otherwise have occurred.

Regional anesthesia permits the patient to place his head, neck, and arms in the most comfortable position possible and allows the patient to maintain his protective airway and eye-closure reflexes. The low sensory level required (below T12) ensures cardiovascular stability during placement in the prone position. Despite these advantages, we find regional anesthesia to be unsatisfactory if the patient is excessively anxious and requires more than minimal sedation (i.e., 10 mg of diazepam and 10 mg of morphine). Furthermore, repeat operations render the epidural technique unreliable because scar tissue formation impairs spread of anesthetic solution. For the same reason, myelographic evidence of lumbar spinal stenosis contraindicates subarachnoid block since subarachnoid injection above the level of stenosis usually requires a high lumber approach (above L2) and runs the risk of having the needle impinge on the spinal cord, with resultant damage to the dorsal columns. Finally, repeat spinal operations take more time than initial procedures so that some patients may not be willing to remain awake in the prone position for more than an hour or two.

Recently, percutaneous injection of the proteolytic enzyme chymopapain has been introduced as a method for dissolving extruded intervertebral disks without surgical intervention (8). Although general anesthesia is not mandatory for chemonucleolysis, the procedure is moderately uncomfortable. Moreover, the presence of personnel familiar with cardiorespiratory support is advisable during chymopapain injection because of a reported 10% to 15% incidence of anaphylactoid reactions and a 1% incidence of overt anaphylaxis. For this reason, all appropriate measures for prompt treatment of anaphylaxis, including reliable intravenous access, airway equipment, bronchodilators, and vasopressors, should be on hand (Table 9.1). Pretreatment with antihistamines and corticosteroids probably is to be recommended, particularly in patients with a history of

Table 9.1   Recommendations for Perioperative Care (70-kg patient)

Available drugs and equipment
   Possibly not use anesthetic with negative inotropic properties
   Large-bore IV
   Usual blood pressure monitoring
   Possibly intubate
   Epinephrine drawn up in syringe 10 ml 1:10,000
   Diphenhydramine
   Cimetidine
   Steroid 1 gm
   Resuscitative drugs (dopamine 400 mg/500 ml D_5W)
   Na Bicarbonate
   Oxygen Source

Patient monitoring
   For 15 minutes after injection of contrast material
   For 15 minutes after injection of chymopapain test dose, if given
   For 2½ to 3 hours after injection of chymopapain

SOURCE: From Chemonucleolysis—anaphylaxis: Recognition and treatment. Smith Laboratories, 1983. (Reprinted by permission.)

atopic reactions or known allergy to papaya products (Table 9.2). Most patients receive general endotracheal anesthesia in the lateral position for this procedure because of discomfort as the herniated disk is localized percutaneously under fluoroscopic control using a paravertebral approach. Once outlined with radiopaque contrast material, the disk is injected with chymopapain solution, which is also a moderately uncomfortable experience. With careful monitoring

Table 9.2   Recommendations for Preoperative Considerations

History
   Females have sixfold increased incidence of reaction
   People with other allergic reactions may be prone to reaction
   Exclude people with history of prior anaphylactic or anaphylactoid reactions
   People with congestive heart failure, coronary artery disease or impaired cardiopulmonary
     physiologic reserve may require special monitoring
   People receiving β-adrenergic blockers should be monitored carefully

Pretreatment
   Possibly H_1 and H_2 blockers (cimetidine 300 mg q 6 h po for 24 hours;
     diphenhydramine 50 mg q 6 h po for 24 hours)
   Hydration

SOURCE: From Chemonucleolysis—anaphylaxis: Recognition and treatment. Smith Laboratories, 1983. (Reprinted by permission.)

Table 9.3   Signs of Anaphylaxis

Cardiovascular
   Hypotension
   Tachycardia
   Supraventricular or ventricular dysrhythmia

Respiratory
   Mild coughing and wheezing from bronchospasm
   Râles
   Frank pulmonary edema

Cutaneous
   Piloerection
   Localized or diffuse urticaria

SOURCE: From Chemonucleolysis—anaphylaxis: Recognition and treatment. Smith Laboratories, 1983. (Reprinted by permission.)

for anaphylactoid response (Table 9.3), the general anesthetic is then discontinued and the patient is allowed to recover, with meticulous attention to cardiorespiratory function over the ensuring hour. Should an anaphylactic reaction occur, the treatment protocol outlined in Table 9.4 should be followed. Analgesics are usually required in the postinjection period because of a 30% to 50% incidence of residual back pain and/or muscle spasm.

Delayed allergic reactions such as rash, itching, or urticaria may occur as long as 15 days after injection.

Table 9.4   Anaphylaxis Treatment Protocol

1.	Stop administration of allergen
2.	Maintain airway with 100% oxygen
3.	Discontinue all anesthetic agents
4.	Restore volume (1 to 2 liters IV; 25 ml/kg for hypotension)
5.	Administer ephinephrine (0.05 to 0.10 mg IV bolus with dropping blood pressure; 0.1 to 0.5 mg IV bolus with cardiovascular collapse)
6.	Administer H_1 and H_2 blockers—(diphenhydramine hydrochloride or chlorpheniramine—1 mg/kg; cimetidine—4 mg/kg)
7.	Administer aminophylline (7 to 9 mg/kg)
8.	Administer catecholamines (isoproterenol; use cautiously in hypotension)
9.	Administer steroids (hydrocortisone—1 gm)
10.	Administer norepinephrine/dopamine

SOURCE: From Chemonucleolysis—anaphylaxis: Recognition and treatment. Smith Laboratories, 1983. (Reprinted by permission.)

SPINAL CORD COMPROMISE

Compression of the spinal cord by an extruded intervertebral disk, tumor mass, or displaced vertebral body can create a host of potential problems for the anesthesiologist. Acute transection of the cord is accompanied by denervation of the sympathetic outflow below the level of damage, causing arterial hypotension and impaired thermoregulation if the lesion is in the cervical or high thoracic region. Similarly, lesions above C5 cause respiratory insufficiency, as loss of intercostal nerve function is accompanied by impaired innervation of the phrenic nerve (C2-3-4) (9). Autonomic hyperreflexia, which is considered in greater detail in Chapter 17, occurs in the later stages in most patients who have sustained spinal cord transections below T5.

Succinylcholine is contraindicated in any patient with acquired spinal cord dysfunction of more than a week's duration, since massive release of intramuscular potassium occurs whenever denervated muscle end-plates become depolarized (10). The resultant hyperkalemia has caused severe arrthythmias and even cardiac arrest in patients with both lower and upper motor neuron dysfunction. The etiology of succinylcholine-induced hyperkalemia is thought to involve extension of the functional muscle end-plate over a wide area of the muscle membrane after motor nerve impulses are interrupted and normal acetylcholine-mediated neuromuscular transmission is minimized. When succinylcholine reaches the enlarged area of the muscle end-plate, massive efflux of intracellular potassium occurs as the process of muscle depolarization is initiated (10). There is evidence that a "defasciculating" dose of nondepolarizing muscle relaxant (i.e., gallamine, 20 mg intravenously, or curare, 3 mg intravenously) will prevent succinylcholine-induced hyperkalemia (11), but many practitioners prefer to use only nondepolarizing drugs when muscle relaxation is required. Still another alternative is to avoid muscle relaxants altogether, since intubation can be performed easily under local anesthesia (see below) and ventilation can be readily controlled with just 60% to 70% nitrous oxide in oxygen and supplemental intravenous narcotics.

General anesthesia for a patient with an unstable cervical spine is one of the most challenging problems in anesthesiology. Since endotracheal intubation is required for almost all cervical operations, the problem relates to placing an endotracheal tube in a patient whose cervical spine is held immobile, either in traction or in a neck brace. Usually, removal of the orthopedic device is contraindicated since any excessive flexion or extension may increase spinal cord damage. In this situation it is wise to confer with the neurosurgeon to assess the stability of the patient's neck and to determine from the patient whether slight movement of the neck results in paresthesias or other symptoms. Endotracheal intubation usually can be managed by using liberal amounts of local anesthetic solution (4% lidocaine) sprayed into the nose and throat, often followed by transtracheal instillation of an additional 2 to 4 ml injected with a 23-gauge needle through the cricothyroid membrane. After gradual sedation with opiates and/or tranquilizers (morphine, 0.20 mg/kg, and diazepam, 0.2 mg/kg, or Innovar, 0.05 to 0.1 ml/kg), an endotracheal tube can usually be placed reasonably easily by one of a variety of techniques that do not require movement of the head and neck:

1. "Blind" passage of the tube via the nose or mouth, listening for breath sounds and manipulating the tube until it enters the larynx.
2. Use of a fiberoptic laryngoscope (or "light wand") to visualize the larynx and pass the tube over the laryngoscope into the trachea (Fig. 9.4).
3. Retrograde passage of an epidural or long central venous catheter after puncturing the cricothyroid membrane with a large-bore 16-gauge needle. When the catheter emerges from the nose or mouth, the endotracheal tube is then introduced using the retrograde catheter as a guide until the tube is securely placed in the trachea. Then the catheter can be gently withdrawn.
4. In extreme situations, jet ventilation through the cricothyroid membrane may be done, although this author has no personal experience with this technique.

Once the endotracheal tube is secured, the patient can, if necessary, help to roll himself into the prone position (Fig. 9.5) for posterior cervical fusion, either with the cervical collar still in place or while an assistant maintains continuous cervical traction.

After the patient is properly positioned, he is asked to move his feet to verify that spinal cord function is still intact. The endotracheal tube is then con-

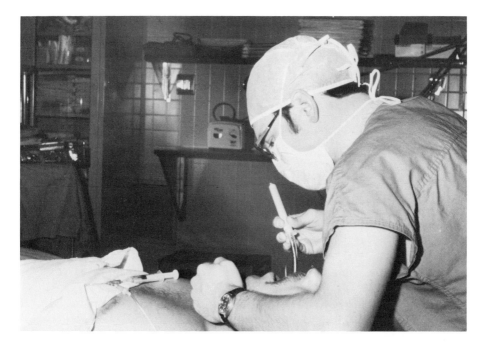

Figure 9.4 "Light wand" is used for orotracheal intubation without laryngoscopy. The anesthesiologist uses his left hand to create a shadow over the patient's neck while the patient opens his mouth wide. Entry of the endotracheal tube into the larynx is indicated by a bright red glow in the midline of the neck.

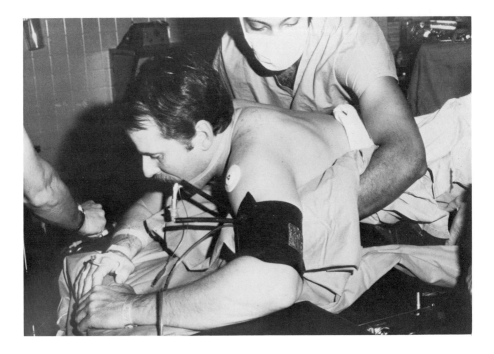

Figure 9.5 Patient moving himself into prone position after intubation. Because he is awake he is still able to protect his eyes, neck, and arms. (Used with permission.)

nected to the anesthetic circuit and general anesthesia is induced, usually with a small dose of Na thiopental (50 to 100 mg). Only then is the patient removed from his protective collar or traction device. If it becomes obvious that spinal cord function has become impaired during this time, additional traction is applied and prompt surgical decompression is undertaken.

Postoperative pain management often can be difficult in patients who have undergone spinal surgery. This is not so much because of excruciating postoperative discomfort (as occurs after cholecystectomy or thoracotomy, for instance), but rather is because many patients are tolerant to analgesics that have been given preoperatively. Many patients with disorders of the spine have been receiving relatively large doses of opiates, tranquilizers, antidepressants, or "muscle relaxants" (i.e., diazepam) preoperatively and may appear to require inordinately high doses of narcotics for postoperative pain relief. My practice is to adminsiter opioid medication postoperatively in divided doses until a satisfactory analgesic state has been achieved, and then to maintain this over the next 24 hours until the immediate pain of the operation begins to diminish and appropriate weaning from medications can begin. Narcotic withdrawal probably should not be attempted preoperatively.

DISK DISEASE

Herniation of an intervertebral nucleus pulposus is the most common degenerative disease of the spinal column requiring operative intervention. The cervical and lumbar spines are the sites most frequently involved.

Cervical disk disease usually presents as neck pain and unilateral arm weakness and/or numbness caused by nerve root compression from the herniated nucleus pulposus. At the cervical level the spinal cord may also be compromised, with attendant symptoms of bladder, bowel, or lower extremity dysfunction. As mentioned earlier, succinylcholine is contraindicated in patients with recent onset of spinal cord symptoms. Some clinicians also feel that the seated position should not be used in patients with myelopathy, since a decrease in arterial perfusion pressure above the level of the heart might result in cord ischemia and increase the degree of spinal cord compromise if the lower limit of cord perfusion autoregulation is exceeded. Occasional instances of acute quadriplegia have been reported after operations performed in the seated position. Usually, these lesions are localized at the C6 level, the watershed area for the anterior spinal artery and the site most likely to suffer from impaired perfusion. Whether overzealous electrocautery in this area or postoperative hematoma plays a role in this phenomenon is not yet entirely clear.

Excessive neck flexion may occur during positioning for cervical laminectomy and cause occlusion of venous outflow from the face and tongue with resultant massive postoperative swelling (12,13). This can be prevented by ensuring that two fingers can be inserted between the chin and suprasternal notch while the neck is being anteroflexed.

Since many patients undergoing cervical discectomy are relatively elderly, we prefer to use a light anesthetic technique in order to maintain a stable blood pressure and optimize perfusion of the cervical cord and brain. Usually, this can be accomplished with 60% to 70% nitrous oxide in oxygen and a sizable dose of pancuronium (0.1 mg/kg). Addition of intravenously administered narcotic (morphine, 0.2 mg/kg, or fentanyl, 3 to 5 μg/kg) usually prevents hypertension and tachycardia, but if this provides inadequate anesthetic depth to prevent excessive cardiovascular stimulation during surgery, then low doses of volatile agents can be added to the inspired gas mixture.

Since venous air embolism is a potential complication of operations performed in the seated position, we routinely use a precordial Doppler monitor and end-tidal carbon dioxide analyzer for detection of air embolism. In addition, it is our usual practice to insert a right atrial catheter for recovery of embolized air from the right heart (14). Whenever the diagnosis of air embolism is suspected, nitrous oxide should be discontinued, as it expands the volume of any air that is entrained into the circulation (15). Fortunately, air embolism occurs less frequently during cervical laminectomy than during posterior fossa operations and usually can be treated promptly by instructing the surgeon to apply bone wax or pack the incision with a soaking-wet sponge as soon as the typical change in Doppler signal is heard. While waiting until signs and symptoms of air embolism have cleared, attempts to recover air bubbles from the right heart should be made by aspirating through the right atrial catheter. Once the embolized air has been exhaled by the lungs and/or recovered from the right heart, circulatory parameters and end-tidal carbon dioxide concentration return to normal, and then additional bone wax can be applied or further cauterization can be carried out until the site of air entry has been occluded. Only rarely, as with repeated episodes of air embolism despite jugular venous compression, is it necessary to lower the head to heart level in an effort to halt entry of air into the circulation.

Lumbar laminectomy for herniated nucleus pulposus is performed in the prone position, and patients may be anesthetized with either regional or general anesthesia. The most usual site of a herniated lumbar disc is at the L4–5 or L5–S1 level. The spinal cord usually ends at L2, so that problems related to cord dysfunction are extremely rare in this condition.

Circulatory instability is not as great a problem in the prone position as it is in the seated position, so that volatile anesthetic agents can be tolerated in higher doses. Nevertheless, as an unconscious patient is rolled into the prone position, there may be a period of "monitoring blackout," during which ECG wires often become disconnected, the blood pressure cannot be measured, and the only vital sign obtainable is a heart beat heard through an esophageal stethoscope. Furthermore, sudden changes in venous capacitance and right heart filling may occur with placement in the prone position, resulting in an acute reduction in blood pressure (16). Because of these hazards, we prefer to induce a state of neuroleptanalgesia and topical upper airway anesthesia as described previously, intubate the patient while still semiconscious, and induce general anesthesia only after the patient has assisted himself into the prone position and stable cardiovascular signs have been achieved. Some patients, of course, are too anxious or uncooperative for this type of approach, and general endotracheal anesthesia must be induced with the patient in the supine position followed by cautious placement in the prone position.

CONGENITAL SPINAL DISORDERS

Meningomyelocele

Meningomyelocele is a congenital failure of normal neural tube development, characterized by absence of skin and bony elements covering the lumbar dural sac. The sac contains neural elements that may or may not be functional. The diagnosis is obvious at birth, and the objective of early surgery in these infants is to close over the exposed dura with cutaneous and areolar tissue before bacterial colonization leads to meningitis (17). Accordingly, these patients usually arrive in the operating suite with an intravenous antibiotic infusion running, which should be continued throughout surgery.

Proper anesthetic management of the patient with meningomyelocele requires an awareness of other important congenital anomalies that may also be present, such as tracheoesophageal fistula, Arnold-Chiari malformation with obstructive hydrocephalus, and patent interatrial septal defect (air bubbles in the intravenous infusion must be avoided) (18).

Because of possible difficulties in maintaining a patent natural airway in anesthetized newborns (receding chin, large head and tongue, floppy epiglottis), awake intubation using a 3.5-mm ID endotracheal tube and a Miller size O laryngoscope blade is preferable. Little resistance is encountered as long as the procedure is performed gently. After the airway has been secured, the infant is placed in the prone position on chest rolls and lightly anesthetized with volatile anesthetic and a nitrous oxide/oxygen mixure sufficient to maintain mean blood pressure above 50 mm Hg. After induction of anesthesia, an arterial blood sample is drawn anaerobically for measurement of gas tensions. Retrolental fibroplasia may develop from excessive oxygenation in infants up to 44 weeks of gestational age, so an arterial oxygen tension (PaO_2) between 60 and 80 mm Hg is desired during surgery. If this cannot be achieved with 70% nitrous oxide in oxygen, then either air or more nitrous oxide is added to the inspired gas mixture until a suitable PaO_2 is achieved (19). Normal arterial carbon dioxide tension ($PaCO_2$) can be maintained by increasing or decreasing the controlled or assisted minute ventilation as appropriate.

As with any other pediatric operation, meticulous attention must be directed toward maintaining the patient's temperature at 37°C. Over and above monitoring rectal or esophageal temperature, appropriate care includes using a warm operating room (24° to 26.5°C), a heating mattress on the operating table, humidified anesthetic gases, and warmed intravenous fluids.

Tethered Cord

"Tethered cord syndrome" is a neurologic symptom complex characterized by progressive sensory or motor changes or pain in the lower extremities, incontinence, and scoliosis. It is most often found in childhood, in conjunction with spina bifida or meningomyelocele. Pathophysiology of the condition derives from a thickened filum terminale, which causes traction on the lower spinal cord and results in dysfunction of the sacral and lower lumbar nerve roots. Surgical correction involves laminectomy and release of the traction forces on the cord (20).

Since these patients are often young children, many of the principles regarding anesthesia for pediatric surgery apply in these cases (such as close attention to fluid and an electrolyte balance, temperature maintenance and assurance of a patent airway with good respiratory exchange). The younger the patient at the time of diagnosis and surgical correction, the better the neurologic outcome will be. Once again, if motor nerve signs are prominent, then succinylcholine should be avoided.

DEGENERATIVE DISEASES OF THE SPINE

Rheumatoid Arthritis

Rheumatoid arthritis is a systemic collagen vascular disorder characterized by chronic inflammation and degeneration of the supportive tissues about articulating joints, including the cervical spine. In advanced cases, the cervical spine may become so unstable that signs and symptoms of spinal cord compromise become evident, necessitating fusion of the cervical vertebrae. As in the case of other disorders that might result in cervical cord compromise, neck motion must be avoided throughout anesthetic induction and patient positioning. A further complicating factor in these patients, however, is that the temporomandibular and intrinsic laryngeal joints may be relatively immobile, resulting in difficult or traumatic endotracheal intubation (21). If blind nasal intubation after sedation and topical anesthetization of the airway is not successful, it is usually necessary to proceed to transtracheal retrograde catheterization with an endotracheal tube passed into the glottis over the catheter via the mouth or nose. Concomitant rheumatoid lung disease may compromise ventilation and/or oxygenation, and arterial blood gas tensions should be determined shortly after anesthetic induction. Many of these patients have been on suppressive doses of corticosteroids preoperatively, and maintenance of steroid coverage is imperative throughout the perioperative period (22).

Cervical fusion may be performed through a posterior approach by wiring the dorsal spines together and placing methylmethacrylate glue between the denuded articular facets. Absorption of this substance may occasionally cause arterial hypotension, but this usually is not as severe a problem during cervical fusion as it is during hip replacement because of the relatively small amount of bone glue and the limited absorptive surface (23). Alternatively, cervical fusion may be performed by an anterior approach, with insertion of a bony plug from the iliac crest between the unstable vertebrae. An unusual complication of this operation is anterior displacement of the bony fragment in the immediate postoperative period, resulting in acute tracheal compression and potentially fatal airway obstruction. Patency of the ipsilateral carotid artery during surgical retraction should be documented by monitoring the superficial temporal artery pulse.

Cord Compression

Acute collapse of a vertebral body may result in sudden spinal cord dysfunction at almost any thoracolumbar level. This usually occurs as a result of either osteoporosis or metastatic tumor, but occasionally may result from a surprisingly minor degree of trauma. Emergency decompression laminectomy for acute cord compression is performed primarily to prevent further cord damage. After only a few minutes of compression-induced symptoms, the possibility of complete return of function becomes remote. Anesthetic induction is best performed using a rapid-sequence intubation (succinylcholine is not contraindicated shortly after cord injury) in order to decrease the risk of regurgitation of gastric contents and pulmonary aspiration. Meticulous hemodynamic monitoring (direct arterial and central venous or pulmonary artery pressure) is necessary with high thoracic or cervical lesions, in which spinal shock may ensue, but low thoracic or lumbar lesions usually do not present this problem (9).

Frequently, decompression laminectomy is combined with vertebral fusion, bone grafts, and Harrington rod insertion to stabilize the spine. The primary problem associated with these stabilizing procedures is that there is brisk bleeding from the denuded bony surfaces of the spine and from the bone graft donor site in the iliac crest. In addition, there may be considerable hemorrhage at the laminectomy site if the vertebral collapse is caused by a vascular metastatic tumor. Accordingly, these operations should be undertaken only after a large-bore cannula has been inserted intravenously and with ample blood available for transfusion. In elective spinal fusion cases, controlled hypotension can be instituted to prevent excessive bone bleeding, but since hypotension may further reduce cord perfusion if a compressing lesion is causing cord ischemia, we feel that the risks of hypotension outweigh the possible advantages of reducing blood loss in these cases.

MASS LESIONS

Arteriovenous Malformation

Arteriovenous malformations (AMV) are congenital vascular lesions found throughout the neuraxis. Within the spinal cord these lesions may present as a mass lesion producing neurologic deficits below the AVM, or they may bleed and produce symptoms typical of intracerebral subarachnoid hemorrhage. The diagnosis is made by selective arteriography, which reveals a tortuous mass consisting primarily of dilated veins and a few feeding arteries. The surgeon's goal is to occlude the feeding vessels to the AVM while maintaining normal perfusion to the spinal cord substance. Once the arterial supply to the AVM has been secured, the veins are no longer under distending pressure, thus reducing both the risk of rebleeding and the bulk of the AVM (23). Excision of these lesions is rarely feasible because of the manner in which the vessels intertwine with normal neural structures. It is, however, advisable to have 4 to 6 units of blood available for transfusion. As this surgery is frequently performed using a microscope, attempts should be made to minimize movement of the spinal contents caused by transmitted thoracic pressure. Such measures include reducing tidal volume and increasing respiratory rate as necessary to maintain adequate gas exchange.

Additional anesthetic considerations for AVM operations include avoidance of succinylcholine in patients with spinal cord symptoms and control of blood pressure to prevent hemorrhage. Controlled hypotensive technique becomes advantageous in this setting because bleeding is minimized during the tedious dissection. Although sodium nitroprusside (SNP) probably is the most frequently used agent for controlled hypotension, it is potentially toxic, since each molecule of nitroprusside is metabolized to five cyanide molecules. Prolonged infusion of SNP produces metabolic acidosis as cyanide binds to cytochrome oxidase and inhibits oxygen uptake in tissues (24). Since AVM surgery is often prolonged and tedious, we prefer to produce hypotension by less toxic means, such as intermittent injections of hydralazine (0.1 mg/kg intravenously) (25) and/or high inspired concentrations of volatile anesthetic agents (26).

Tumors

Tumors of the spinal canal may be either extradural or intradural. Extradural tumors usually are malignant lymphomas or metastatic lesions that present as acute paraplegia and are operated upon on an urgent basis in order to minimize cord damage. Since these often are highly vascular lesions, appropriate precautions should be taken to avoid excessive blood loss (induced hypotension, early blood replacement). Furthermore, attention must be directed toward the possibility of the patient's having a full stomach at the time of anesthetic induction and steps should be taken to avoid vomiting and aspiration. In contrast to the malignant lesions, benign extradural tumors usually present with gradual onset of symptoms suggestive of disk disease and are eminently amenable to surgical resection. Good surgical results usually are obtained after excision of intradural fibromas, angiomas, chondromas, and lipomas.

Intradural tumors of the spine may be extramedullary, such as meningiomas and neurofibromas. These usually are found in the dorsal spine and are easily removed, since the confines of the spinal canal cause symptoms early when the lesions are small. Occasionally, cervical lesions can extend cephalad through the foramen magnum and present with brain-stem compromise and impairment of respiration and swallowing. Intraoperatively, cardiac arrhythmias may occur in response to surgical stimulation and traction on the brain stem, and must be treated appropriately. Atropine, 0.4 to 1.0 mg IV, is given for bradycardia, whereas lidocaine, 1 to 1.5 mg/kg IV, may be required for ventricular premature beats and a combined α, β adrenergic agent such as ephedrine, 10 to 25 mg IV, may be needed for bradyarrhythmias complicated by arterial hypotension. Postoperatively meticulous attention must be paid to ventilatory and airway care during recovery from the localized trauma of tumor excision. Impaired function of the ninth, tenth, and twelfth cranial nerves may allow aspiration pneumonitis to develop because of inability to swallow or cough. Brain-stem compromise may inhibit respiratory drive until postoperative edema has decreased. For these reasons patients usually remain intubated postoperatively until they are awake and demonstrate the ability to ventilate normally and protect their airway with a vigorous cough and normal swallowing function.

Intramedullary tumors of the spine usually are operated upon for tissue diagnosis only, since gliomas and ependymomas usually are diffusely invasive and excision would result in severe cord damage. After a formal laminectomy has been performed, needle-biopsy is performed and further treatment is directed toward radiation therapy. In patients unresponsive to radiation, however, surgical resection of the lesion may be beneficial (27).

Syringomyelia

Syringomyelia is a condition characterized by the development of a fluid-filled glial-lined cavity (syrinx) within the spinal cord substance, usually at the cervical level. The etiology of this condition is uncertain; ischemia, inflammation, and trauma have all been implicated (28). In addition, idiopathic syringomyelia may occur, usually associated with Arnold-Chiari malformation. A common feature of this condition is communication of the syrinx cavity with the fourth ventricle without involvement of the central spinal canal (29). Syringomyelia usually presents as weakness and paresthesia with hyporeflexia of the arms and hyper-reflexia of the legs. Widening of the cord is seen on myelogram. Surgical correction of this condition typically involves a decompression laminectomy at the site of the lesion and, if this is not successful, posterior fossa exploration with plugging of the opening in the fourth ventricle with fat and muscle. Additional procedures such as CSF shunts may be performed in an attempt to prevent further expansion of the syrinx. Anesthetic considerations include the problems of prone or seated positioning, potential increases in intracranial pressure if Arnold-Chiari malformation coexists, and possible hyperkalemia from the use of succinylcholine. Finally, any surgery in the high cervical areas, if it involves dorsal or lateral columns, may result in impairment of normal involuntary respiration (Ondine's syndrome). The patient will be able to take deep breaths on request but will have minimal respiratory drive while asleep. Fortunately, this condition usually is self-limited, and respiratory function returns to normal as postoperative edema subsides.

REFERENCES

1. Garcia-Bengochea F, Munson EJ, Freeman JV: The lateral sitting position for neurosurgery. Anesth Analg (Cleve) 1976;55:326–330.
2. Michenfelder JD, Martin JT, Altenberg BM, et al.: Evaluation of an ultrasonic device (Doppler) for the diagnosis of air embolism. Anesthesiology 1972;36:164–167.
3. Marshall WK, Bedford RF, Miller ED: Hemodynamics in the seated position. Anesth Analg (Cleve) 1982;61:201.
4. Keykhad MM, Rosenberg H: Bilateral footdrop after craniotomy in the sitting position. Anesthesiology 1979;51:163–164.
5. Martin JT: Neuroanesthetic adjuncts for surgery in the sitting position. II: The antigravity suit. Anesth Analg (Cleve) 1970;49:588–593.
6. Tice WP: The use of epidural anesthesia for excision of the lumbar disc. J Neurosurg 1957;14:1–5.
7. Rosenberg MK, Berner G: Spinal anesthesia in lumbar disc surgery: Review of 200 cases. Anesth Analg (Cleve) 1965;44:419–423.
8. Javid MJ, Nordby EJ, Ford LT, et al.: Safety and efficacy of chymopa pain (Chymodiactin) in herniated nucleus pulposus with sciatica. JAMA 1983;249:2489–2492.
9. Quimby CW, Williams RN, Greifenstein FE: Anesthetic problems of the acute quadriplegic patient. Anesth Analg (Cleve) 1973;52:333–340.
10. Gronert GA, Theye RA: Pathophysiology of hyperkalemia induced by succinylcholine. Anesthesiology 1975;43:89–99.
11. Konchigeri HN, Tay CH: Influence of pancuronium in potassium efflux produced by succinylcholine. Anesth Analg (Cleve) 1976;55:474–477.
12. Ellis SC: Massive swelling of the head and neck. Anesthesiology 1975;42:102–103.

13. McAllister RG: Macroglassia—apositional complication. Anesthesiology 1974;40: 199–200.
14. Tinker JH, Gronert GA, Messick JM, et al.: Detection of air embolism, a test for positioning of right atrial catheter and Doppler probe. Anesthesiology 1975;43:104–106.
15. Munson ES: Effect of nitrous oxide on the pulmonary circulation during venous air embolism. Anesth Analg (Cleve) 1971;50:785–793.
16. Smith RH, Gramling ZW, Volpitto PP: Problems related to the prone position for surgical operations. Anesthesiology 1961;22:189–195.
17. Sharrard WJW: Meningomyelocoele: Prognosis of immediate operative closure of the sac. Proc R Soc Med 1963;56:510–513.
18. Whitby JD: Spinal dysraphism and the anaesthetist. Anaesthesia 1961;16:432–438.
19. Betts EK, Downs JJ, Schaffer DB, et al.: Retrolental fibroplasia and oxygen administration during general anesthesia. Anesthesiology 1977;47:518–520.
20. Yamada S, Zinke DE, Sanders D: Pathophysiology of "tethered cord syndrome." J Neurosurg 1981;54:494–503.
21. Funk D, Raymond F: Rheumatoid arthritis of the cricoarytenoid joints: An airway hazard. Anesth Analg (Cleve) 1975;54:742–745.
22. Jenkins LC, McGraw RW: Anaesthetic management of the patient with rheumatic arthritis. Can Anaesth Soc J 1969;16:407–415.
23. Ommaya AK, DiChiro G, Doppman J: Ligation of arterial supply in the treatment of spinal cord arteriovenous malformations. J Neurosurg 1969;30:679–692.
24. Michenfelder JD: Cyanide release from sodium nitroprusside in the dog. Anesthesiology 1977;46:196–201.
25. James DJ, Bedford RF: Hydralazine for controlled intraoperative hypotension. Anesth Analg (Cleve) 1982;61:192–193.
26. Bedford RF: Sodium nitroprusside: Hemodynamic dose-response during enflurane and morphine anesthesia. Anesth Analg (Cleve) 1979;58:174–178.
27. Epstein F, Epstein N: Surgical management of holocord intramedullary spinal cord astrocytomas in children. J Neurosurg 1981;54:829–832.
28. Oakley JC, Ojemann GA, Alvord EC, Jr: Posttraumatic syringomyelia. J Neurosurg 1981;55:276–281.
29. Garcia-Uria J, Leunda G, Carriollo R, et al.: Syringomyelia: Long-term results after posterior fossa decompression. J Neurosurg 1981;54:380–383.

CHAPTER 10

Peripheral Nerve Surgery
Somasundaram Thiagarajah

Surgery on the peripheral nerves may be performed for transposition, release of compression, excision of a nerve tumor, reconstruction of nerves damaged during trauma or by tumor, or for differential sectioning to relieve neuralgia pain or spasm of muscles. A brief review of the anatomy of the peripheral nerves and discussion of the nature of nerve injuries and their complications are presented. The reader is referred to several excellent publications for additional information (1–6).

The nerve cell, including the axon and dendrites, constitutes the neuron (Fig. 10.1A). Each axon is surrounded by Schwann cells (Fig. 10.13). In the medullated nerves the Schwann cells surround the axon, wrapping it in a lipid-protein myelin sheath. In nonmedullated nerves, Schwann cells enclose the axon without forming a myelin sheath. Surrounding the Schwann sheath of each axon is a collagen layer, the endoneurium, which forms a bilaminar limiting membrane (Fig. 10.1B). Collections of axons, each surrounded by endoneurium, are bound together into fascicles enclosed by a loose fibrous tissue, the perineurium, which is enclosed in turn by a loose areolar tissue, the epineurium (Fig. 10.2). The fascicles consist of motor and sensory nerves and connective tissue. The quantity of axonal tissue in each fascicle is variable but is less than 50% (Fig. 10.2).

Nerve injuries may be classified into three types. *Neuropraxia* is the term applied when the nerve injury is a physiologic block. It usually follows minor injury and is transient, with complete recovery occurring in six weeks. A nerve injury is referred to as *axonotmesis* when it results from compression or traction. The axis cylinder is damaged but continuity of the sheath is not disrupted, and regeneration occurs over several weeks or months. *Neurotmesis* describes the situation when the nerve is completely or partially divided. This is usually associated with an incision or laceration, fracture, or blast injury. Surgical intervention is indicated only in this last type of injury.

221

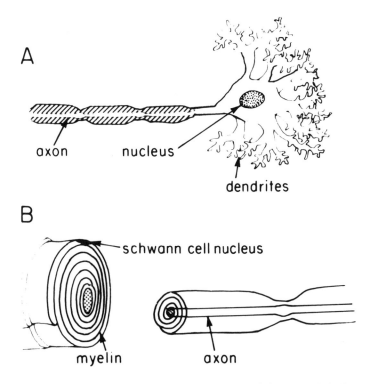

Figure 10.1 (*A*) The nerve cell with its axon and dendrites. (*B*) The Schwann cell spins the myelin (medullary) sheath around the axon. The myelin sheath is interrupted at intervals known as *nodes of Ranvier.*

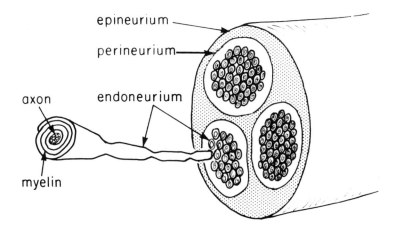

Figure 10.2 Section through a nerve displaying the structural arrangements.

Sunderland(1) has recently classified the nerve injuries based on structural change into five groups:

Sunderland's Classification	*Corresponds to:*
1. Conduction block	Neuropraxia
2. Axis cylinder damaged without breach of endoneurium	Axonotmesis
3. Endoneurium damaged	
4. Perineurium damaged	Neurotmesis
5. Epineurium damaged	

When a nerve is severely contused or the damage causes discontinuity, degeneration of the axon and myelin sheath occurs distal to the site of damage. Moreover, degenerative changes take place in a small segment of the nerve proximal to the site of injury. The process of degeneration, fragmentation, and phagocytosis of nerve tissue is termed *Wallerian degeneration*. This process takes three weeks and leaves behind only the empty connective tissue framework of the peripheral nerve. The neuron, situated in the anterior horn cell of the spinal cord, which is connected to the damaged axon, also undergoes a reaction. If this neuron survives, then the axon reestablishes continuity by growing from it into the intact framework, over approximately three weeks, at the rate of 2 mm per day. If the connective tissue framework is disrupted or scarred, reestablishment of structural and functional activity is impaired or prevented.

Differential diagnosis of the type of nerve injury is made from history, examination, and electromyographic studies (7). In denervated muscles, fibrillatory action potentials are seen in two to three weeks, and with clinical correlations a structurally damaged nerve can be differentiated from one that has sustained axonotmesis.

SURGERY FOR NERVE TRAUMA

When nerve continuity is disrupted, surgical intervention is necessary. Although controversy exists as to the appropriate time for neurorrhaphy (2,3), the consensus is that if the nerve injury is clearly demarcated and is due to a sharp object, and if the patient presents within three to four hours of trauma, the nerve can be successfully repaired without delay. Early surgery avoids the problem of bridging the gap caused by retraction and scarring of the severed nerve ends that occur with time. It also shortens the disability period.

If, at the time of injury, the extent of nerve damage cannot be delineated, and if the wound is grossly contaminated, a sling stitch is placed to prevent retraction of the nerve and neurorrhaphy is delayed for one month. By that time, the amount of nerve damage will be clearly demarcated and the perineurium and epineurium will be thicker and can withstand suturing better. Also, the transected nerves will have undergone Wallerian degeneration and be regenerating, which is an optimal time to reestablish growth along the framework.

The first step in the delayed nerve suturing procedure is to locate the nerve and reduce the gap between the two segments that has resulted from scarring and retraction. In certain cases the nerve will have to be stripped back to its point of origin from the main trunk. For the ulnar nerve, the gap can be closed by anterior transposition. Use of an autograft or frozen irradiated graft is another means of reducing the gap. Sensory nerves of similar caliber (i.e., lateral femoral cutaneous and saphenous nerve) are taken as autografts. Once the resection is completed and the method of filling the gap between the two nerve ends is decided, the proximal and distal nerve segments are dissected free of scar tissue, exposing the fascicular pattern. The two ends are then meticulously approximated and sutured using microscopic techniques (3).

ANESTHETIC CONSIDERATIONS

Preoperative Evaluation

Primary Repair

In the preoperative evaluation of patients undergoing emergency surgery for repair of a damaged nerve, adverse effects of trauma on other vital organs should be excluded. Head injury, pneumothorax, hemothorax, fracture of cervical vertebrae, cardiac contusion, hemopericardium or major bleeding—either intra-abdominal, thoracic, or associated with bone fractures—should be diagnosed and treated. Sometimes these injuries may not be obvious initially and may progress intraoperatively, causing diagnostic problems and even catastrophe (Table 10.1). In particular, any coagulopathy associated with head injury should be identified and treated as absolute hemostasis is essential to good outcome of nerve repair (Chapter 15).

Table 10.1 Possible Consequences of Injuries Associated with Major Trauma

Injury	Effect	Result
Head trauma	Increased intra-cranial pressure	Cerebral hypoxia
Fractured cervical vertebrae	Cord compression	Quadriplegia
Pneumothorax	Tension pneumothorax	Cardiac arrest
Hemopericardium	Cardiac tamponade	Cardiac arrest
Occult major bleed	Cardiovascular collapse	

These patients may have eaten recently and are liable to aspirate in the perioperative period. The current trend is to use cimetidine preoperatively to increase the gastric pH above 2.5 in individuals at risk for aspiration or in those who have decreased gastric pH (8). But the literature on the use of cimetidine in emergency situations for such patients is scant, and the oral dose may be ineffective. Cimetidine, 300 mg, given intramuscularly or as a slow intravenous infusion over 15 minutes (Fig. 10.3) has been advocated (9). Intravenous cimetidine, if given rapidly, will induce arrhythmias, hypotension (9), or even cardiac arrest (10). Therefore, the intramuscular route, which is equally effective (Fig. 10.4), is preferred. The risk of aspiration can be further minimized by continuing to give cimetidine every six hours and by decreasing gastric volume by suctioning with a stomach tube. Vigilance and a safe anesthetic technique are nevertheless mandatory in preventing aspiration during the perioperative period when the upper airway reflexes are obtunded.

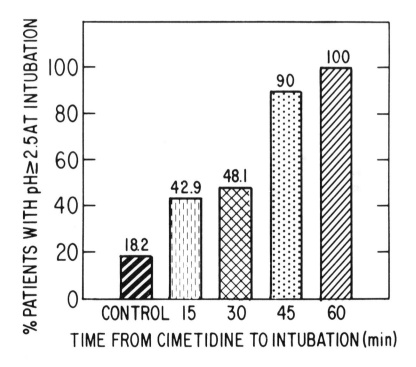

Figure 10.3 Frequency of "safe" gastric pH (>2.5) in five groups of patients at induction of anesthesia. Control groups received no cimetidine (placebo) while the other four groups received cimetidine prophylaxis, 300 mg intravenously, at variable times up to an hour prior to anesthetic induction. (Adapted with permission from Coombs et al., courtesy of International Anesthesia Research Society.)

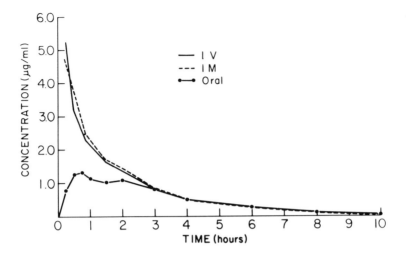

Figure 10.4 Mean blood levels after administration of 300 mg of cimetidine by various routes. Clinically effective drug levels of 0.5 μg/ml are achieved and maintained by any route of administration. (Adapted with permission from Walkenstein SS, Dubb JW, Randolf WC: Bioavailability of cemetidine in man. Gastroenterology 1978;74:360–365.)

Delayed Repair

Patients who are scheduled for reconstructive surgery after four weeks may experience potentially serious problems related to hyperkalemia, causalgia, or immobility.

One possible consequence of nerve injury is supersensitivity of denervated muscles to depolarizing muscle relaxants (11,12). In normal patients following a conventional bolus dose of succinylcholine, the serum potassium increases by 0.5 mEq per liter, which is usually without adverse sequelae. In certain groups of patients with neuromuscular disease (e.g., paralysis from spinal cord injuries, peripheral nerve trauma, or nerve degeneration), succinylcholine may produce severe hyperkalemia (Fig. 10.5), leading to cardiac arrest. The end-plate, a small specialized structure adherent to the muscle fiber at the neuromuscular junction, is the specific site of action for acetylcholine and succinylcholine. During the depolarization stage, the end-plate is permeable to ionic fluxes (potassium efflux). When a muscle is denervated, however, the ionic permeability of potassium is not restricted to the end-plate but instead spreads to involve the entire muscle membrane (13). This efflux of potassium is about 30% higher in denervated nerves than in the damaged nerves of paraplegic animals (7) (Fig. 10.5).

This change in response of the muscle membrane occurs within a day following denervation, is maximal within 10 days, and persists up to 6 to 12 months until the denervated muscle is gradually reduced by fibrous tissue, thus diminishing the

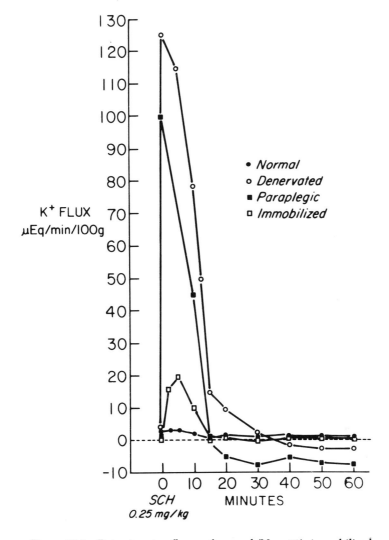

Figure 10.5   Potassium ion fluxes of normal (N = 10), immobilized (N = 5), paraplegic (N = 7) and denervated (N = 5) canine skeletal muscle after injection of succinylcholine (SCH). Efflux indicated by positive values, influx by negative. Unpaired *t* tests indicate that the first portions of the curves are different from each other. (Adapted with permission from Fig. 1, Ref. 11.)

potassium content (14). During the supersensitivity period, severe hyperkalemia will occur within two to four minutes after administration of a depolarizing relaxant, causing ventricular arrhythmias. Ventricular tachycardia or fibrillation may result. The hyperkalemic response is transient, lasting five to ten minutes, and the excess potassium is rapidly taken up by the liver. The degree of hyperkalemia will be proportional to the severity of neuromuscular dysfunction.

If a patient who has had extensive nerve trauma is scheduled for neurorrhaphy, the use of a depolarizing relaxant should be avoided. In the event of cardiac arrest owing to administration of succinylcholine in a susceptible patient, cardiopulmonary resuscitation should be begun immediately to maintain adequate oxygenation to the vital organs until the hyperkalemic period is over. If conventional means of cardiopulmonary resuscitation are ineffective, open-chest massage may be necessary. Prior dose of a nondepolarizing relaxant attenuates the hyperkalemic response but does not block it completely (10,11).

Causalgia develops in fewer than 5% of patients who sustain a definite transection injury to a large peripheral nerve (above the knee or elbow). Characteristically, these patients experience continuous burning pain beginning immediately or within a week of the injury. Other features are hyperesthesia and vasomotor disturbance with vasodilation in the early phase and vasoconstriction in the late stages of the disease. Trophic changes develop, leading to atrophy of skin and subcutaneous tissue and osteoporosis of bones. The physical discomfort is so severe that these patients become psychologically disturbed.

A small number of patients with causalgia achieve spontaneous remission. For the others, regional sympathetic block with local anesthetic will, in most instances, produce complete relief, and 90% of those who achieve only temporary relief may benefit from surgical sympathectomy. Both the pain and the patient's psychological status should be given due consideration in the preoperative preparation, during positioning and handling of affected limbs, and in selection of medications.

If a patient has been immobilized because of major nerve damage involving the lower extremities, the possibility of pulmonary infection and deep vein thrombosis should be considered. The most common site of origin of venous emboli is from the ileofemoral venous system. Clinical signs and symptoms are elicited in only 50% of these patients. The most accurate test to detect deep vein thrombosis is contrast venography, which is invasive. The combination of three minimally invasive techniques—iodine-125 fibrinogen study, phleborheography, and Doppler ultrasound studies—will identify 95% of the patients with deep vein thrombosis (15,16). Pulmonary embolism in the perioperative period, although rare, frequently proves catastrophic.

Choice of Anesthetic

Nerve trauma usually involves the extremities. The surgery is precise and time-consuming. An immobile field with minimum bleeding is ideal, and functional integrity of the nerve may have to be tested intermittently throughout the operation. General anesthesia probably best achieves these goals. Selection of a narcotic or an inhalation technique will be dictated by the anesthesiologist's preference and the patient's condition.

The use of regional techniques for nerve surgery in the extremities requires careful consideration. Well-performed spinal or epidural anesthesia for procedures involving a lower extremity may be suitable provided it is appropriate to the duration of the operation, and the positioning of the patient during surgery does not compromise his comfort.

For surgery on the upper extremity, if block of the brachial plexus by a supraclavicular, interscalene, or axillary approach is contemplated, one should keep in mind both the inherent complications and the 2.8% incidence of postanesthetic nerve lesions associated with the technique. Common complications are

1. Pneumothorax
2. Total spinal anesthesia
3. Hoarseness
4. Horner's syndrome
5. Phrenic nerve palsy
6. Hematoma
7. Nerve damage
8. Axillary artery compression
9. Vascular insufficiency

Trauma caused by the injecting needle while paresthesia is being elicited to perform the block has been cited as the cause of subsequent nerve lesions (17). Correct position of the needle should be determined by loss of resistance as the sheath is penetrated rather than by direct nerve stimulation. Use of short, beveled needles, inserted with the bevel in the long axis of the nerve, and avoiding the use of epinephrine with the local anesthetics are further maneuvers recommended to minimize nervous tissue damage.

Common sense would seem to dictate that nerve blocks not be performed for repairing injured nerves. Soetens and colleagues (18), however, claim to have performed 2755 nerve blocks without causing any nerve injuries. The sympathetic block, which is associated with regional techniques, is a recognized treatment for sympathetic dystrophy.

Intravenous regional anesthesia (Bier's block) is an alternative for upper and lower extremity surgery. A disadvantage of this technique is that it requires the use of a pneumatic tourniquet, which limits the duration of surgery. A large dose of local anesthetic drug is necessary, which decreases the safety margin.

SURGERY FOR COMPRESSIVE LESIONS AND MISCELLANEOUS CONDITIONS

Entrapment Syndromes

Carpal tunnel syndrome, thoracic outlet syndrome, cubital tunnel syndrome, and peroneal nerve compression are the commonly seen clinical entities that require surgical decompression.

Carpal tunnel syndrome (19) is due to compression of the median nerve at the wrist, under the transcarpal ligament, along the course from the forearm into the hand. It is seen mostly in middle-aged women, although it may be a troublesome complication of pregnancy and fluid retention. The symptoms are pain, paresthesia, and numbness in the hand along the distribution of the median nerve. Eighty percent of patients are temporarily relieved of symptoms by injections of lidocaine and hydrocortisone, but the majority suffer an exacerbation of symptoms. If muscle wasting occurs, surgical excision of the transcarpal ligament is required.

Of all the nerve injuries, carpal tunnel syndrome probably lends itself best to regional anesthetic technique for correction. Bier's intravenous or an axillary brachial plexus block using 30 ml of 0.5% to 1% lidocaine affords good anesthesia without motor paralysis for one to two hours. A local technique may also be satisfactory, although infiltration of the tissues causes distortion.

Thoracic outlet syndrome (20) results from compression of the brachial plexus and subclavian artery at the thoracic outlet by a cervical rib tumor or fascial band in the scalenus anticus muscle. The syndrome is seen most commonly in middle-aged women and has also been reported in 24% of patients following injury to the neck (21). Pain, weakness, paresthesia in the arm, and color change in the hand are the common presenting features. Resection of cervical ribs or the medial part of the first rib may be necessary to alleviate symptoms. Surgical encroachment onto the pleura intraoperatively can cause a pneumothorax, which may progress to a tension pneumothorax.

Cubital tunnel syndrome is caused by compression of the ulnar nerve in the ulnar groove at the elbow and is associated with incapacitating symptoms of pain and paresthesia along the distribution of the nerve. If conservative treatment is ineffective, anterior transposition of the nerve away from the groove usually relieves the symptoms. Again, a brachial plexus block, by either the axillary or interscalene approach, is often satisfactory for this procedure, which requires approximately 45 minutes.

Nerve Tumors

Peripheral nerve tumors are rare (22). Jenkins (23) has classified them as false neuroma, neurofibroma, neurilemmoma, and neurofibrosarcoma. Multiple neurofibromas (von Recklinghausen's disease) is a Mendelian dominant inherited disorder.

When the tumors cause symptoms from compression, surgical excision is required. In the rare event of coexisting neurofibromatosis and pheochromocytoma, safe resection of the latter tumor is the primary therapeutic goal. From 5% to 10% of neurofibromas undergo sarcomatous change (24).

Miscellaneous Group

Neuralgic pain (25), facial muscle spasm (26), blepharospasm, and reconstructive surgery on the facial nerve following tumor or Bell's palsy (27,28) are some of the other causes for surgical intervention.

PNEUMATIC TOURNIQUET

The pneumatic tourniquet is widely used in limb surgery, particularly in orthopedic procedures and not infrequently in operations to correct peripheral nerve lesions. The use of pneumatic tourniquets in patients with sickle-cell anemia is claimed to be safe provided the limb is exsanguinated as completely as possible prior to inflation of the tourniquet (29).

Complications

The advantage of the tourniquet technique is achievement of a bloodless field, which makes the surgery easier, quicker, less traumatic, and improves healing. There are, however, a number of complications related to this technique such as:

1. Nerve palsy
2. Tissue ischemia
3. Hypertension during inflation of cuff
4. Hypotension during deflation of cuff, leading to brain-stem ischemia, pulmonary embolism, arterial emboli
5. Local irritation and damage
6. Inadvertent deflation of the cuff

These complications can be grouped into four major categories. The first group results from ischemia to tissues distal to the tourniquet (30–32). Secondly, the high pressure of the tourniquet on structures directly underneath causes compression. A third group of complications are related to inflation and deflation of the pneumatic cuff. Finally, problems arise from faulty equipment and technique.

When a limb is isolated from the rest of the circulation by application of a pneumatic tourniquet, the only circulation to that limb is via the intramedullary blood vessels of the long bones, and is estimated to be less than 1% of the limb's normal allocation (33). Therefore, if the ischemic period is prolonged, permanent damage to structures in the area can result (34). Muscle tissue, when rendered ischemic, will show histologic changes that are reversible in 24 hours, but muscle power may take a week to return to normal (31).

Injury to the peripheral nerves, although rare, is claimed to be due to direct pressure of the pneumatic tourniquet on the nerves rather than a result of ischemia (35,36). The documented incidence is around 0.15%, but such cases are not usually reported, and therefore this figure probably is underestimated (36). Redness, bruising, blistering, and chemical burns of the skin are other adverse effects of pressure of the tourniquet. These complications may be avoided by gentleness in application of the Esmach bandage and by placing the pneumatic tourniquet with cotton pads at the proximal end of the limb, where the muscle mass protects the nerves and vessels. Chemical burns can be prevented by not allowing antiseptic solutions to pool under the tourniquet.

Thromboembolic complications have been associated with the use of the pneumatic tourniquet. Dislodgment of venous emboli can cause pulmonary embolism (37). The use of a pneumatic tourniquet does not increase the risk of deep vein thrombosis, but rather decreases the incidence of venous thrombosis resulting from increased fibrinolytic activity (38,39). Dislodgment of atheromatous plaques causing ischemia to the extremity has also been reported (40).

Hemodynamic problems may occur during inflation and deflation of the cuff. A blood pressure increase of more than 30% occurred in 11% of elderly patients during inflation of the tourniquet (41). Brain-stem ischemia with cortical blindness immediately following release of the tourniquet from the upper arm has been reported (42); and hypotension caused by reactive hyperemia in the ischemic limb following release of the cuff was cited as the reason for the ischemia. Such an ischemic episode is likely to occur if the patient is upright or if there is an obstructive lesion in the subclavian artery (subclavian steal syndrome) (42).

The most common complications of the tourniquet system itself relate to errors in the pressure-regulating mechanism. The actual pressure in the tourniquet in one reported case averaged 150 to 400 mm Hg more than the recorded pressure (31). Frequent calibration of the aneroid pressure gauge is required to prevent this complication.

Duration of Tourniquet Occlusion

The suggested critical period for the development of irreversible ischemia with use of the pneumatic tourniquet has been debated. At present the most widely accepted maximum limit is two hours, although longer periods have been used without outward effects in the upper extremities (43). Critical pressures for adults are 300 mm Hg for the upper limb and 500 mm Hg for the lower limb; in children the respective values are 150 and 250 mm Hg. Ideally, the tourniquet pressure should be maintained at 60 to 70 mm Hg above systolic pressure. If occlusion time is to be exended beyond the two-hour limit, the tourniquet should be released for 20 minutes before being reinflated. The pressure should then be maintained for no longer than an additional 30 to 45 minutes (31,44). Cold irrigating solutions increase tolerance of ischemic periods.

Recently, microprocessor-based tourniquets with audiovisual alarms and digital displays of time and pressure have been introduced (45). This equipment maintains a constant pressure difference between systemic arterial pressure and tourniquet cuff pressure.

REFERENCES

1. Sunderland S: Nerves and nerve injuries. Edinburgh, Livingstone, 1968, pp 127–137.

2. Rosen JM: Concepts of peripheral nerve repair. Ann Plast Surg 1981;7(2):165–171.

3. Brown HA, Brown BA: Treatment of peripheral nerve injuries. Review of Surgery 1967;24:1–8.

4. Chare RA: Reconstructive procedures after irreversible nerve damage in the upper extremity. Clin Neurosurg 1970;17:142–159.

5. Sunderland S: Anatomical features of nerve trunks in relation to nerve injury and nerve repair. Clin Neurosurg 1970; 17:38–62.

6. Campbell JB: Peripheral nerve repair. Clin Neurosurg 1970;17:77–99.

7. Howard FM: The electromyogram and conduction velocity studies on peripheral nerve trauma. Clin Neurosurg 1970; 17:63–75.

8. Manchikanti L, Kraus JW, Edds SP: Cimetidine and related drugs in anesthesia. Anesth Analg (Cleve) 1982;61(7):595–608.

9. Coombs DW: Clinical use of cimetidine, in Hershey SG(ed): Refresher courses in anesth. Philadelphia, Lippincott, 1982, vol 10, pp 37–50.

10. Shaw R, Mashford M, Desmond P: Cardiac arrest following bolus cimetidine. Med J Aust 1980;2:629–630.

11. Gronert GA, Theye RA: Pathophysiology of hyperkalemia induced by succinylcholine. Anesthesiology 1975;43:89–99.

12. Tobey RE, Jacobsen PM, Kagle CT, et al.: The serum potassium response to muscle relaxants in neural injury. Anesthesiology 1972;37:332–337.

13. Axelsson J, Thesleff S: A study of supersensitivity in denervated mammalian skeletal muscle. J Physiol (London) 1959;147:178–193.

14. Hines HM, Knowlton GC: Changes in the skeletal muscle of the rat following denervation. Am J Physiol 1933;104:379–391.

15. Konigsberg SF, Rosenberg N, Finkelstein NM: A multiphasic approach to screening for venous thrombosis, in Dietrich EB (ed): Noninvasive cardiovascular diagnosis, current concepts. Baltimore, University Park Press, 1978, pp 493–504.

16. Yao JS, Henkin RE, Bergen JJ: Venous thromboembolic disease. Evaluation of new methodology in treatment. Arch Surg 1974;109:664–670.

17. Selander D, Edshage S, Wolff T: Paresthesia or no paresthesia? Acta Anaesthesiol Scand 1979;23:27–33.

18. Soetens M, Van Craeyvett H, Vaes L, et al.: Brachial plexus block. Acta Anaesthiol Belg 1981;4:301–315.

19. Hamlin E, Lehman RAW: Current concepts in carpal tunnel syndrome. N Engl J Med 1967;276:849–850.

20. Brown HS, Smith RA: First rib resection for neurovascular syndromes of the thoracic outlet. Symposium on surgical anatomy and embryology. Surg Clin North Am. Philadelphia, Saunders, 1974;54(6):1277–1289.

21. Woods WW: Thoracic outlet syndrome. West J Med 1978;128:9–12.

22. Pilgaard S: Tumor of the ulnar nerve. Acta Orthop Scand 1968;39:332–335.

23. Jenkins AS: Solitary tumors of peripheral nerve trunks. J Bone Joint Surg [Am] 1952;34B:401–411.

24. Richardson EP, Adams RD: Degenerative disease of the nervous system, in Isselbacher, Adams R, Braunwald E, et al. (eds): Harrison's principles of internal medicine, ed 9. New York, McGraw-Hill, pp 2206–

25. Teng P: Meralgia paresthetica. Bull Los Angeles Neurol Soc 1972;37(2):75-83.
26. Crumley RL: Recent advances in facial nerve surgery. Advances in Facial Nerve Surgery 1982;4(3):233-236.
27. Britton BH: Surgery in Bell's palsy. Symposium on diseases and injury of the facial nerve. Otolaryngol Clin North Am 1974;7(2):511-515.
28. Hitselberger WE: Hypoglossal-facial anastomosis. Symposium on diseases and injury of the facial nerve. Otolaryngol Clin North Am 1974;7(2):545-550.
29. Yates SK, Hurst LN, Brown WF: The pathogenesis of pneumatic tourniquet paralysis. J Neurol Neurosurg Psychiatry 1981;44:759-769.
30. Klenerman L: Tourniquet time—how long? Hand 1980;12:231-234.
31. Flatt AE: Tourniquet time in hand surgery. Arch Surg 1972;104:190-192.
32. Klenerman L, Crawley J: Limb flow in the presence of a tourniquet. Acta Orthop Scand 1977;48:291-295.
33. Rorabeck CH, Kennedy JC: Tourniquet-induced nerve ischemia complicating knee ligament surgery. Am J Sports Med 1980;8(2):98-102.
34. Ochoa J, Fowler T, Gilliatt RW: Anatomical changes in peripheral nerves compressed by a pneumatic tourniquet. J Anat 1972;113:433-455.
35. McEwen JA: Complications of and improvements in pneumatic tourniquets used in surgery. Med Instrum 1981;15(4):253-257.
36. Estrera AS, King RP, Platt MR: Massive pulmonary embolism: A complication of the technique of tourniquet ischemia. J Trauma 1982;22(1):60-62.
37. Fahmy NR, Patel DG: Hemostatic changes and postoperative deep-vein thrombosis associated with use of a pneumatic tourniquet. J Bone Joint Surg [AM] 1981;63-A(3):461-455.
38. Simon MA, Mass DP, Zarins CK, et al.: The effect of a thigh tourniquet on the incidence of deep venous thrombosis after operations on the fore part of the foot. J Bone Joint Surg [AM] 1982;64-A(2):188-191.
39. Ginnestras NJ, Cranley JJ, Lentz M: Occlusion of tibial artery after a foot operation under tourniquet. J Bone Joint Surg [AM] 1977;59-A(5):682-683.
40. Kaufman RD, Walts LF: Tourniquet-induced hypertension. Br J Anaesth 1982;54:333-336.
41. Carney AL, Anderson EM: Tourniquet subclavian steal: Brainstem ischemia and cortical blindness—clinical significance and testing, in Carney AL, Anderson EM (eds): Advances in neurology. Vol 30, Diagnosis and treatment of brain ischemia. New York, Raven Press, 1981, pp 283-290.
42. Joza L, Renner A, Santha E: The effect of tourniquet ischemia on intact tenotomized and motor nerve injured human hand muscles. Hand 1980;12(3):235-240.
43. Kolstad MK, Wigren A: Systemic reaction to tourniquet ischemia. Acta Anaesthesiol Scand 1978;22:609-614.
44. Stein RE; Urbaniak J: Use of the tourniquet during surgery in patients with sickle cell hemoglobinopathies. Clin Orthop 1980; No 151.
45. McEwan JA; McGraw RW: Adaptive tourniquet for improved safety in surgery. IEEE Trans on Biomedical Engineering 1982;29:122-128.

CHAPTER 11

Pediatric Neurologic Surgery
Carlos U. Arancibia and
Kenneth Shapiro

Pediatric neuroanesthesia is a unique challenge in that it combines the demands of neuroanesthesia with the special problems of the pediatric patient.

In large pediatric medical centers, neurosurgical operations comprise 12% of all operations performed (1). In a general neurosurgical practice, pediatric cases constitute about 10% of the total case load. In addition, more than 200,000 children are hospitalized annually in the United States because of head injury, so that the problems of caring for the immature nervous system become ubiquitous.

More than numbers should be considered, however. The first preoperative visit commonly initiates a long association between the patient, parents, and the surgical team; the first operation often is only the beginning of a lengthy treatment experience (correction of some neural tube defects, such as spina bifida, require multiple neurosurgical, orthopedic, and urologic procedures). A similar relationship develops with children with hydrocephalus because the high incidence of shunt dysfunction requires frequent surgical correction. An awareness of some special problems such as particular fears, drug reactions, or anatomic abnormalities can help the clinician to establish a special bond with the young patient.

This chapter deals with some of the common problems in pediatric neuroanesthesia. Unfortunately, solutions to every problem are not available: nevertheless, we aim to provide a framework for the continuous improvement in neuroanesthetic care of "our children."

CRANIOSYNOSTOSIS

The heading of craniosynostosis includes a large variety of clinical syndromes, from abnormalities of a single suture of the skull to complex craniofacial syndromes with abnormalities of the skull base and other parts of the body. Normally, the skull grows passively in response to enlargement of the cerebral mass. The skull of the newborn has a capacity for considerable deformation, which enables it to conform to the changes necessary for delivery. The brain of a normal newborn weighs approximately 330 gm and is encased by bones held together at the sutural lines by fibrous connective tissue. The weight of the brain doubles in the first six months of life and by the age of 2 years usually weighs approximately 1000 gm, which is about 80% of the weight of the adult brain. The rate of increase of brain weight decreases after age 2, and the final weight is achieved about the age of 12 (2). The skull and the base of the cranium increase appropriately with expansion of the brain. The cranium of the newborn demonstrates considerable mobility, especially along the sagittal and coronal sutures. The posterior fontanelle closes around the third month of life, but the anterior fontanelle may remain open until the eighteenth month. It is necessary to differentiate functional closure from radiologic closure of the normal sutures. Functional closure is evident at age 2 and is completed at age 10. Radiologic closure occurs only in the third decade of life or even later.

Classification

If one of the cranial sutures closes prematurely, the normal growth of the skull is modified and the shape becomes deformed. This intrinsic abnormality of the cranium is termed *primary craniosynostosis*. The growth of the brain is affected only if more than one suture closes prematurely. It is necessary to differentiate this picture from secondary craniosynostosis, which occurs when the growth of the brain is impaired. In this condition, the shape of the skull may appear normal, but growth of the head falls below the relation between standard curves: that is, head and body size are disproportionate.

Craniosynostosis has a higher association with other congenital malformations. The craniofacial abnormalities of Crouzon's disease and Apert's syndrome are characterized by bilateral synostosis of the coronal sutures associated with different abnormalities of the face and digits, such as syndactyly and midface hypoplasia. Other associated anomalies include hypertelorism. Although the etiology of primary craniosynostosis is unknown, both Crouzon's disease and Apert's syndrome are inherited abnormalities (the original description of Crouzon's disease was based on two patients, mother and son [3]).

Incidence

Although craniosynostosis is seen frequently in neurosurgical centers, the incidence of primary craniosynostosis in the population is unknown. An indication is obtained from the experience of the Children's Hospital of Boston, where between 1927 and 1966, 530 patients were treated for craniosynostosis. Of this group, 519 patients were treated surgically (4). This study, among others, indicates the relative frequency of compromise of the sutures. The most common form of craniosynostosis is premature closure of the sagittal suture, and occurs in about 50% of cases. The coronal suture is involved in 35% of the cases, and in 5% of the cases the suture involved is the metopic. Unilateral or bilateral compromise of the lambdoid suture probably occurs less frequently.

Evaluation

In the newborn with primary craniosynostosis, the diagnosis is made clinically. As a general rule, any abnormal shape of the cranium that does not disappear within the first week of life must be investigated. Usually all that is necessary to visualize the sutures are skull films. Once the diagnosis is made, the urgency of

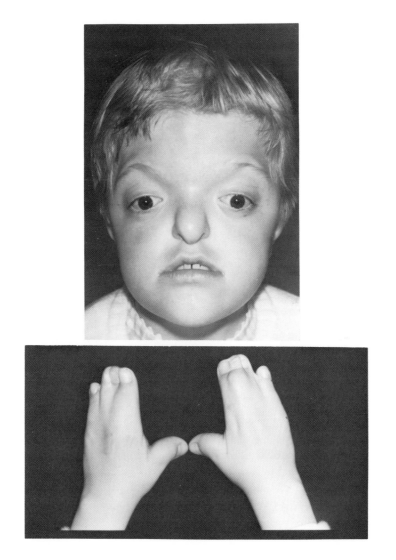

Figure 11.1 This 3-year-old female has Apert's syndrome, with bilateral coronal synostosis, secondary proptosis, syndactyly, and mental retardation. Craniofacial reconstruction consists of early coronal synostectomy, bilateral orbital advancement, and delayed mid-face advancement.

management will be determined by two factors: the presence or absence of increase in intracranial pressure (ICP) and the presence of other malformations.

In the syndromes associated with midface hypoplasia, especially Crouzon's disease and Apert's syndrome, careful examination of the mouth and upper airway are performed to assess potential compromise of the airway. Computed tomography (CT) provides a noninvasive examination of brain and skull bone anatomy and may reveal unexpected anomalies of the intracranial compartment. Special attention must be given to the eye examination since it is not uncommon for a certain degree of exophthalmos to be present due to shallow orbits formed in bicoronal synostosis (Fig. 11.1). Narrowing of the optic foramina can also lead to optic atrophy. Since growth of the skull can still take place at the unfused sutures, generalized raised ICP is most unusual but may occur even in the absence of total suture closure. There is no doubt that in every case of primary craniosynostosis there is a certain degree of compression of the brain. There is no evidence, however, that the abnormality of one suture produces significant neurologic damage. The situation is quite different when two or more sutures are compromised and the risk of intracranial hypertension increases, as does the possibility of late complications such as optic atrophy and mental retardation. There is no known medical treatment for this malformation. When the abnormality involves only one suture the surgical decision is essentially cosmetic, and although the risk of the operation is low, it should be carefully evaluated. Surgery must be accomplished relatively early in life in order to allow the rapidly growing brain to expand and reshape the skull. Most neurosurgeons operate on these infants between 1 and 2 months of age. When two or more sutures are closed, surgical intervention is directed to prevent the complications of cerebral compression. The need for surgery is emergent in the cases of increased ICP and ulcerative keratitis. The surgical correction of extensive craniofacial malformations is usually staged to allow for the differing rates of bone growth between skull and facial bones, with opening of cranial sutures early in life and correction of the facial anomalies later.

Preoperative Management

The anesthetic preoperative visit must include careful chart review. In patients younger than 10 years, the preoperative visits are best conducted with the relatives present. In older children it is often convenient to ask the parents to leave for a few minutes to allow the establishment of better personal contact between the anesthesiologist and the patient and to allow the patient to formulate questions that he may be hesitant to ask in front of relatives. Patients usually remember only the unpleasant part of previous operations. With verbalization and patience, these fears, normal or abnormal, may be eliminated or greatly decreased. The preoperative visit should also include an explanation of the logistic details that will surround the operation. It is often not realistic to tell the parents and the patient that surgery will be completed at a specific hour. Rather, explanations should be directed to the sequence of events from preoperative preparation to awakening in the recovery room.

The physical examination must be very careful and detailed. In newborns and infants, simple observation reveals significant information. Some of the aspects that deserve special attention are:

1. Clinical evaluation of ICP using the tension of the fontanelle in infants and an examination of the fundi in children and teenagers.
2. Careful examination of the upper airway to determine, a priori, possible difficulties with intubation, since choanal atresia and narrowed airways are associated anomalies. Special attention should be directed to the relation between head and body size in small infants, since it may cause compromise of the airway during anesthetic induction.
3. Examination of the extremities to identify veins useful for cannulation.
4. Whenever there are associated musculoskeletal abnormalities it is important to determine the degree of limitation of the joints, since this may create a significant problem in the positioning of the patient in the operating room.

The laboratory testing needed is within normal requirements for the age of the patient and includes hematologic evaluation with coagulation profile, serum electrolytes, and tests of liver and renal function. Except in cases of primary craniosynostosis of only one suture, the minimal requirement of available blood for transfusion should equal the estimated blood volume of the patient.

The preoperative orders for patients up to 6 months of age include administration of normal feeding formula until midnight, continuing with solutions of 5% glucose until four hours before the operation. Between the ages of 6 months and 2 years, nothing is administered by mouth in the six hours preceding surgery. In patients older than 2 years of age, the regular preoperative fasting routine is used. In rare cases where the surgery is planned for the afternoon this protocol may be modified. Anticholinergic drugs are not ordered routinely. Should there be an indication for such medication (bradycardia, secretions), the same, if not better, results may be obtained by giving these drugs parenterally in the operating room, avoiding the extremely unpleasant sensation of a dry mouth. Normally, premedication is not given to patients below the age of 6 months. In patients older than 6 months, pentobarbital, 2 mg/kg intramuscularly, may be given one hour before surgery. Alternative medications include diazepam, 1 mg/10 kg, or diphenhydramine hydrochloride elixir, 12.5 mg/10 kg (5 ml), both given orally one to one-and-a-half hours preoperatively.

Intraoperative Management

Normal essential intraoperative monitoring equipment includes continuous electrocardiogram, precordial stethoscope, blood pressure cuff and temperature. Maintenance of anesthesia is accomplished with halothane in oxygen and nitrous oxide, and additional amounts of pancuronium bromide are given according to the response to the nerve stimulator. Although an increase in cerebral blood flow, and therefore ICP, is associated with inhalation anesthetics in the spontaneously breathing patient (least so with isoflurane), this technique is preferable to proceeding with an intravenous induction, as it is better to avoid struggling with a patient who is crying and moving. Rectal barbiturates offer a reasonable alternative that permits smooth induction, less increase in ICP, prompt establishment of hypocapnia, and early, safe introduction of low-concentration inhalation anesthesia.

Certain aspects that deserve special mention include the need to provide a second fixation of the endotracheal tube, control of body temperature, the care necessary for the positioning of the patient on the operating table, and fluid replacement. In those cases where the patient is placed supine with neck flexion, the position of the endotracheal tube must be checked once all the preoperative movements have been accomplished (Fig. 11.2). Because of the small size of the trachea, movements of the chin away from the carina, which cause the tube to move up the trachea, make accidental extubation possible. Also, as the chin is moved toward carina, the tube may enter the right main-stem bronchus. When the patient is in the prone position, it is necessary to ensure that the eyes

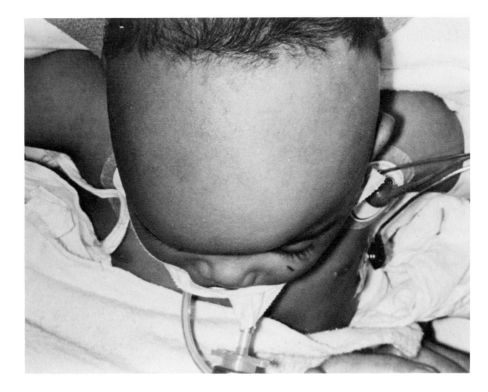

Figure 11.2 This 4-month-old infant has left sided coronal synostosis with secondary plagiocephaly. Note flattening of the left forehead and retrusion of the left orbit.

are not compressed and that the endotracheal tube is patent. In every position it is necessary to make sure that the degree of flexion of the neck is such that the chin of the patient is not compressed against the thorax.

The induction technique is simplified if intravenous cannulation has been performed preoperatively. An intravenous induction uses 2.5% thiopental in doses of 3 to 5 mg/kg. The remainder of the anesthetic course is similar.

Craniectomy is associated with considerable blood loss. The use of invasive monitoring probably is not justified in simple craniosynostosis. We do employ the oscillometric automatic method for measuring the blood pressure, which affords accurate recordings and provides the additional advantage of allowing the anesthesiologist to perform other tasks at the same time. It is necessary to quantify the magnitude of the bleeding: we employ a combination of techniques, such as measuring blood in suction bottles with a scale graduated in milliliters and weighing all sponges used during the procedure. All of these techniques, however, must be considered only a help and in no way a replacement for careful observation of the surgical field (Fig. 11.3). Blood transfusion is started at the

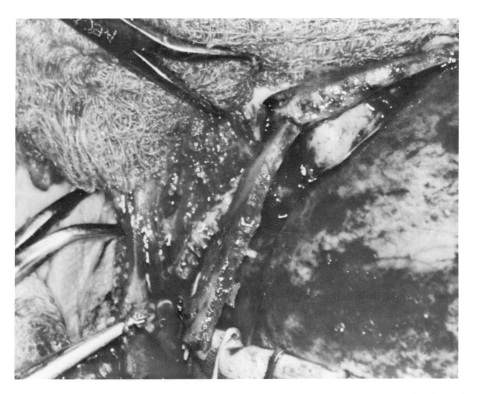

Figure 11.3 This intraoperative picture was taken during advancement of the left lateral canthus and left coronal synostectomy. The supraorbital vein has been advanced and held in place by a bone strut, achieving an immediate cosmetic improvement.

time of the incision, and blood is replaced as lost. We prefer to use packed red cells administered by syringe in increments of 10 ml. We infuse 0.25% N saline in 5% glucose solution in patients up to 6 months of age. In patients over 6 months of age we use Ringer's lactate with 5% glucose. Reasonable replacement is 3 to 5 ml/kg/hr. Initial deficit caused by the fasting condition should be calculated and replaced at the rate of one-half during the first hour and one-quarter over each of the next two hours.

The anesthetic system most commonly used is that described by Bain (Fig. 11.4), with mechanically controlled ventilation, humidified gas, an electric thermometer located near the connection of the endotracheal tube, a capnograph, and an inspired oxygen analyzer (5,6,7). At the end of the procedure, once the bandage of the head has been completed, muscle relaxant action is reversed and the trachea extubated.

The situation is completely different when the operative plan involves multiple sutures or is directed to the correction of a craniofacial abnormality. Craniofacial reconstructive surgery received impetus with the work of Tessier and colleagues (8,9), Converse and associates (10), and Epstein and co-workers (11). Essentially, these operations require a bifrontal craniotomy with extensive extradural dissection along the wings of the sphenoid bones and sometimes separation of the dura covering the cribriform lamina. Multiple osteotomies of the orbits and maxillae are needed to reconstruct the upper face. Final fixation is achieved using rib grafts. Dural tears created during dissection are repaired primarily or with pericranial grafts. These procedures are often performed in children 1 to 2 years of age who frequently have compromised upper airways. The extensive intracranial and extracranial dissections often require two teams of surgeons and demand extensive monitoring. We use an intraarterial cannula in-

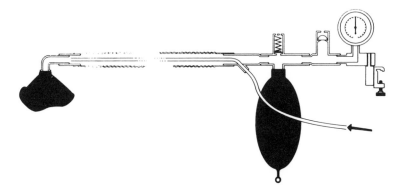

Figure 11.4 Modified Mapleson "D" circuit (Bain breathing circuit.) (From Bain JA, Spoerel WE, Low flow anesthesia utilizing a single limb circuit-in-low flow and closed system anesthesia, in JA Aldrete, HJ Lowe, RW Virtue, (eds.) New York: Grune & Stratton, 1979, pp 151–164.)

serted percutaneously in the radial, dorsal pedal, or posterior tibial artery. Central venous cannulation helps guide volume replacement and may assist treatment of air embolism should this occur.

While certain groups advocate routine tracheostomies (12), we have encountered many children with practically normal upper airways. In those cases it is possible to proceed with an intravenous induction as usual; however, all patients with craniofacial malformations may be subjects of anatomic abnormalities of the airway. In these cases, alternatives include (a) to proceed with topical anesthesia of the mouth and the pharynx and continue with an awake intubation or (b) to utilize an inhalation induction using halothane, with tracheal intubation at deeper planes. Whichever technique is selected, the upper airway must be maintained patent. We prefer an awake intubation unless the patient cannot tolerate this procedure, when inhalation induction is employed with the surgeon prepared to perform emergency tracheostomy. Fixation of the tube is essential; in those cases where the bony structures of the face will be displaced, the endotracheal tube can be sutured in place.

The selection of anesthetic agents is not of crucial importance. Since postoperative intubation is usual, we have used a technique based on fentanyl, 25 to 50 μg/kg, oxygen and nitrous oxide (1:2) and muscle relaxants, especially pancuronium bromide. Ventilation is mechanically controlled, maintaining arterial carbon dioxide tension ($PaCO_2$) around 30 mm Hg. This is achieved by incremental doses of fentanyl and/or pancuronium according to clinical evaluation and nerve stimulator. Sometimes it is necessary to produce periods of deliberate hypotension to reduce the loss of blood, especially during the osteotomies. We prefer to use small concentrations of halothane added to the gas mixture, on the order of 0.25% to 0.5%. Along with others (13), we believe that attention to all the details of the anesthetic management is essential, including use of the smallest flows of fresh, warmed, humidified gas that is possible. During the intracranial part of the operation, brain retraction is facilitated by administering furosemide, 1 mg/kg, or mannitol, 1 gm/kg intravenously. In larger children, a catheter is placed in the lumbar subarachnoid space at the outset to drain cerebrospinal fluid (CSF). The maneuver decreases or avoids the need for diuretic agents. One of the possible complications in this type of operation is damage of the endotracheal tube during the osteotomies. Accordingly, it is mandatory to have replacement tubes available.

Quantitative evaluation of blood loss is vital, since blood loss is constant and may reach 10 ml/kg/hr. All the problems associated with massive transfusion can occur and should be treated according to the specific deficits. Two other complications commonly arise. The oculocardiac reflex, related to traction on the intrinsic muscles of the eye and globe, may require judicious doses of atropine. Blood that originates from bleeding in the oropharyngeal cavity may pool in the stomach in large amounts. For this reason it is mandatory at the end of the operation to insert a nasogastric tube that will remain for at least 24 hours or until the trachea is extubated. At the end of the operation, the patient is transported to the intensive care unit, intubated and receiving 100% oxygen.

Postoperative Care

Mechanical ventilation at an inspired oxygen concentration of 40% using humidified gases is appropriate for several hours.

In all patients where wire fixation has been used for the mandible, a wire cutter must be placed at the head of the bed. A tray with all the equipment necessary for an emergency intubation and tracheostomy must be readily available. Analyses of hematocrit, coagulation profile, electrolytes, creatinine, and liver function are obtained. The frequency of arterial blood gas sampling depends on the clinical setting. A chest film is used to verify the position of the endotracheal tube and the central venous pressure cannula and to exclude pneumothorax, which may occur while harvesting rib grafts. Close monitoring continues for at least 24 hours after extubation.

CRANIAL AND SPINAL DYSRAPHISM

Defects in closure and differentiation of the neural tube, usually occurring in the fourth week of embryonic life, lead to conditions of cranial and spinal dysraphia. Closure normally starts in the midportion and extends in cephalad and caudal directions, so that defects of closure are more common in the lumbosacral area and head than in the midspinal segment. The spectrum of these defects ranges from anencephaly, with absence of cerebral hemispheres, to spina bifida occulta, where there is normal nervous tissue with absence of midline bone formation. In some cases the cranial and spinal defects may coexist in the same patient.

Cranial Dysraphism (Encephalocele)

The clinical picture ranges from the absence of a small area of the scalp to cranium bifidum with encephalomeningocele (Fig. 11.5). Most of these lesions are located in or around the midline in the occipital area. The incidence of occipital encephalocele is low, occurring in approximately 1 in every 5000 live births in the United States. This incidence is significantly less than similar lesions in the spine. Matson, drawing from 40 years' experience in Boston, cited 265 cases of which more than 85% were in the occipital area (14).

There is a large variety of presentations, and except for very small flattened lesions, the diagnosis usually is obvious at birth. The defect may present as a sessile protuberance or, more commonly, as a pedunculated mass projecting in the midline, often associated with malformations of the occipital lobes or the cerebellum, which may be incorporated in the sac. The size of the sac does not correlate with the amount of nervous tissue within it. It may be partially or totally covered by skin, which is important in determining the urgency of surgical intervention. The initial evaluation should include roentgenograms of the skull, transillumination of the sac, and a CT scan that will help delineate the contents of the sac and the presence of other associated malformations.

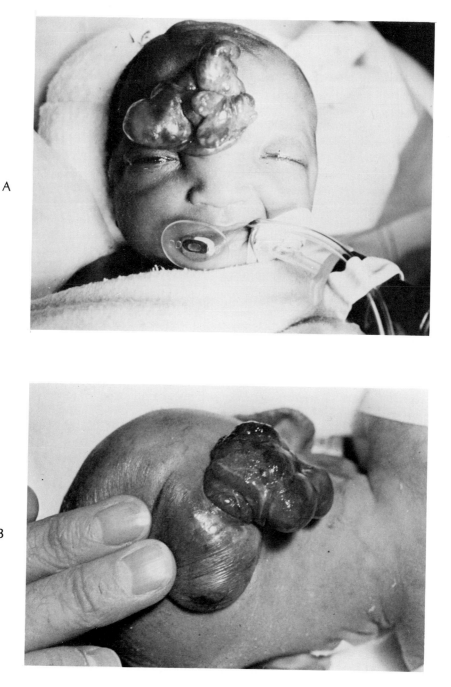

Figure 11.5   These newborn infants have encephaloceles. *A,* frontal encephalocele; *B,* occipital encephalocele; both were repaired within the first 24 hours of life.

Surgery is directed at closing the defect to prevent infection, preserve viable neural tissue, and facilitate nursing care.

Since the majority of the defects are occipital, operations are performed with the patient in the prone position in a cerebellar frame. An elliptical incision is made in the base of the lesion trying to preserve skin for closure. The sac is dissected to the bone edges. If the sac contains neural tissue, it is dissected free and those parts that are grossly abnormal are amputated. Viable tissue is replaced in the intracranial compartment and a water-tight closure of dura performed. When excessive, apparently viable cerebral tissue is present, this area of the brain may be covered with a dural graft. Aside from preserving brain tissue, this maneuver avoids bradycardia associated with brain replacement under tension.

Prognosis for intellectual development depends on the amount of neural tissue in the sac and the presence of hydrocephalus. Of 31 patients operated on at the Hospital for Sick Children in Toronto during a 10-year period, 10 recovered completely and 21 survived with residual abnormalities (15). Frontal encephaloceles, considerably less common than those of the occiput, carry a better prognosis for long-term outcome.

Spinal Dysraphism

As is the case with cranial dysraphism, the extent of the malformation at the spinal level varies considerably. Minor defects of the posterior neural arches are very common, affecting approximately 10% of the population. This picture of spina bifida occulta frequently is an incidental finding in routine radiologic studies at the lumbar level. But when this occult form of dysraphism is associated with cutaneous abnormalities of the lumbar area, at least 20% of patients will have an intraspinal tumor (dermoids, lipomas) or other abnormalities such as tethering of the cord (Fig. 11.6). It is not uncommon to see the appearance of urologic, motor, and sensory symptoms as growth progresses (16).

The other extreme of spinal dysraphism, myelomeningocele, is protrusion of a meningeal sac through a defect of the spine (Fig. 11.7). The incidence of myelomeningocele is about 2 per 1000 live births, and epidemiologic studies have shown a familial incidence. The risk in subsequent offspring in a family where one member is affected is 5% and increases to about 10% when two or more members are affected (17). Approximately 80% of myelomeningoceles occur in the lumbosacral area. The diagnosis usually is obvious at birth, with presentation of a partially skin-covered sac with a plaque of neural tissue in the center. If the sac ruptures during delivery, the resultant CSF leak requires emergency operation. The neurologic examination is usually consistent with the level of myelomeningocele, ranging from relatively normal intact lower extremity function in sacral sacs to paraplegia in thoracolumbar lesions. Often other malformations coexist, most frequently the Chiari type II malformation, which includes kinking of the lower brain stem and cerebellar hypoplasia. Laryngeal stridor and airway obstruction are complications of this syndrome (18) that usually occur

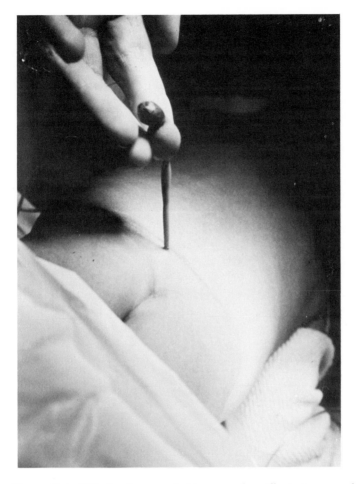

Figure 11.6 This lumbar sacral skin appendage illustrates one of many cutaneous signs of underlying spinal dysraphism. Myelography disclosed an intra- and extradural lipoma.

later in infancy or in childhood. As many as 80% of the infants will have hydrocephalus accompanying the myelomeningocele.

The management of patients with myelomeningocele remains controversial and depends on both medical and ethical issues (16). Often these infants are referred to centers experienced in dealing with the initial decision for long-term treatment of children with myelomeningocele.

Because of the risk of infection and possible increased neurologic deficit with drying out of neural elements, the myelomeningocele should be repaired within 24 hours of birth. This is only the first step in a long journey that will involve constant specialized care and, frequently, multiple surgical procedures to correct complications and the sequelae of other malformations.

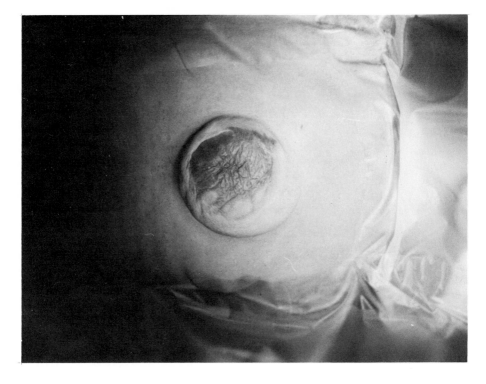

Figure 11.7 This newborn infant has a lumbar sacral myelomeningocele with distal paresis of her lower extremities.

Anesthetic Considerations

Before transporting the infant to the operating room, the anesthesiologist must make certain that the temperature of the operating room is at least 24°C, with heating blanket on the surgical table and the anesthetic equipment and drugs ready. We prefer the use of a non-rebreathing system, either a Jackson Rees modification type or a Bain circuit, with a source of humidification, more for control of temperature than to prevent the deleterious effect of dry gases in the tracheobronchial tree. A variety of masks, tubes, and laryngoscope blades, lubricated stylets, and intravenous infusion equipment should be available. Cotton tissue is used to wrap the baby's extremities. The anesthesiologist should adopt a semi-sterile technique (hand washing, gloves, gowns) to minimize the risk of infection.

The patient should be transferred to the operating room in a portable incubator. Electrocardiographic leads, blood pressure cuff, and cotton wrappings can all be placed while the patient is still in the transporter. If the patient has a nasogastric tube in place, we aspirate gently and leave it patent. Once all this has been accomplished, the baby is transferred to the operating table, in the lateral position with the right side up. The patient is covered with a warm blanket and placed under radiant heat lamps. A temperature probe is placed and attached to a recording device.

Because of the malformation, positioning of these patients for intubation may be a problem. We prefer an awake intubation in the lateral position, using small, clear plastic, disposable endotracheal tubes. When unable to intubate patients in this position, an assistant can hold the baby in his stretched arms or the baby may be placed with the defect protruding through a ring cushion. The trachea can usually be intubated without difficulty in this modified supine position. Frequently umbilical cannulation has been performed. If not, a secure intravenous route must be established before any surgical manipulation is attempted. We prefer a 20- or 22-gauge needle inserted to the dorsum of the hand. If this is not possible, our next choices are the feet, ankles, and the antecubital areas. Scalp vessels should not be overlooked. Rarely is it necessary to resort to surgical means. If, because of associated abnormalities, central venous cannulation is indicated, the subclavian route is used. A bladder catheter or a urine collector is placed to measure collected urine and to minimize the chances of urine contaminating the surgical field.

Induction of anesthesia is achieved with a mixture of nitrous oxide and oxygen, to which increasing concentrations of halothane are added. When the infant arrives in the operating room with an intravenous route secured, we administer 3 to 5 mg/kg of sodium thiopental prior to intubation and proceed with general inhalation anesthetic maintenance. We do not use muscle relaxant drugs routinely, as they would interfere with the use of nerve stimulators in the operating field. The stimulators are extremely useful as identification devices in preservation of as much functional nervous tissue as possible.

The operation is done in the prone position. The head of the patient rests in a cerebellar frame or on the table. When a cerebellar frame is used, extreme care must be exercised in preventing the compression of the eyes against the frame. We prefer to bring the endotracheal tube through the central opening of the frame. It is necessary to make sure that the tube is well secured, so that secretions do not loosen the tape, and the weight of the connections of the delivery system do not exert undue traction or cause kinking of the tube. When the head rests on the table, we prefer to use a well-padded "doughnut" type head ring. To avoid compression of the abdomen, rolls of towel are placed under the shoulders and upper thighs. After placement of these rolls, the position of the head and neck must be rechecked to ensure that changes in the degree of flexion or extension of the neck have not resulted in displacement of the tip of the endotracheal tube and the chin is not compressed against the chest or the table. Great care must be taken with the position of the lower extremities. It is our practice to use appropriate sized tape to secure the patient to the table, passing the tape across the buttocks and across the shoulders to both sides of the table.

Problems include control of ventilation, maintenance of temperature, and blood loss. Ventilation is controlled either manually or mechanically, maintaining normocapnia with an inspired oxygen concentration of not more than 40%.

Wrapping the infant in the adhesive plastic sheets used to define the surgical field has been a useful means of maintaining body heat. Blood loss can be considerable. Schroeder and Williams reported that in 100 cases, 48 had losses of less than 10% of the estimated blood volume, 44 lost between 10% and 20% of their estimated blood volume, and in 8 cases the blood loss was more than 20% (19). Of all the methods available for quantifying the blood loss, none is more valuable than direct observation and communication.

After completion of surgery, the baby is returned to the lateral position. After careful evaluation and extubation of the trachea, the patient is returned to the portable incubator in the lateral position or prone and transferred back to an intensive care unit, where nursing will be done in the prone position in heated incubators with high humidification. Since active hydrocephalus often becomes apparent after the initial operation, careful attention should be given to the clinical evaluation of ICP and head circumference measurements in order to minimize the chances of a CSF leak from the site of repair. As many as 80% of these infants will require a ventriculoperitoneal shunt to control ICP. Other serious complications are wound infection, meningitis, and wound dehiscence.

This is only the beginning of a long process that must involve a multidisciplinary group. With early aggressive treatment at least 80% of these patients will be alive at age 7. Most of these survivors will require many operations, orthopedic and urologic as well as neurosurgical.

HYDROCEPHALUS

Among the many causes of macrocrania in children, one of the most common is hydrocephalus. Although hydrocephalus has many causes, the common denominator is excessive accumulation of CSF in the ventricles. Depending on the rate of ventricular enlargement, age of the child, and associated disease processes, hydrocephalus may present with a variety of symptoms and signs.

Approximately 0.35 ml/min of CSF is produced within the cerebral ventricles, both from the choroid plexuses and by the brain parenchyma, and circulates from the lateral ventricles to the third ventricle, the Sylvian aqueduct, and the fourth ventricle. From here the CSF passes to the subarachnoid space through the foramina of Magendie and Luschka. The fluid in the subarachnoid space can flow caudally into the spinal subarachnoid space or may move cephalad through different pathways to terminate at the level of the dural sinuses, where reabsorption takes place across the arachnoid villi. There is considerable debate as to the various mechanisms that propel the CSF and the alternative sites of absorption (20).

Incidence

The incidence of congenital hydrocephalus is about 1 per 1000 live births. If all infantile hydrocephalus presenting in the first three months of life are grouped together, the incidence approximates 3 to 4 per 1000 births, with congenital cases occurring three times more frequently than acquired (21).

Etiology and Classification

While excess production of CSF, as seen in choroid plexus papilloma, and impaired venous return have been associated with hydrocephalus, the usual cause is relative obstruction of CSF absorption. This may occur within the ventricular system, leading to so-called noncommunicating hydrocephalus, or may be secondary to obstruction outside the ventricles, producing communicating or external hydrocephalus.

Clinical Picture

The signs and symptoms are those of increased ICP, but the manifestations depend on age, expansibility of the skull, and the type and duration of hydrocephalus.

In infancy the first manifestation is an accelerated rate of head growth. The ability of the cranial sutures to separate in response to increased ICP explains why small infants may not develop symptoms until later and underscores the importance of serial measurement and plotting of the head circumference.

When present, eye signs, including setting-sun sign and abducens nerve palsy, usually indicate advanced hydrocephalus with raised ICP. Papilledema is rare; vomiting of a projectile nature is an overrated sign that can be seen in many other conditions. Lethargy and instability are seen more commonly.

The evaluation and treatment of patients has changed dramatically since the introduction of the CT scan. All children suspected of having hydrocephalus have skull roentgenograms to document the presence of suture separation or of increased ICP, together with CT scan. The entire anatomic configuration of the ventricular system is shown by the CT scan, a noninvasive procedure that normally can be performed without general anesthesia. The need for angiography, ventriculography, and pneumoencephalography has been reduced to a minimum.

Treatment

Although medical therapy has been directed to decrease CSF production (22,23) or lower ICP (24), the only effective treatment to date is diverting CSF from the brain to another part of the body. Most hydrocephalic children will require a functioning shunt for life (25). The ventriculoatrial (V/A) shunt is difficult to maintain in the years of rapid growth, because adequate function usually depends on the position of the distal tip. This is partially the reason why these patients require significantly more revisions than those with ventriculoperitoneal shunts.

While atrial placement of the distal catheter remains useful, V/A shunts appear to have a higher incidence of late complications of a more serious nature than the ventriculoperitoneal route. The most common complications of V/A shunts are mechanical obstruction, infection, and thromboembolism leading to cor pulmonale. V/A shunts have been associated also with a specific form of glomerulonephritis (shunt nephritis) (26) caused by antibody formation to low-grade shunt infections. In ventriculoperitoneal shunts the most common complication is also obstruction, followed by infection. Peritonitis is an uncommon complication of these shunts. The incidence of infection is similar for both types of shunt (27,28).

Ventriculopleural and lumboperitoneal shunts are other means of diverting CSF. Distal placement in the pleural cavity is useful when other peritoneal or atrial placement proves difficult. Lumboperitoneal shunts can be used when ventricles are small or in a situation of "communicating" hydrocephalus.

Anesthetic Considerations

In active pediatric neurosurgical services, operations for correction of hydrocephalus are among the most common. The problems that can be encountered can be separated into those related to the cause of the hydrocephalus, those directly related to the hydrocephalus, and those that arise secondary to the treatment (29).

As already mentioned, hydrocephalus is often associated with spinal dysraphism. As neonatal care has improved, an increasing number of low-birth-weight, premature infants with respiratory distress are surviving intraventricular hemorrhage and require shunting procedures. Obviously, the existence of these associated pathologies affects the anesthetic management of the patient. The main anesthetic issue in relation to hydrocephalus is the existence of elevated ICP. This will vary depending on the setting: infants undergoing an initial shunt may have minimally elevated ICP, while older children with acute malfunction may have life-threatening intracranial hypertension. Usually premedication is not necessary in these patients, who are often somnolent because of their hydrocephalus. A relatively small percentage of these patients will be scheduled for surgery electively, another small percentage will come as a life-saving emergency, and the vast majority will be urgent cases that do allow for some hours to correct biochemical problems. Except for those cases scheduled electively, we consider all other patients to have elevated ICP and full stomachs. If the patient has an intravenous infusion already in place or has reasonably adequate veins, we proceed with an intravenous induction using generous doses of barbiturates and intubation with short-acting relaxants monitored with nerve stimulator and cricoid pressure. After adequate hyperventilation, halothane can be added to the gas mixture in concentrations of not more than 1 MAC (minimum alveolar concentration). In the absence of intravenous cannulation, inhalation induction is performed using halothane at low concentration and establishing an intravenous route as soon as possible. This approach minimizes the elevations of ICP that occur with multiple attempts to secure an intravenous route in a crying and struggling child. Since these children probably will have several shunt procedures, surgical intervention is avoided wherever possible to preserve future intravenous routes. In critically ill patients, however, we do not hesitate to secure a route in the most expeditious manner to administer drugs and to reduce increased ICP. The maintenance of anesthesia is usually with halothane in oxygen and nitrous oxide, with the patient paralyzed and ventilation mechanically controlled to produce a $PaCO_2$ of about 30 mm Hg.

The large head of these children may complicate maintenance of the airway and may add to the difficulty of intubation. Since the head is disproportionately large compared to the body, a large surface area is exposed during shunting procedures so that maintenance of body temperature may be difficult. Evaporation from the exposed skin during cleansing may also contribute to hypothermia. Every effort should be made to maintain temperature as close to normal as possible. Ambient temperature should be increased; as much area of the body as possible should be covered; humidifiers, vapor condensers, and warm washing solutions should be used. Alcohol preparation must be avoided.

Since these are short procedures, we aim to have the patient awake as soon as possible. Our experience has shown us that we can accomplish these goals successfully using minimal concentrations of halothane. Positioning these patients on the operating table may also be difficult because of joint deformities in older children. Rotating the head to facilitate insertion of the shunt may be enough to occlude flow in the internal jugular vein (30).

Dramatic systemic changes can occur during shunt placement. Insertion of the atrial catheter can induce transient arrythmias, which usually respond to withdrawal of the cardiac end of the shunt. Bradycardia and cardiac arrhythmias as well as gasping respiration or Cheyne-Stokes pattern have been precipitated by rapid changes of intracranial volume. These changes probably result from brain-stem movement following decrease of CSF volume. These latter alterations have been reversed by reexpanding ventricular volume and elevating the foot of the operating table, thereby decreasing CSF flow through the shunt. Bridging cortical veins may be formed as a result of rapid CSF drainage and ventricular collapse. Tearing may create a subdural hematoma. While usually not an acute complication, the distal end of a peritoneal shunt can perforate the bowel, leading to peritonitis. Also, an infected peritoneal shunt can be confused with acute appendicitis. Children with pleural shunts can have large amounts of CSF in the pleural cavity, so that careful evaluation of respiratory status should be performed prior to anesthetizing this group for shunt or other surgical procedures.

On average, children shunted during infancy will require 2 or 3 shunt revisions during the first decade of life. Despite this, as many as 60% to 80% of these children will have a reasonably normal intellectual outcome, making the early investment in their care extremely rewarding.

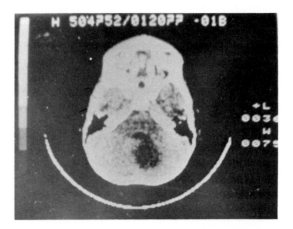

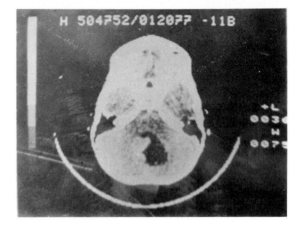

Figure 11.8 This CT scan shows a cystic cerebellar astrocytoma in a 4-year-old. This tumor, histologically benign, was removed without sequelae.

TUMORS

Incidence

The most common form of neoplasm in the pediatric population is leukemia, followed by primary intracranial tumors. About 20% of all intracranial neoplasms occur before the age of 20 years. There are significant differences in the relative incidence of different tumors in relation to age. Until age 3, there is roughly the same percentage of tumors above as below the tentorium. After that age, the incidence of infratentorial neoplasms is double that occurring in the supratentorial region. This distribution begins to reverse in adolescence, resembling the adult distribution of 70% supratentorial, 30% infratentorial.

The types of tumor also are different in the pediatric group. Of the infratentorial tumors, about 60% to 70% are either cerebellar astrocytomas or medulloblastomas. Gliomas of the brain stem account for about 20%. Ten percent of the tumors are ependymomas. In the supratentorial area, 70% to 80% of the tumors are gliomas, 1% to 3% are tumors of the pineal gland, 2% to 3% are choroid plexus papillomas, and 10% to 15% are classified as parasellar tumors (31–33). Brain tumors in childhood differ in many ways from those found in adults. At least half of the tumors in children are found in the posterior fossa. Since the tumors arising from the cerebellum usually obstruct CSF pathways, these tumors present with obstructive hydrocephalus and cerebellar signs. Many childhood tumors are thought to be congenital in origin, making the histology and prognosis considerably different from tumors found in adulthood. Although tumors in children may arise from glial origins as in adults, these tumors often grow in the brain stem, presenting the cranial nerve paresis that may lead to respiratory compromise. Like tumors in adults, brain tumors in children may also present with seizures and focal neurologic deficit. The differential diagnosis of brain tumors in children can usually be made on the basis of the location and chronicity of symptoms. A CT scan usually suffices to confirm the location and give important clues as to the histologic nature of these tumors (Fig. 11.8). Since the calvarial sutures are not fused until late in the first decade of life, the appearance of many of the symptoms of brain tumors in children may be delayed by the expansibility of the skull.

Anesthetic Management

Operations for infratentorial tumors in children under age 2 years usually are performed in the prone position. This is due to the small size of the patient and difficulty in securing the seated position on the operating table. Since these children usually have hydrocephalus, the possibility of ventricular collapse and subdural collections is decreased by the prone position. All the precautions already described for this position must be taken. Children over 2 years often are operated on in the sitting position, although some neurosurgeons prefer to do all posterior fossa operations in a modified prone position.

Premedication with atropine is given if there are excess secretions, often found when there are decreased pharyngeal reflexes. Otherwise this drug is avoided because of its drying effects. In the absence of an established intravenous route, induction with rectal thiopental or isoflurane is used. The establishment of a large-bore intravenous route is necessary as blood replacement is frequent. If required, cannulation of the interior jugular vein is preferable to and easier than subclavian puncture. Direct measure of blood pressure by arterial cannulation should be undertaken where possible. Frequently it is easier to insert a small scalp vein needle in the dorsalis pedis or posterior tibial artery rather than in the radial artery in the small infant. Routine urinary catheterization is not essential in babies and may be harmful because of the small meatus. Usually credéing these infants intraoperatively is sufficient.

Many children will come to the operating room maintained on corticosteroid medication, usually dexamethasone. Since this medication has been used in pharmacologic doses to reduce brain swelling, the drug must be continued according to the preoperative schedule. In children with posterior fossa tumors and obstructive hydrocephalus a ventriculostomy usually is inserted preoperatively or intraoperatively. Some pediatric neurosurgeons prefer placement of a shunt preoperatively to reduce intracranial hypertension. In the event that the ICP remains high despite these maneuvers or ventricular cannulation is not possible, either mannitol (1 gm/kg) or furosemide (1 mg/kg) may be given to reduce ICP. Furosemide may be preferable for infants because of the relatively small volume needed to produce a diuretic effect. Depending on the state of preoperative hydration, fluids are administered at the rate of 2 to 5 ml/kg/hr using 0.25% N saline in 5% dextrose solutions. These solutions must be warmed, as should the irrigating solutions used by the surgeon, to minimize hypothermia. As detailed earlier, the surgeon must be cautioned to avoid alcohol or acetone skin cleansing, which leads to excessive heat loss.

At the conclusion of the operation, the patient should be responsive. The endotracheal tube may be removed when the patient is fully conscious with stable cardiovascular and respiratory function. Usually the patients are nursed in the position in which they have been operated. A child operated on in the sitting position should be nursed with the bed at a 60-degree angle. This is done to ensure that the hemostasis achieved in the operating room is maintained in the postoperative period. A nasogastric tube should be passed at the end of the procedure to empty the stomach, especially if the cranial nerve reflexes have been depressed in the preoperative period. In children with brain-stem tumors, a laryngoscope may be used to check the movement of the vocal cords. Feeding should be withheld until gag reflexes have been reestablished.

The management of patients with supratentorial tumors is similar to that employed in adult patients. Special care must be taken with those patients having procedures in the sellar and parasellar area, since they may present transient or permanent diabetes insipidus and pituitary insufficiency. Children with diabetes insipidus prior to the operation will already have been treated with pitressin. This drug is usually continued during the operative period with judicious administration of maintenance intravenous fluids. In this setting, a careful and frequent intraoperative monitoring of serum osmolarity, serum electrolytes, and urinary output must be maintained. In children with craniopharyngiomas, who may develop diabetes insipidus intraoperatively or postoperatively, it has been our practice not to administer pitressin in the preoperative or intraoperative period. While some have advocated this policy, the preoperative administration of pitressin may lead to fluid overload, especially in those children who are not destined to develop diabetes insipidus. Also, diabetes insipidus is usually transient and onset may be delayed for several hours, not occurring until such time as the child is fully awake and can cooperate enough to be given vasopressin by nasal insufflation. Onset of action is within a few minutes. On the other hand, continued unnecessary administration of pitressin may lead to delayed complications.

VASCULAR DISORDERS

The incidence of vascular disorders of the central nervous system in the pediatric population is low. Until recently interest in these pathologic disorders was essentially academic. The picture is changing now because of several factors, among them improved techniques of radiologic diagnosis and surgical treatment and the significant improvement in the perioperative anesthetic management of these patients. In general, it can be said that the clinical presentation is dependent on the age of the patient (34).

Intracranial Bleeding of the Newborn

Intraventricular hemorrhage (IVH) originates in the subependymal germinal matrix and usually ruptures into the ventricles of the low birth weight premature infant (35,36). Almost invariably associated with respiratory distress syndrome of the newborn, there is increased ICP, frequently increased muscle tone, convulsions, and depending on the amount of bleeding, anemia. CT scan or ultrasonography confirms the diagnosis. Although the prognosis was considered poor in the past with a mortality in the range of 80% to 90%, earlier treatment coupled with increasing diagnosis of less severe hemorrhages has increased the number of survivors. The anesthesiologist's involvement is twofold: the need for immediate resuscitation and ventilatory assistance, both for the respiratory distress syndrome as well as for the elevated ICP, and during the operative management of survivors who develop hydrocephalus.

Aneurysm of the Vein of Galen

The low incidence of this condition is exemplified by the discovery by Gold, Ransohoff, and Carter in 1964 of only 34 case reports in the literature (37). Twelve years later, review by Yasargil and colleagues yielded only 177 cases (38). Such aneurysms, however rare, are extremely challenging because of the complexity of their diagnosis and management. This entity is a clear example of the relationship between age and clinical presentation.

There are basically three clinical pictures:

1.	The newborn with severe congestive heart failure, symptomatic in the first hours of life. Usually these patients have macrocrania, and cranial bruit is easily heard over the fontanelle. It is not uncommon for these babies to undergo cardiac catheterization for possible congenital heart malformation. Suspected diagnosis depends on high oxygen saturation of the blood in the superior vena cava and jugular veins, narrow arteriovenous oxygen difference, pulmonary hypertension, peripheral unsaturation, and wide pulse pressures (39,40). Definitive diagnosis is made by cerebral angiography.

2. In some newborns the cardiac failure is mild and may escape detection until, as infants, they are studied for macrocrania. The hydrocephalus is due to obstruction of the third ventricle or the Sylvian aqueduct by the aneurysm. A loud cranial bruit usually is present. In this group of patients, bleeding from the aneurysm is uncommon (41).

3. In older children and adolescents the initial symptom frequently is a migrainelike headache that may or may not be associated with hydrocephalus. Usually there is no evidence of cardiac failure, although sometimes they have episodes of exercise syncope (42). Spontaneous subarachnoid hemorrhage is uncommon.

The treatment for the newborn in severe congestive heart failure must be prompt. Without treatment the result is uniformly fatal. Since these patients are in congestive heart failure, angiographic studies with contrast media have an increased risk. The operation in itself is a major "tour de force." Craniotomy with potential for considerable bleeding may be done in a modified sitting position with significant risk of air embolism, in a patient in congestive heart failure that may be aggravated by a too rapid occlusion of the malformation. The procedure should be undertaken with full monitoring support, for sudden, rapid changes can occur during obliteration of the malformation. While controlled hypotension would appear useful, this technique coupled with the low diastolic pressure found in these infants leads to myocardial ischemia and cardiac arrest. Close communication with the surgeon is needed, for obliteration of a large feeding vessel may significantly alter hemodynamics and cause sudden high-output failure. In contrast to others, we have not used profound hypothermia and extracorporeal circulation (43).

Arteriovenous Malformation

The most frequent presentation of arteriovenous malformation is intracranial hemorrhage; however, about 20% to 30% of patients present with seizures. A smaller percentage may come to attention because of headache, and a few cases of vascular disorders are incidental findings. Of children presenting with subarachnoid hemorrhages, leakage from arteriovenous malformations is a more common cause than ruptured aneurysms (Fig. 11.9).

Arteriovenous malformations become manifest clinically more frequently in the adolescent years. They generally are located in the cerebral hemispheres and present with bleeding. Aneurysms occur more commonly in children with essential hypertension, coarctation of the aorta, and polycystic kidneys. They

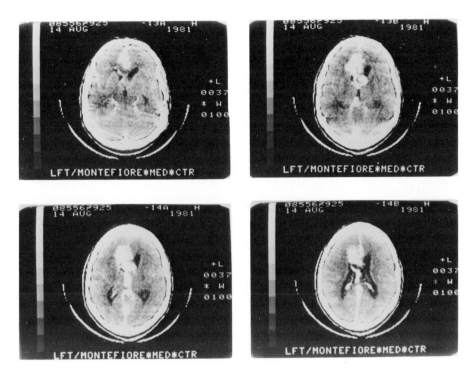

Figure 11.9 This CT scan, taken after injection of contrast, shows an arteriovenous malformation of the corpus callosum. Blood density in the third ventricle (*bottom left*) indicates recent hemorrhage.

tend to be larger than in adults. Compared with adults, their initial presentation is more often as a mass than as subarachnoid bleeding. Clinical aspects and surgical treatment of aneurysms have been reviewed by Matson (44), Patel and Richardson (45), and Amacher and Drake (46), and arteriovenous malformations by Moyes (47), Long et al. (48), and Kelly, Mellinger, and Sundt (49).

The anesthetic management of patients with vascular disorders is similar to that used in the adult population (50). Some minor differences include the use of heavier preoperative sedation (pentobarbital 3 mg/kg intramuscularly one hour before surgery) and use of the internal jugular veins for central venous cannulation, as there is less risk of hemothorax. The technique of monitoring is the same as in the adult patient.

Long-term follow-up of pediatric patients operated for vascular disorders is not available. In experienced hands the perioperative mortality for aneurysms and arteriovenous malformations, with the exception of vein of Galen malformation, is less than 5%. For patients with aneurysms of the vein of Galen, the mortality is still extremely high (about 75%).

The incidence in childhood of cerebrovascular accidents owing to occlusive disease is very low. Characteristically, intracranial vessels are involved as opposed to the involvement of large extracranial vessels seen in adults (51,52). Among the occlusive disorders, moyamoya disease is characterized by multiple progressive involvement of the intracranial part of the internal carotid, anterior, and middle cerebral arteries (53). Different treatments have been attempted, such as bilateral cervical sympathectomies (54) and extracranial-intracranial bypass surgery. These efforts have not been critically evaluated, however.

HEAD TRAUMA

Incidence

Trauma is the most common cause of death below the age of 14; about 25% of these deaths are caused by head trauma (34). Perinatal trauma causes one-third of the neonatal deaths occurring within the first 14 days of life (55).

It can be said that all children will sustain head trauma of different intensity at one time or another, and one child in ten will be rendered unconscious by the injury. In the United States this represents more than 200,000 hospital admissions per year (56). In Glasgow, one-third of the cases of severe head trauma and half of the admissions with depressed skull fracture were patients of 16 years of age or less (57). Among the causes of head trauma in children are motor vehicle accidents (usually as pedestrian victims), falls, injuries during play, and the syndrome of the battered child. It is fortunate that the mortality rate in children after severe head trauma is less than in the adult population and that the incidence of disability is also less. The exact reasons for this are not known.

Management

While the general principles of management of pediatric head injury parallel those described elsewhere in this volume for adults (see Chapters 15–17), certain differences exist. First, the immature brain apparently responds to injury with hyperemia, resulting in a higher incidence of intracranial hypertension in severe head injury (58,59). If diuresis is indicated, furosemide is preferable to mannitol, which initially increases blood volume. The raised ICP in these children appears more responsive to barbiturate therapy than in adults. Second, surgical lesions in head-injured children are less frequent than in adults. Because of the disproportionate size of the head of infants relative to body size, however, a significant percentage of circulating volume can be lost intracranially prior to operation. Blood must be available for transfusion prior to operating on large intracranial hematomas in infants and small children (Fig. 11.10). Also, because of the flexible calvarium, depressed skull fractures can occur in infants and young children without scalp laceration. Since these injuries are not compound, surgical treatment is less urgent than in adults.

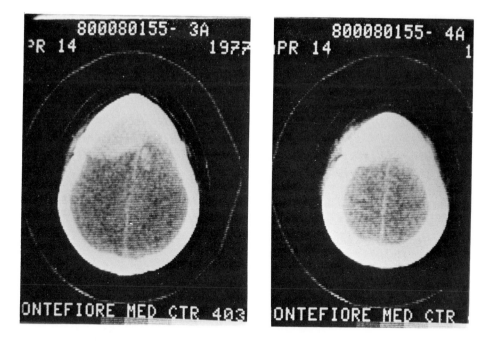

Figure 11.10 This CT scan shows a left frontal epidural hematoma in a young child. Falling hematocrit was the earliest clinical sign of the nature of this child's lesion.

Prognosis

In cases of cerebral contusion, the long-term prognosis is a function of the severity of the injury as well as its location. In cases of extradural hematoma without signs of brain-stem compression, and if there is prompt evacuation of the mass, the patient usually returns to normal. Unfortunately, the mortality for acute subdural hematomas associated with cerebral contusion is still greater than 50%.

Overall, the chances of recovery after severe head trauma are better in children than in adults. Children have a remarkable ability to recover, and it is difficult to make a prognosis in the first few days of coma. Long-term studies by Brink and co-workers (60) have shown that 87% of children who sustained head trauma severe enough to be in a coma for an average of seven weeks were able to recover sufficient motor function to be independent in ambulation and self-care. Unfortunately, the motor recovery does not parallel intellectual recovery, and significant deficits were found in intelligence test scores. Heiskanen and Kaste (61) studied school performance in 36 children after a period of four to ten years following a severe head trauma. Only 50% of the patients recovered enough to be classified as "doing fairly normal," and about 25% were unable to return to normal schools. However pessimistic these results may be, it is necessary to remember that intellectual improvement may continue for years following the injury.

REFERENCES

1. Smith RM: Anesthesia for infants and children, ed 4. St. Louis, CV Mosby, 1980.
2. Coppoletta JM, Wolbach SB: Body length and organ weights of infants and children. Am J Pathol 1933;9:55-70.
3. Crouzon MO: Dysostose craniofaciale héréditaire. Bull Mem Soc Med Hop Paris 1912;33:545-555.
4. Shillito J, Matson DD: Craniosynostosis: A review of 519 surgical patients. J Pediatr 1968;41:829-853.
5. Bain JA, Spoerel WE: A streamlined anaesthetic system. Can Anaesth Soc J 1972;19:426-435.
6. Bain JA, Spoerel WE: Flow requirements for a modified Mapleson D system during controlled ventilation. Can Anaesth Soc J 1973;20:629-636.
7. Henville JD, Adams AP: The Bain anaesthetic system. Anaesthesia 1976;31:247-256.
8. Tessier P, Guiot G, Rougerie et al.: Ostéotomies cranio-naso-orbito-faciales: Hypertélorisme. Ann Chir Plast 1967;12:103-118.
9. Tessier P: The definitive plastic surgical treatment of the severe facial deformities of craniofacial dysostoses: Crouzon's and Apert's disease. Plast Reconstr Surg 1971; 48:419-442.
10. Converse JM, Wood-Smith K, McCarthy JG, et al.: Craniofacial surgery. Clin Plast Surg 1974;1:499-557.
11. Epstein FJ, Wood-Smith D, Converse JM, et al.: Radical one-stage correction of craniofacial anomalies. J Neurosurg 1975;42:522-529.
12. Matthews DN: Experiences in major craniofacial surgery. Plast Reconstr Surg 1977;59:163-174.
13. Davies DW, Munro IR: The anesthetic management and intraoperative care of patients undergoing major facial osteotomies. Plast Reconstr Surg 1975;55:50-55.
14. Matson DD: Neurosurgery of infancy and childhood. Springfield, Ill, Charles C Thomas, 1969.
15. Creighton RE, Relton JS, Meridy HW: Anaesthesia for occipital encephalocele. Can Anaesth Soc J 1974;21:403-406.
16. Milhorat TH: Pediatric neurosurgery. Philadelphia, FA Davis, 1978, pp 155-157.
17. Carter CO, Roberts JA: The risk of recurrence after two children with central nervous system malformations. Lancet 1967;1:306-308.
18. Fitzsimmons JS: Laryngeal stridor and respiratory obstruction associated with myelomeningocele. Dev Med Child Neurol 1973;15:533-536.
19. Schroeder, HG, Williams NE: Anesthesia for meningomyelocele surgery. Anaesthesia 1966;21:57-65.
20. Milhorat TH: The third circulation revisited. J Neurosurg 1975;42:628-645.
21. Milhorat TH: Congenital hydrocephalus, in Sano K, Ishii S, LeVay S (eds): Recent progress in neurological surgery. Amsterdam, Excerpta Medica, 1973, pp 67-73.
22. Rubin RD, Henderson ES, Ommaya AK, et al.: The production of cerebrospinal fluid in man and its modification by acetazolamide. J Neurosurg 1966;25:430-436.
23. Schain RJ: Carbonic anhydrase inhibitors in chronic infantile hydrocephalus. Am J Dis Child 1969;117:621-625.
24. Lorber J: Isosorbide in the medical treatment of infantile hydrocephalus. J Neurosurg 1973;39:702-711.
25. Hemmer R, Bohn B: Once a shunt, always a shunt? Dev Med Child Neurol 1976; 18:69-73.

26. Wald SL, McLaurin RL: Shunt-associated glomerulonephritis. Neurosurgery 1978;3: 146–150.

27. Schoenbaum SC, Gardner P, Shillito J: Infections of cerebrospinal fluid shunts: Epidemiology, clinical manifestations and therapy. J Infect Dis 1975;131:543–552.

28. George R, Leibrock L, Epstein M: Long-term analysis of cerebrospinal fluid shunt infections. J Neurosurg 1979;51:804–811.

29. Rockoff MA: Anesthesia for children with hydrocephalus. Anesth Rev 1979;6: 28–34.

30. Watson GH: Effect of head rotation on jugular vein blood flow. Arch Dis Child 1974;49:237–239.

31. Oakes WJ, Wilkins RH: Neurosurgical considerations, in Filston HC: Surgical problems in children. Recognition and referral. St. Louis, CV Mosby, 1982, pp 382–409.

32. Milhorat TH: Pediatric neurosurgery. Philadelphia, FA Davis, 1978, pp 211–283.

33. Hooper R: Intracranial tumors in childhood. Med J Aust 1976;1:624–627.

34. Oakes WJ, Wilkins RH: Neurosurgical considerations, in Filston HC: Surgical problems in children. Recognition and referral. St. Louis, CV Mosby, 1982, pp 488–547.

35. Larroche JC: Hémorrhagies cérébrales intra-ventriculaires chez le prémature. I. Anatomie et physiopathologie. Biol Neonatol 1964;7:26–56.

36. Towbin A: Cerebral hypoxic damage in fetus and newborn. Arch Neurol 1969; 20:35–43.

37. Gold AP, Ransohoff J, Carter S: Vein of Galen malformation. Acta Neurol Scand 1964;40:5–31.

38. Yasargil MG, Antic J, Laciga R, et al.: Arteriovenous malformations of vein of Galen: Microsurgical treatment. Surg Neurol 1976;6:195–200.

39. Levy AM, Hanson JS, Tabakin BS: Congestive heart failure in the newborn infant in the absence of primary cardiac disease. Am J Cardiol 1970;26:409–415.

40. Holden AM, Fyler DC, Shillito J, et al.: Congestive heart failure from intracranial arteriovenous fistula in infancy. Pediatrics 1972;39:30–39.

41. Amacher AL, Shillito J: The syndromes and surgical treatment of aneurysms of the great vein of Galen. J Neurosurg 1973;39:89–98.

42. Milhorat TH: Pediatric neurosurgery. Philadelphia, FA Davis, 1978, pp 311–345.

43. Hood JB, Wallace CT, Mahaffey JE: Anesthetic management of an intracranial arteriovenous malformation in infancy. Anesth Analg (Cleve) 1977;56:236–241.

44. Matson DD: Intracranial arterial aneurysms in childhood. J Neurosurg 1965;23: 578–583.

45. Patel AN, Richarson AE: Ruptured intracranial aneurysms in the first two decades of life. J Neurosurg 1971;35:571–576.

46. Amacher AL, Drake CG: Cerebral artery aneurysms in infancy, childhood and adolescence. Childs Brain 1975;1:72–80.

47. Moyes PD: Intracranial and intraspinal vascular anomalies in children. J Neurosurg 1969;31:371–378.

48. Long DM, Seljeskg EL, Chore SN, et al.: Giant arteriovenous malformations of infancy and childhood. J Neurosurg 1974;50:304–312.

49. Kelly JJ, Mellinger JF, Sundt T: Intracranial arteriovenous malformations in childhood. Ann Neurol 1978;3:338–343.

50. Arancibia CU, Babinski MF, Albin MS, et al.: The experts opine. Induced hypotension during neurosurgical procedures. Surv Anesthesiol 1981;25:406–413.

51. Chiofalo N, Madsen J, Fuentes A, et al.: Occlusive arterial disease of the child and young adult. Childs Brain 1978;4:1-14.
52. Solomon GE, Hilal S, Gold P, et al.: Natural history of acute hemiplegia of childhood. Brain 1970;93:107-120.
53. Susuki J, Takaku A: Cerebrovascular moyamoya disease. Arch Neurol 1969;20: 288-299.
54. Susuki J, Takaku A, Kodama N, et al.: An attempt to treat cerebrovascular "moyamoya" disease in children. Childs Brain 1975;1:193-206.
55. Natelson SE, Sayers MP: The fate of children sustaining severe head trauma during birth. Pediatrics 1973;51:169-174.
56. Milhorat TH: Pediatric neurosurgery. Philadelphia, FA Davis, 1978, pp 41-89.
57. Jennett B: Head injuries in children. Dev Med Child Neurol 1972;14:137-147.
58. Bruce DA, Schut L, Bruno LA, et al.: Outcome following severe head injuries in children. J Neurosurg 1978;48:679-688.
59. Shapiro K, Marmarou A: Clinical applications of the pressure volume index in treatment of pediatric head injuries. J Neurosurg 1982;56:819-825.
60. Brink JD, Gareett AL, Hale WR, et al.: Recovery of motor and intellectual function in children sustaining severe head injuries. Dev Med Child Neurol 1970;12:565-571.
61. Heiskanen O, Kaste M: Late prognosis of severe brain injury in children. Dev Med Child Neurol 1970;12:565-571.

CHAPTER 12

Surgery for Seizures
Philip L. Gildenberg

Hughlings Jackson was the first to recognize that seizures might originate in a focal area of abnormality of the brain (1). At his recommendation the neurosurgical management of epilepsy was introduced in 1886 by Horsley, who excised a posttraumatic cortical scar under general anesthesia from a 22-year-old man who had no further seizures following the operation (2). Surgical management of epilepsy during the subsequent 65 years, however, was confined to the resection of demonstrable lesions, such as meningiomas or arteriovenous malformations, or recognized areas of focal scarring.

Electrical stimulation of the cortex to elicit manifestations of epilepsy was initiated in 1925 by Foerster (3), who also reported the first electrical recordings from the exposed cerebral cortex, electrocorticography, to identify an epileptic focus (4). After working with Foerster, Wilder Penfield began his studies on epilepsy in Montreal in 1928. He and Jasper (5) improved the technique of intraoperative recording and began what has become the standard approach to epilepsy surgery.

It was not until 1951, when Bailey and Gibbs (6) reported resection of the anterior portion of the temporal lobe based solely on preoperative electroencephalographic evidence, that it became feasible to plan surgery based on presurgical electrical localization in the absence of an anatomic abnormality. This report was soon followed by others from the Montreal Neurological Institute, which refined the techniques for localization of foci of partial seizures and for subtotal temporal lobectomy, procedures that form the basis of present-day seizure surgery. Additional refinements have been made to provide more accurate localization of the origin of epileptogenic electrical activity as well as functionally important areas of the brain, so the seizure focus may be identified by preoperative or intraoperative recording and the extirpation of that focus and adjacent brain tissue can be accomplished without neurologic impairment (5,7,8).

Localization of electrical foci has been further enhanced by the use of depth electrodes (9,10,11), since not all epileptogenic foci can be identified by scalp or sphenoidal electrodes alone. Computed tomography (CT) makes it possible to identify abnormal areas of the brain, which previously would have been undetected prior to resection (12). Future developments will undoubtedly include detection of abnormal areas of cerebral metabolism (13), alterations in cerebral blood flow (14,15) and identification of seizure foci by nuclear magnetic resonance (16).

EPILEPSY

The most common form of epilepsy is manifested as partial complex seizures that originate in a focal or circumscribed region of the brain and may be expressed with automatisms or automatic psychomotor activity, with psychosensory or ideational symptoms, affective or visceral symptoms, or impaired consciousness only, usually resulting from a focus or a lesion in the mesial part of the temporal lobe.

Focal symptoms and signs may be the only clinical manifestation, or initially there may be focal abnormalities that ultimately spread to produce generalized convulsions or other signs of widespread cerebral involvement. In contrast, generalized seizures almost instantaneously involve widespread areas of the brain or the entire cortex.

The incidence of epilepsy in the United States is approximately 5:1000, or an estimated 1.1 million patients. About 70% are managed satisfactorily with anticonvulsant medications (17); 30% of those managed medically may achieve complete seizure control, 50% have only occasional seizures, and the remainder achieve only borderline control. About 10% of patients will have no success with medical management. One must also consider that anticonvulsant drugs have serious side effects, especially with long-term usage, such as bone marrow suppression, gingival hyperplasia, unsteadiness, drowsiness, difficulty with concentration, or personality changes.

Recent evidence suggests that the occurrence of seizures may cause progressive neurologic impairment, so that one should be aggressive in trying to obtain complete seizure control in any patient who may be a candidate for treatment. Consequently, many patients with epilepsy can be managed in an optimal fashion only with carefully selected neurosurgical procedures (18). Although it has been estimated that between 25,000 and 100,000 patients in the United States with intractable partial seizures would be candidates for surgical therapy if they were evaluated, only about 200 procedures are performed in this country per year.

In order to be considered for surgery, several basic criteria must be met:

1. The seizure disorder must be partial, except in those patients who may have seizures secondary to a focal cicatrix after head injury.
2. The patient must have had an adequate trial of medical management without satisfactory control.
3. An underlying etiology such as a brain tumor or arteriovenous malformation must be ruled out, since treatment in those cases is directed toward the underlying lesion rather than the seizures per se.
4. Preoperative electrical studies should allow identification of the epileptogenic focus and localization in a resectable area, such as the temporal lobe.

5.   The patient should not have excessive diffuse cerebral damage, as evidenced by mental retardation or psychosis. Success is far less likely in such patients, especially if the IQ is below 70, and control of seizures is not likely to improve such underlying neurologic deficits or disability.

If it can be determined that the origin of the seizures is unilateral and the origin is a single focus in a resectable area, preferably the temporal lobe, en bloc resection of the anterior temporal lobe is indicated.

Fortunately, the anterior 5 to 6 cm of either temporal lobe or up to 8 to 10 cm of the nondominant temporal lobe can be resected unilaterally without significant neurologic deficit. Such resection may lead to seizure control, and it is the combination of these factors that makes it possible to treat epilepsy with temporal lobe surgery.

The original concept was that an epileptogenic lesion was limited to a small discrete area of the cortex, and if the focus were excised, control of epilepsy would result (19). Rasmussen has demonstrated that the epileptogenic area may be fairly extensive, a zone rather than a focus, and the success of the surgery is related to the completeness of the excision of the epileptogenic cortex (20–22). He demonstrated also that it is possible to convert a poor result into complete seizure control by repeating the surgery and extirpating additional temporal lobe tissue.

PREOPERATIVE EVALUATION

Patient selection involves screening a large number of epilepsy patients and providing optimal medical management in order to identify those patients who defy medical control and meet the above criteria. The details of preoperative evaluation vary from institution to institution, based to some extent on the experience and sophistication of the treatment team. At the minimum, the team should include a neurologist with an interest in epilepsy, who can screen the large number of patients to identify those who might be candidates for surgery and provide sophisticated medical management in order to identify those patients best treated conservatively. An electroencephalographer must also be available in the operating room at the time of surgery and should be the same individual who supervises the preoperative electroencephalograms. The ability to perform prolonged electroencephalographic (EEG) studies is important, and telemetered 24-hour recordings may be ideal. For those patients in whom scalp recording is not definitive, the surgeon should be familiar with and have access to the use of subdural electrodes and should have the capability for stereotactic insertion of depth electrodes for subcortical recording.

The preoperative evaluation is begun with an attempt to localize the seizure focus or origin with repeated scalp EEGs. If a unilateral interictal focus of epileptiform activity can be identified, the patient may be considered for surgery. If an interictal focus is not identifiable, it often is helpful to record a seizure in order to note the site from which the seizure activity originates and from where it is propagated. If a seizure does not occur during a recording session, it may be necessary to perform 24-hour monitoring with EEG telemetry. Since many patients have their seizures while asleep, random EEG sampling during the usual hours of operation of the electrophysiologic laboratory may not be adequate. Seizures originating from the mesial surface of the temporal lobe are most difficult to identify with a scalp EEG, although such seizures are among the most successfully treated with surgery. It may be helpful to record from sphenoidal leads in patients undergoing electroencephalography to evaluate epilepsy (7,8,10).

If a unilateral temporal focus of epileptogenic activity cannot be identified on scalp and sphenoidal EEG or 24-hour monitoring, subdural electrodes may be employed. Since the scalp diffuses and averages electrical activity from beneath, much sharper localization can be obtained by recording from the cortex. Subdural electrodes can be readily inserted through small burr holes, left in place for one to two weeks and removed at the time of temporal lobe resection.

If the localization still is not discrete, electrodes may be implanted stereotactically into the temporal lobes for direct subcortical recording. The electrodes are placed through twist drill holes and emerge through the scalp for direct access. They can be left in place for one to two weeks or more. Localization from a discrete subcortical site, particularly from the amygdaloid area, may identify a focus that can be resected by temporal lobectomy. Insertion of such electrodes is not entirely without risk; there is a 2% to 4% rate of complications, primarily involving hemorrhage or occlusion of blood vessels. The risk can be minimized by identifying the stereotactic coordinates of the major vessels and planning the insertion of the electrodes.

Preoperative CT scanning should include the use of intravenous contrast material and may provide corroborative demonstration of areas of abnormal cortex (12), particularly if a high dose of contrast agent and delayed scanning are employed. CT should rule out anatomic lesions that may produce seizures and should be treated primarily.

Four-vessel cerebral angiography should be done to evaluate the vasculature in the area of potential resection and to rule out vascular abnormalities in those areas. At the time of angiography, the opportunity should be taken to perform the Wada test in order to evaluate cerebral dominance (23). While the catheter is in the carotid artery, sodium amobarbital is injected to "anesthetize" a single hemisphere. The patient lies with both arms upraised, speaking, counting, or reciting while the injection is made. The dropping of the contralateral arm indicates that the injected hemisphere is anesthetized. If speech simultaneously abruptly halts, the injected hemisphere may be considered dominant for speech. If not, it is recognized that the noninjected hemisphere participates in speech. Since there may be mixed dominance with both hemispheres participating in speech, it is necessary to test both sides, since knowledge of dominant hemispheres is important in anticipating how much brain tissue can be safely resected.

Some centers also perform positron emission tomography (PET) scanning or cerebral blood flow measurements, but the use of these techniques is still investigational (14).

Prognosis

Some institutions have elaborate preoperative evaluation protocols. For instance, the presurgical protocol used at the University of California at Los Angeles involves two phases. Phase one includes 24-hour scalp and sphenoidal EEG telemetry and videotape monitoring for one to two weeks. Patients with clearly defined and consistent focal electrical characteristics and focal cerebral dysfunction in the same area are considered for surgery without further investigation. Phase two involves telemetry with stereotactically implanted depth electrodes. Since the two-phase protocol was instituted in 1977, one-third of those patients identified with the phase one protocol (the best candidates) are rendered seizure free or almost seizure free with surgery. Most patients who underwent the phase two depth electrode evaluation followed by surgery had only occasional seizures (7), demonstrating that results of surgery can be improved with this conscientious sophisticated approach.

It can be stated conservatively that after temporal lobe resection in carefully selected patients, one-third of the patients will be seizure free without medication, one-third will have significant reduction in the frequency of seizures and/or reduction in medication requirements, and one-third will be unchanged or, rarely, worse. It should be noted that improvement in electrophysiologic localization techniques has produced more favorable results. The surgery is relatively safe, but 2% of patients suffer some major complication, infection being the most common surgical problem, and hemiparesis from interruption of blood vessels to the internal capsule the greatest neurologic risk. It is common for patients to have a small visual field deficit following temporal lobe extirpation, usually a superior quadrantanopsia, which is only rarely a problem or even symptomatic. An occasional patient will suffer a minor verbal memory deficit, particularly if there was a preoperative memory problem, presumably because the opposite temporal lobe may be partially impaired and unable to compensate.

In the experience at the Montreal Neurological Institute, 20% of 1902 patients operated for seizures had tumors or vascular malformation, leaving 1515, of whom 1407 were followed for at least two years (24). Of that group 33% were seizure free and 32% had a marked reduction of seizure tendency. In the entire series, there were 18 postoperative deaths. Of the entire group, there were 18 postoperative deaths (less than 1%).

ANESTHETIC CONSIDERATIONS

Ideally, craniotomy and temporal lobe resection for epilepsy are performed under local anesthesia, so that intraoperative electrical recording can be done and the patient tested for areas of neurologic importance, such as speech. This presents a challenge for both surgeon and anesthesiologist. Preanesthetic assessment should determine whether there are any complications of the long-term administration of anticonvulsants. Liver function studies should be performed to assess any hepatic damage. A complete blood count, including reticulocyte count, should be done to document bone marrow depression. The mouth and teeth should be inspected for gingival hyperplasia that may be associated with loose dentition or a difficult airway.

Anesthetic goals in seizure surgery are as follows:

1. The patient should have sufficient sedation or analgesia to tolerate the craniotomy and remain immobile on the operating table for the necessary time, often six to eight hours. Nervous or apprehensive patients may require psychic as well as pharmacologic sedation.
2. Medications should have minimal interference with electrocortography or depth electrical recordings.
3. Pharmacologic agents should not interfere with EEG response to electrical or drug-induced stimulation of seizure activity.
4. The patient should be alert and cooperative enough to participate in verbal and motor testing.

The local anesthetic agent must meet several criteria:

1. It must provide local insensibility of tissues lasting for at least six to eight hours.
2. It should have sufficiently prompt onset of action.
3. Since greater absorption of most parenterally administered local anesthetics influences the EEG, particularly by increasing seizure activity, doses must be small enough to avoid these changes.

The local anesthetic combination recommended is lidocaine 1%, bupivacaine 0.25%, and epinephrine 1:200,000. Up to 40 cc may be used. This concentration may be obtained by mixing equal amounts of lidocaine 2% containing 1:100,000 epinephrine with bupivacaine 0.5%.

Although lidocaine may have an anticonvulsive effect at blood levels of 0.5 to 4.7 ug/ml(25), even 1:200,000 epinephrine in 0.5% lidocaine allows only a transient elevation of blood lidocaine levels, which returns to less than 0.2 ug/ml by the end of 10 minutes (26). Sudden intravascular administration of large doses may cause seizures, however.

A minimum dose of pharmacologic agents should be employed to achieve adequate analgesia or sedation, but, when it is necessary to employ those agents to meet the above goals, a knowledge of the effect of those agents on the recording of electrical activity is mandatory.

In estimating the required dose of drug or anesthetic agent, it is important to recognize that long-term anticonvulsant administration may lead to enzyme induction, which increases the rate of detoxification, so the dose may be adjusted upward accordingly or more frequent doses administrated.

The recommended sedation—intravenous droperidol, 2.5 mg, and fentanyl, 0.05 mg (27)—or other narcotics provide both analgesia and sedation and have minimal effects on the EEG (28). This combination of drugs may be repeated as necessary during the procedure, particularly during the initial stages of the craniotomy and elevation of the bone flap (29).

Nitrous oxide/oxygen at usual anesthetic doses does not appear to have any effect on limbic neuronal firing, even in patients with limbic epileptogenic foci

(30), which makes it a valuable agent during intraoperative recording of cortical and subcortical activity. If used alone, it does not suppress awareness sufficiently to be considered a general anesthetic, but it may be combined with other agents that have minimal effect on electrical recording. It does, however, have an analgesic effect similar to that of narcotics (31).

Diazepam is an effective anticonvulsant. Consequently, it should be avoided prior to the electrical recording session since it may mask seizure activity. Nevertheless, it may be a valuable drug if a frank seizure occurs during surgery, in which case it should be given slowly intravenously at the rate of 1 to 2 mg/min. The infusion is stopped as soon as there is a decrease in seizure activity and should not be continued until the seizure stops completely, since the patient's level of consciousness will continue to diminish. Respiration should be observed closely throughout administration. Although the duration of anticonvulsant activity is relatively short and electrical recording can be resumed within 30 minutes of administration of diazepam, it should not be used unless necessary.

Barbiturates, on the other hand, should be avoided. Although the short-acting barbiturates, such as thiopental, may cause prompt control of a seizure, the seizure may recur immediately after the short-acting barbiturate is metabolized. The longer-acting barbiturates may interfere with electrical recording throughout the procedure. In addition, the respiratory depressant effects of the barbiturates for a given anticonvulsive effect may be greater than that of diazepam.

Ketamine hydrochloride, a rapidly acting injectable anesthetic that produces a catatonic state associated with analgesia, may cause profound alterations in the EEG. During normal routine EEG, ketamine may produce alternating high-amplitude delta complexes and periods of fast activity. If abnormal focal paroxysmal activity exists, the effect of ketamine on the abnormality is variable (32). The EEG effects of ketamine have been interpreted as depression of the thalamo-neocortical system with activation of the limbic system (33–36). Consequently, it is generally recommended that ketamine be avoided in epileptic patients for fear of promoting frank seizures (37) and because the induced EEG changes may make interpretation difficult.

In general, it is advisable to avoid antihistamines in patients with focal epilepsy, since small doses can activate focal seizures, even at doses below those required for sedation, Also, antihistamines may cause excitement and hyperventilation rather than sedation in some patients (38).

Patients who are too young to have surgery under local anesthesia or patients who are too anxious or unable to cooperate for other reasons may require general anesthesia, and are candidates for surgery only if preoperative electrical localization is unquestionable. Some centers use general anesthesia with an intraoperative period of awakening to allow electrical recording and/or psychomotor testing, but the variability of patient response to anesthetic agents and the difficulty with testing a drowsy patient often make this procedure unsatisfactory.

If the seizure focus is well documented from preoperative studies, routine general anesthesia may be employed if no intraoperative recording is contemplated. If intraoperative electrocorticography is to be done, however, nitrous oxide/oxygen may be employed, supplemented as necessary with intravenous narcotics. Intratracheal instillation of 4% lidocaine through the lumen of a cuffed endotracheal tube may prevent coughing, even when anesthesia is quite light (39). Halothane, 0.25% to 1%, may be used with nitrous oxide/oxygen if the halothane and nitrous oxide are discontinued five minutes prior to the electrocorticography. If the recording session is not too long, the halothane is sufficient to prevent coughing (40). In addition, methohexital (20 to 25 mg) or other barbiturates may be given by intravenous bolus to activate the seizure focus during the brief interruption of halothane (41). Methohexital may also be used as a continuous intravenous infusion to maintain anesthesia, and may be used with a muscle relaxant (42,43), such as pancuronium.

Enflurane probably should be avoided as it has been identified as a cause of seizure patterns in a dose-related fashion (>2.5%), enhanced by hyperventilation (44). It has been suggested that EEG changes may persist for up to 30 days after enflurane anesthesia in patients who exhibit epileptiform activity preoperatively (45).

One anecdotal report of two cases suggested the development of generalized seizures six to eight days postoperatively related to enflurane or its byproducts (46). The authors conceded, however, that postoperative ischemic or embolic phenomena could not be ruled out, and in a subsequent study one of the authors was unable to confirm any long-term EEG or behavioral abnormalities in animals (47). A recent study on the use of enflurane in patients with a known history of seizures did not show any obvious changes or correlations between the vapor concentrations and intraoperative EEG findings and concluded that the use of this technique was not contraindicated for epileptics (48). Nevertheless, as there are other agents available (isoflurane or halothane) that do not interfere with recording, their use would appear more appropriate.

SURGICAL PROCEDURE

As surgery proceeds by steps, the anesthetic requirements vary from one stage to another. The surgery is ideally performed under local anesthesia, and since anesthetic management of a craniotomy in an awake patient presents a particular challenge, that technique will be considered primarily.

Anesthetic considerations begin prior to surgery. Since it is the anesthesiologist who has the most personal contact with the patient during the operation, it is helpful for the patient to meet the anesthesiologist prior to the stressful operative period. Much of the "sedation" consists of verbal assurance and reinforcement. Describing the procedure allows the patient to anticipate each step and decreases anxiety associated with the unknown. A calm manner is important, especially the reassurance that there is little pain associated with the surgery and that local anesthesia can be supplemented if required. A personal assessment of the patient's level of anxiety and of the requirement for intraoperative sedation should involve the anesthesiologist who will be with the patient throughout the procedure.

No premedication should be given unless the patient specifically requires it. If necessary, small doses of chlorpromazine (2.5 mg) and/or a narcotic may be administered. Sedatives that might interfere with recording or could mask seizure activity should be avoided, as should barbiturates.

The first important step in the operating room is positioning the patient on the operating table in the lateral decubitus position. The arm on which the patient is lying must be sufficiently padded to allow the patient to be comfortable for the long surgical procedure. It is helpful to put a pad under the ribs to relieve some of the pressure on the shoulder.

The type of head holder will vary with the individual surgeon. The patient's head must be secured firmly, however, since the patient may have a seizure during surgery. The author prefers to use the three-pin Mayfield head holder, infiltrating the sites of pin placement with local anesthesia at least 10 minutes before application. The patient should be warned that he will have a constricting sensation about the head, but that it will last for only 5 to 10 minutes. Not only are patients able to tolerate this very well, but the head remains secure even during a grand mal seizure with the brain exposed.

Drapes must be placed in such a way as to allow access to the face to permit the anesthesiologist to converse with the patient. An overhead instrument table is ideal. The drapes may be sutured to the edge of the surgical exposure, using appropriate local anesthetic injection, and can extend from the incision to the overhead table. This creates an area underneath the table where the anesthesiologist can talk to the patient and administer appropriate sensory and motor tests.

A fairly large craniotomy incision is required, extending down to the zygoma for maximum visualization of the tip of the temporal lobe and the inferior temporal gyrus. It is important that the temporalis muscle be well infiltrated with local anesthetic or retraction will cause pain. The local anesthetic should be injected into both the subcutaneous plane and the plane deep to the temporalis fascia, which serves as a barrier to the diffusion of anesthetic.

The patient should be warned beforehand about the noise involved with creating a craniotomy bone flap. The sound of a power drill is distressing, so generally a Hudson brace and Gigli saw are preferred when the patient is awake.

Intracranial structures that are painful to touch include the dura and blood vessels. The dura cannot be anesthetized prior to its exposure, but local anesthetic should be used to irrigate the dura as soon as it appears within the burr hole.

The most painful part of the craniotomy is stripping the dura from the inner table of the bone, since both the dura and middle meningeal artery are manipulated before they can be anesthetized. It may be necessary to provide the patient with additional sedation at that point in the procedure, either with a narcotic or the combination of fentanyl and droperidol. Since physiologic testing occurs soon after the dura is opened, it is inadvisable to use a long-acting agent or one that may interfere with testing.

The dura should be irrigated lightly with local anesthetic agent several minutes prior to opening. Only local anesthetics with epinephrine should be used in order to minimize diffusion to underlying brain tissue. A modest dose should be employed, and the dura should be washed thoroughly with saline before opening to avoid contamination of the cortex with the drug. When the brain is exposed, a direct cortical recording is performed. The electrode array is secured to the craniotomy opening, and recordings may be done with 16 to 24 electrodes to verify the focus of the epileptogenic activity. The most commonly used electrode array consists of a horseshoe-shaped holder that attaches to a post at the edge of the craniotomy opening. The electrodes that contact the cortex are saline-soaked cotton wicks suspended from metal rods attached to the horseshoe. They rest lightly on the cortex to maintain contact atraumatically despite brain pulsation.

Following the recording of spontaneous electrical activity from the cortex, it may be desirable to stimulate the exposed cortex to map out neurologically important areas, particularly if the surgery is on the dominant hemisphere. Because an attempt is made to identify the motor cortex, the anesthesiologist will be asked to observe the patient's face and extremities for involuntary movement provoked by stimulation. The area representing the face and mouth is at the inferior portion of the precentral gyrus or motor cortex, just above the temporal lobe, so it is the motor area most likely to be stimulated. As the stimulating electrode is placed higher on the exposed motor cortex, the contralateral hand may move. Although the patient is usually aware of such involuntary movements, direct observation is important.

As various areas of the temporal or parietal lobe are stimulated, the patient may report thoughts or sensations. Again, it is important to instruct the patient prior to the procedure to report any unusual feelings, and to maintain verbal contact with the patient throughout this portion of the procedure. Obviously, the patient must be awake in order to perceive and report sensations that may be vague or unfamiliar.

The patient may be asked to perform certain tasks so the surgeon can assess the effect of stimulation. The most usual is to test the effect of stimulation on speech. The patient is asked to recite, count, or answer questions. Stimulation of the speech area is signaled by an abrupt interruption in speech, which may be resumed immediately upon cessation of the stimulation. Again, it is important to have an alert patient instructed in the procedure prior to surgery. Occasionally, cortical stimulation will provoke a seizure, which may require small doses of intravenous diazepam (2.5 to 5.0 mg), repeated as necessary.

If localization of the seizure focus is still in doubt after cortical recording, it may be desirable to record from depth electrodes. One or several electrodes may be inserted into the brain by hand or with a micromanipulator. The anesthetic requirements are the same as for recording spontaneous cortical activity, that is, no agent should be used that interferes with spontaneous electrical activity or that might suppress a seizure focus.

After the epileptogenic focus is electrically identified and functional areas of the exposed brain have been mapped out, the anterior portion of the offending temporal lobe is resected. The brain itself has no sensation, but pain is experienced when there is traction or coagulation of blood vessels. It is not always possible to identify blood vessels prior to putting traction on them, and it is desirable to minimize the amount of local anesthetic applied directly to the brain, so the patient may require more sedation for this part of the procedure. It may or may not be necessary to record from the surrounding area after the temporal resection has been completed. The presence of seizure activity in the brain adjacent to the resected brain immediately after resection probably has no prognostic value (49). If it is agreed that postresection recording will not be done, sedation may be used more generously, bearing in mind that ventilation is not controlled so drugs causing respiratory depression should be avoided.

It is usually not necessary to have the patient alert enough to participate in neurologic testing following resection of the temporal lobe. Since, by this time, the patient has been lying still for several hours, sufficient medication may be given to allow the patient to doze throughout the remainder of the procedure.

Following resection of the temporal lobe and establishment of strict hemostasis, the craniotomy incision is closed. The dura is usually closed tightly and the bone flap secured in place prior to closure of each layer of remaining tissues.

POSTOPERATIVE CARE

Even patients who eventually have complete relief from seizures may experience them during the initial postoperative period, and they should be treated like any other patient with this condition. It is sometimes desirable to withhold anticonvulsant medications for one or several days prior to surgery in order to identify the epileptogenic focus more accurately. Since it takes several days for the blood level of anticonvulsants to become established, and the threshold for seizures may be decreased immediately following the resection, the patient may be at additional risk for seizures during the first few days after surgery. In consultation with the neurologist or neurosurgeon, it may be advisable to increase the amount and frequency of intravenous doses of anticonvulsants beginning immediately after the completion of the recordings.

Personnel in the recovery room and nursing unit should be instructed and appropriate orders written for immediate management in the event that the patient has a seizure postoperatively, including management of the immediate problem with intravenous anticonvulsants, such as diazepam, and maintenance of the airway and ventilation.

Usually there is little postoperative pain associated with craniotomies such as this. The major source of pain is the temporalis muscle. Most patients do well on moderate doses of codeine or small doses of narcotic.

The patient should be maintained on the preoperative dose of anticonvulsant medications for three months, and, if no seizures occur during that time (except for the initial postoperative period), the medication can be decreased over an additional 3 to 12 months, as directed by the patient's neurologist.

SUMMARY

A number of patients with partial seizures intractable to medical management are candidates for surgical management. Patients in whom an epileptogenic focus can be localized to a single temporal lobe can be treated successfully with minimal neurologic complications by resection of that temporal lobe. Patient selection depends on preoperative EEG evaluation. The surgery should be done under local anesthesia, if at all possible, in order to identify the source of abnormal electrical activity by intraoperative recording and to identify functionally important areas during the resection. Patients who are too young or cannot cooperate during this extensive stressful procedure may require general anesthesia. A knowledge of the effect of pharmacologic agents on EEG is necessary to afford the patient optimal sedation and/or anesthesia with minimal interference with intraoperative recording and brain resection.

REFERENCES

1. Jackson JH: Selected writings of John Hughlings Jackson. Vol 1, On epilepsy and epileptiform convulsions. London, Hodder and Stoughton, 1931.
2. Horsley V: Brain surgery. Br Med J 1886;2:670–675.
3. Foerster O: Zur Pathogenese und chirurgischen Behandlung der Epilepsie. Zentralbl Chir 1925;52:531–549.
4. Foerster O, Altenburger H: Electrobiologische Vorgange an der menschlichen Hirnrinde. Dtsch Z Nervenheilkd 1935;153:277–288.
5. Penfield W, Jasper HH: Epilepsy and the functional anatomy of the human brain. Boston, Little Brown & Co, 1954.
6. Bailey P, Gibbs FA: The surgical treatment of psychomotor epilepsy. JAMA 1951;145:365–70.
7. Engel J, Rausch R, Lieb JP: Correlation of criteria used for localizing the epileptogenic foci in patients considered for surgical therapy of epilepsy. Ann Neurol 1981;9:215-224.
8. Gloor P: Contributions of electroencephalography and electrocortiocography to the neurosurgical treatment of epilepsies. Adv Neurol 1975;8:59–106.
9. Talairach J, Bancaud J: Stereotactic approach to epilepsy. Prog Neurol Surg 1973;5:297–354.
10. Ajmone-Marsan C: Depth electroencephalography and electrocorticography, in Aminoff MC (ed): Electrodiagnosis in clinical neurology. New York, Churchill Livingstone, 1980, pp 167–196.
11. Crandall PH, Walter RD, Rand RW: Clinical application of studies on stereotactic implanted electrodes in temporal epilepsy. J Neurosurg 1963;20:827–840.
12. Oakley J, Ojemann GA, Ojemann LN: Identifying epileptic foci on contrast-enhanced computerized tomographic scans. Arch Neurol 1979;36:699–671.
13. Kuhl DE, Engel J, Phelps ME, et al.: Epileptic patterns of local cerebral metabolism and perfusion in humans determined by emission computed tomography of ^{18}FDG and $^{13}NH_3$. Ann Neurol 1980;8:348–360.
14. Kuhl DE, Barrio JR, Huang HC: Quantifying local cerebral blood flow by N-isopropyl-p-^{123} I-iodoamphetamine (Imp) tomography. J Nucl Med 1982;23:196–203.

15. Meyer JS, Hayman LA, Amano T: Mapping local blood flow of the human brain by CT scanning during stable xenon inhalation. Stroke 1981;12:421-436.

16. Hawkes RC, Holland GN, Moore WS, et al.: Nuclear magnetic resonance (NMR) tomography of the brain: A preliminary clinical assessment with demonstration of pathology. J Comput Assist Tomog 1980;4:577-586.

17. Sypert GW: New concepts in the management of epilepsy: Medical and surgical. Clin Neurosurg 1977;24:600-641.

18. Rodin EA: The prognosis of patients with epilepsy. Springfield, Ill, Charles C Thomas, 1968.

19. Walker AE: Surgery for epilepsy, in Magnus O, Lorentz de Hass AM (eds): The epilepsies. In Desmedt JE (ed), Handbook of clinical neurology. Basel: Karger, Vol 15;1974, pp 739-757.

20. Rasmussen T, Marino R (eds): Functional neurosurgery. New York, Raven Press, 1979.

21. Rasmussen T: The role of surgery in the treatment of epilepsy. Clin Neurosurg 1969;16:288-314.

22. Rasmussen T: Cortical resection and the treatment of focal epilepsies. Adv Neurol 1975;8:131-154.

23. Wada J, Rasmussen T: Intracarotid injection of sodium amytal for lateralization of cerebral speech dominance: Experimental and clinicial observations. J Neurosurg 1960;17:266-282.

24. Rasmussen T: Cortical resection for medically refractory focal epilepsy: Results, lessons and questions, in Rasmussen T, Marino R: Functional neurosurgery. New York, Raven Press, 1979. pp 253-269.

25. Julien RM: Lidocaine in experimental epilepsy: Correlation of anticonvulsant effects of blood concentrations. Electroencephalogr Clin Neurophysiol 1973;34:639-645.

26. Stoelting RK: Plasma lidocaine concentrations following subcutaneous or submucosal epinepherine lidocaine injection. Anesth Analg (Cleve) 1978;57:724-726.

27. Gilbert RGB, Brindle GF, Galindo A. Anesthesia for neurosurgery. Boston, Little Brown & Co, 1966, pp 132-137.

28. Nilsson EE, Ingvar DH: EEG findings in neuroleptanalgesia. Acta Anaesthesiol Scand 1967;11:121-127.

29. Brindle GG: The use of neuroleptic agents in the neurosurgical unit. Clin Neurosurgery 1969;16:234-250.

30. Babb TL, Ferrer-Brechner T, Brechner VL, et al.: Limbic neuronal firing rates in man during administration of nitrous oxide oxygen or sodium thiopental. Anesthesiology 1975;43:402-409.

31. Berkowitz BA, Ngai SH, Finck AD: Nitrous oxide "analgesia": Resemblance to opiate action. Science 1976;194:967-968.

32. Rosen I, Hagerdale M: Electroencephalographic study of children during ketamine anesthesia. Acta Anaesthesiol Scand 1976;20:32-39.

33. Corssen G, Miysaka M, Domino EF: Changing concepts in pain control during surgery: Dissociative anesthesia with CI-581. A progress report. Anesth Analg (Cleve) 1968;47:746-759.

34. Winters WD: Epilepsy anesthesia with ketamine. Anesthesiology 1972;36:309-312.

35. Ferrer-Allado T, Brechner VL, Dymond A, et al.: Ketamine-induced electroconvulsive phenomenon in the human limbic and thalamic regions. Anesthesiology 1973;38:333-344.

36. Kayama K, Iwama K: EEG, evoked potentials and single unit activity during ketamine anesthesia in cats. Anesthesiology 1972;36:316-328.

37.   Bennett DR, Madsen JA, Jordan WS, et al.: Ketamine anesthesia in brain damaged epileptics. Electroencephalographic and clinical observations. Neurology (Minneap) 1973;23:449–460.

38.   Melville KI: Antihistamine drugs, in Schacter M (ed): Histamines and antihistamines. International encyclopedia of pharmacology and therapeutics. Oxford, Pergamon, 1973, section 74, pp 127–171.

39.   Ingvar DH, Jeppsson ST, Nordstrom L: A new form of anesthesia in surgical treatment of focal epilepsy. Acta Anaesthesiol Scand 1959;3:111–121.

40.   Gordon E, Widen L: General anesthesia with halothane for surgical interventions and electrocorticography in cases of focal epilepsy. Acta Anaesthesiol Scand 1962;6:13–28.

41.   Campkin TV, Turner JM: Neurosurgical anesthesia and intensive care. Boston, Butterworths, 1980, pp 142–147.

42.   Paul R, Harris R: A comparison of methohexitone and thipentone in electrocortigraphy. J Neurol Neurosurg Psychiatry 1970;33:100–104.

43.   Ford EW, Morrell F, Whistler WW: Methohexital anesthesia for treatment of uncontrollable epilepsy (Sci Prog Abstr) Anesth Analg (Cleve) 1982;61:185.

44.   Neigh JL, Garman J, Harp JR: The electroencephalographic pattern during anesthesia with Ethrane: Effects of depth of anesthesia, $PaCO_2$ and nitrous oxide. Anesthesiology 1971;35:482-487.

45.   Burchiel KJ, Stockard JJ, Rowe MJ, III, et al.: EEG abnormalities following enflurane anesthesia, abstracted. Am Soc Anesthesiol Scientific Papers, Annual Meeting 1975, pp 335–336.

46.   Ohm WE, Cullen BR, Amory DW, et al.: Delayed seizure activity following enflurane anesthesia. Anesthesiology 1975;42:367–368.

47.   Heavner JE, Amory DVM: Brain excitability after multiple enflurane exposures, abstracted. Am Soc Anesthesiol Scientific Papers, Annual Meeting 1976, p 193.

48.   Opitz A, Oberwetter WD: Enflurane or halothane anaesthesia for patients with cerebral convulsive disorders? Acta Anaesthesiol Scand 1979; suppl 71:43–47.

49.   Ojemann G, Ward AA, Jr: Stereotaxic and other procedures for epilepsy. Adv Neurol 1975;8:241–263.

CHAPTER 13

Percutaneous Cervical Cordotomy
Philip L. Gildenberg

There are several aspects of percutaneous cervical cordotomy that are of particular interest to the anesthesiologist. It is an important ablative procedure in the management of cancer pain, and anesthesiologists concerned with such programs should be familiar with its capabilities. It has supplanted surgical cordotomy in most cases, and knowledge of the percutaneous procedure is necessary for anyone who may be in a position to recommend a cordotomy. Since it is performed at cervical levels, the complications, particularly respiratory, are of interest to anesthesiologists involved in the management of respiratory problems. Although it is generally performed under local anesthesia, sometimes with an anesthesiologist in attendance, preoperative and intraoperative sedation are critical and sometimes difficult to manage, especially as most patients are maintained on large doses of narcotics prior to the procedure and are debilitated from their disease. In some parts of the world, particularly in Europe, the procedure is performed by anesthesiologists.

Despite the percutaneous and nonsurgical nature of the procedure, it is important to recognize that it produces a major physiologic change in the patient's sensory system and involves a moderate risk of untoward side effects (1–3). Consequently, the indications should be the same as those for surgical cordotomy. During the early years of percutaneous cervical cordotomy, it was often used inappropriately for chronic pain of benign origin, partly because the procedure was so easy to perform that it invited misuse and partly because the philosophy in those years promoted the liberal use of ablative procedures (1,4–6). It was to a large extent through the experience gained by long-term follow-up of patients after percutaneous cervical cordotomy that a more conservative attitude about ablative procedures for pain other than cancer pain evolved.

The major indication for percutaneous cervical cordotomy is unilateral cancer pain involving the trunk and/or lower extremity (and occasionally the arm) that has become intractable to pharmacologic management. Patients with bilateral pain may be candidates for bilateral percutaneous cervical cordotomy performed in two separate procedures (4,5,7,8), but midline or perineal pain responds less well to this maneuver, which is true also for surgical cordotomy. Occasionally, a patient with chronic pain of benign origin may be a candidate for cordotomy, but only if the patient has been investigated within a chronic pain clinic program, has a specific etiology that defies treatment, is not receiving or dependent on narcotics, is emotionally stable, and all behavioral and stimulation approaches have been exhausted.

Even with strict selection criteria, it must be recognized that pain relief may be only temporary, as with any other ablative procedure. It is important to inform the patient not only of the nature of the procedure, but of the potential drawbacks and risks. The patient should be warned that, even with cancer pain, pain relief may be only temporary. It should be pointed out that cordotomy is not intended to replace pain with normal sensation, but to replace pain with the absence of pain perception, which might leave the body part unprotected.

Potental risks of percutaneous cervical cordotomy performed at the level of the second cervical vertebra include those of sleep-induced apnea and hemiparesis or hemiplegia (1,3,5,7–10). The anterior approach to the lower cervical spinal cord does not affect respiration, but may leave the patient with monoparesis of the hand ipsilateral to the lesion, or a hemiparesis or hemiplegia on that side. Patients with pelvic cancer who already have some impairment of bladder function may have additional difficulty, particularly after bilateral cordotomy, possibly to the point of urinary retention, but the incidence of this complication appears to be less than after surgical cordotomy. Patients who have pulmonary carcinoma may present a particular problem. If the upper chest, shoulder, or arm is involved, it is necessary to perform the cordotomy at the C2 level in order to have analgesia at an adequate level. But if there has been unilateral pulmonary involvement and there is little respiratory function on the painful side, the patient may suffer sleep-induced apnea after a unilateral cordotomy on the contralateral side, so that cordotomy may be contraindicated (5).

ANESTHETIC CONSIDERATIONS

It is advantageous to discuss the procedure in detail with the patient. Since it is necessary to test for sensation and motor function while the lesion is being made, it is far better to instruct the patient during the preoperative discussion than during the stress of the procedure and its associated sedation. Not only should the patient be instructed to indicate on testing with a pin or pinwheel whether the pain is sharp or dull, but also to compare degrees of sharpness between left and right at ascending dermatome levels. A hypodermic needle, particularly the disposable type designed for painless insertion, is too sharp and slippery to provide an adequate stimulus for pinstick sensation, and may cause considerable tissue damage. For testing pinstick sensation, a Wartenberg pinwheel is preferable to a safety pin. Not only does it provide appropriate sharpness, but it allows a consistent stimulation, and the dermatomes may be tested successively to identify the level at which sensation changes. Motor function should be tested in all four extremities with hand grasp, flexion at the elbow, straight leg raising, and dorsiflexion and plantar flexion at the ankle.

There is considerable debate about whether it is better to discontinue pain medications prior to or following pain-relieving procedures such as cordotomy. Some of the confusion results because of different patient requirements. Patients with chronic pain of benign origin should be withdrawn from medications prior to any procedure as part of a conservative program, and cordotomy considered only for those patients who have completed participation in a multidisciplinary pain clinic protocol. On the other hand, patients with cancer pain do not tolerate being withdrawn from analgesic medication, sometimes because of the severe pain that is unmasked and sometimes because of withdrawal symptoms. Therefore, as percutaneous cervical cordotomy should usually be considered only for patients with cancer pain, generally patients receive narcotics until after the cordotomy.

Consequently, cordotomy patients present particular problems with preoperative medication. The procedure is not without discomfort. Patients already have considerable pain from their cancer and may have difficulty lying still. Tolerance to narcotics makes response to premedication somewhat unpredictable. A single general protocol that addresses all these issues involves the administration of twice the dose of narcotic that the patient would receive in a four-hour period, given one half hour prior to initiation of the cordotomy procedure. The most reliable way to calculate the dose is to average the patient's total daily narcotic dose for the past three or four days and divide this amount by three. Thus, patients who receive 100 or 150 mg of meperidine in a four-hour period should receive a single dose of 200 to 300 mg. Patients who receive 15 or 20 mg of morphine every four hours will be administered 30 to 40 mg of morphine preoperatively. These doses are invariably questioned by the nurse responsible for their administration, but patients who have been receiving large doses of narcotics for a time and require cordotomy because they have become tolerant to those medications generally tolerate these doses without complications. They tend to be reasonably comfortable and may doze during the nonpainful parts of the procedure, but are alert enough when motor and sensory function are tested.

Patients who are particularly apprehensive may benefit by the addition of diazepam, 5 to 10 mg, to their dose of narcotic, recognizing that the response of patients who have been taking large doses of medications may be atypical. Even if tranquilizers are given, it is best to administer the full dose of narcotics to prevent withdrawal symptoms during the procedure.

Patients who have impaired pulmonary function secondary to pulmonary carcinoma or lung resection might be given the narcotic in divided doses to assure that it does not cause undue respiratory depressant effects. Since the recommended dose is geared to the patient's own dosage schedule, which takes tolerance into account, respiratory depression has not been a problem. Patients whose pulmonary function may be so impaired that they are candidates only for lower cervical cordotomy may be evaluated with pulmonary function tests prior to the procedure, and the effect of the intended dose of narcotic on pulmonary function can be assessed at that time. The application of the radiofrequency current is often sufficiently painful to arouse the patient for the sensory testing that follows immediately thereafter. It is far better to have patients moderately well sedated for the procedure than to have a patient who is in so much pain that he is unable to lie still and to participate meaningfully in motor and sensory testing, in which case the procedure is more often unsatisfactory or carries a higher risk.

Atropine, 0.4 mg, should be administered as part of preoperative medications to patients about to undergo lower cervical cordotomy to avoid a carotid sinus reflex when the carotid artery is manipulated in preparation for insertion of the needle. The recommended sedation schedule is sufficient so patients do not complain of a dry mouth.

Although there is no evidence that the administration of steroids decreases or prevents the edema that may occur at the site of lesion production, some surgeons administer steroids prophylactically on the day before and for perhaps three days following production of the lesion. A usual dose would be dexamethasone, 24 mg/day. This author has not noticed any link between improved recovery of patients and steroid administration.

It must be emphasized that percutaneous cervical cordotomy requires knowledge, skill, and practice and represents a major procedure. It should not be undertaken by anyone without adequate instruction and practice.

PROCEDURE

Percutaneous cervical cordotomy as done at the C2 level (6,10,12,13) differs significantly from the anterior cordotomy at lower cervical levels (1,5). In the former case, the procedure is done using biplane fluoroscopy or a C-arm fluoroscope, since the needle is introduced transversely and the trajectory can be identified directly on anteroposterior (AP) and lateral views. In the lower cervical procedure, however, the needle is introduced obliquely and is not visible on either view, so it is necessary to obtain both AP and lateral radiographs to calculate the angle of trajectory.

It is advantageous to use a head holder with triplane microdrive for the C2 cordotomy to support and advance the needle electrode under precise control. In the lower cervical procedure, the intervertebral disk holds the needle adequately, so no other device is required (6).

C2 Percutaneous Cervical Cordotomy

Most physicians prefer to use the C2 approach for unilateral procedures since it is easier than the lower cervical approach. It should not be used for bilateral procedures, however, because of the risk of respiratory complications, although it can be combined with a lower cervical procedure on the other side. Because the progressive nature of cancer makes it possible that any patient may later require C2 cordotomy on the contralateral side, this author prefers initially to use the anterior approach to the lower cervical spinal cord.

An intravenous route should be established prior to the procedure, preferably before the patient arrives in the x-ray room, to allow administration of additional medication. The patient should be fasting for at least eight hours. An electrocardiogram monitor may be used, but it should be turned off during application of the radiofrequency current to avoid damage to the monitor. Blood pressure should be monitored prior to and immediately following production of each lesion and during the immediate postoperative period, since the sympathetic fibers within the spinal cord may be interrupted by the lesion.

For C2 cordotomy, the patient is placed in the supine position on the operating or x-ray table (13). The C-arm fluoroscope is angled upward by 15° to 20°, and the AP view can be taken through the open mouth. The x-ray apparatus should be arranged so that AP and lateral views can be taken without moving the patient or disturbing the electrode.

The side of the neck and earlobe on the side of the lesion, that is, the side opposite the pain, are cleansed. Under guidance of lateral fluoroscopy, a point is noted on the skin which directly overlies the anterior half of the crotch between the arch of the C1 vertebra and the lamina of C2. The skin and underlying muscle are infiltrated with local anesthetic solution. The 18-gauge needle that constitutes part of the electrode is inserted directly laterally, aiming toward a point approximately one-third of the way back from the anterior border of the spinal canal at the C1-2 level. It is advanced with repeated fluoroscopic guidance until it enters the subarachnoid space just anterior to the attachment of the dentate ligament. It is important that the needle is in the subarachnoid space, and not subdural as signified by a flow of cerebrospinal fluid. Care must be taken not to advance the needle so far as to traumatize the spinal cord.

The location of the dentate ligament may be verified by withdrawing 2 ml of spinal fluid and shaking it vigorously in a syringe with 2 ml of Pantopaque and then reinjecting the emulsified fluid. A few droplets will lie on the dentate ligament, identifying its position.

The needle tip is positioned just inside the dura and the electrode stylet inserted through the needle pointing to the spinal cord, usually 2 mm anterior to the dentate ligament. For pain lower in the body, a position immediately anterior to the dentate ligament is preferred. The needle is advanced until the tip of the electrode lies within the spinal cord. It may be necessary to enter the pia with a sharp thrust, since frequently it is fairly tough. Entry into the spinal cord can be verified by monitoring electrical impedance (1).

The target for sacral pain lies 6 mm lateral, and for thoracic pain the tip of the electrode should be 4 mm lateral. Stimulation may be employed for precise localization of the tip of the electrode (12,13). The negative lead is attached to the electrode and the positive lead to the shaft of the needle. In most instances, stimulation at 50 or 60 Hz provides sensation projected to that part of the body which will be rendered analgesic when a lesion is made. Occasionally, a patient will not demonstate the appropriate sensation but will, nevertheless, obtain good analgesia from application of the radiofrequency current.

The patient should be tested for motor function and analgesia after insertion of the electrode. Not infrequently, the mechanical presence of the electrode will cause an area of analgesia or even analgesia of the total contralateral side of the body and extremities, which is generally followed by good permanent analgesia with a relatively small lesion.

The current necessary to produce a lesion varies somewhat, depending on the individual electrode configuration (4,10,11). The literature provided by the manufacturer should be consulted. The ideal temperature for lesion production is 80°C, and some electrodes are available to monitor the temperature directly. It is possible to obtain an estimation of the temperature generated by a particular current by holding the assembled electrode in egg white, attaching the leads, and noting how much current causes a protein coagulum to form at the tip of the electrode. This represents the current that should be employed to make the lesion clinically. The electrodes employed by the author require a current between 50 and 60 mA.

If at the time of lesion production during the percutaneous cordotomy there is a sudden drop in current, one should assume that the current is too high, in that the tip of the electrode has exceeded 100°C and a gas bubble has formed around the electrode, which increases the impedance. In the event of a sudden decrease in current, the current should be stopped, the stylet wiped clean of any coagulum and reinserted, and a lesion produced with a lower current.

With the electrode in position, a small test lesion is made for 10 or 15 seconds. The patient should be warned that the application of current may cause pain, but that it will last for only a short time during current application. Following the test lesion, the patient is tested for the development of analgesia. If the area of analgesia is too low, the electrode may be advanced another millimeter. If it is too high, the electrode may be withdrawn a millimeter.

If the lesion indicates that the electrode tip is in the right position, a permanent lesion is made by applying the same current for 30 to 60 seconds. The patient is again tested for the presence of motor function and analgesia, and the electrode repositioned or the lesion enlarged accordingly.

When adequate analgesia has been obtained, AP and lateral films verify the final position of the electrode prior to electrode withdrawal.

Postoperatively, the patient may resume activity as soon as his condition permits. Discontinuation of narcotics depends on the amount of dependency and the success of pain relief, but the patient should not be withdrawn so abruptly that withdrawal symptoms are intolerable.

An interesting phenomenon in patients with widespread cancer is that the successful alleviation of pain on one side of the body may be followed immediately by the appearance of pain on the opposite side. This appears to be true release from inhibition of pain and not merely an unmasking of lesser pain. Both the physician and the patient must be aware of the possibility that it might occur.

Lower Cervical Percutaneous Cordotomy

The technique of percutaneous cervical cordotomy at a lower cervical area differs markedly from that of the C2 cordotomy (1,5).

The target point can be selected according to the area of the patient's pain. Since the lateral spinothalamic fibers often are somatotopically widely distributed in the anterolateral quadrant of the spinal cord at lower cervical levels, it is frequently possible to render analgesic only that part of the body or extremity involved with the pain, minimizing the loss of sensation and potential side effects (14).

The dimensions of the spinal cord in the lower cervical area at the usual magnification, that is, with an 80- to 95-cm tube-to-cassette distance, is 18 mm in transverse diameter and 10 mm in AP diameter. Since the spinal cord lies against the posterior wall of the cervical canal in a supine position, AP measurements may be made from the posterior wall of the cervical canal, and lateral measurements are made from the midline of the bony canal. The sacral fibers lie 7 to 8 mm lateral to the midline at the point at which the dentate ligament attaches to the spinal cord, which is 5 mm anterior from the posterior wall of the cervical canal. If pelvic pain predominates, it is often best to insert the electrode to a target point 4 mm anterior from the posterior wall of the cervical canal, or 1 mm behind the dentate ligament, to assure dense analgesia at sacral levels. The lower cervical and upper thoracic areas are represented by fibers 3 mm lateral to the midline and 7 mm anterior to the posterior wall of the cervical canal.

Because of current spread to incoming segmental sensory fibers, stimulation in the lower cervical area is helpful for localization of the electrode in only half of the patients. Those patients will, indeed, have projection of sensation to the area of the body about to be rendered analgesic on application of 50 or 60 Hz stimulation at low voltages, but other patients will have such intense segmental sensation at very low currents that the stimulation cannot be increased sufficiently to obtain projected sensation to the body.

The patient is placed in the supine position on the x-ray table. AP and lateral x-ray tubes are arranged so that AP and lateral films can be taken with identical magnification without the necessity of moving the patient. Ideally, two x-ray tubes should be employed, so each film is taken with identical projection and magnification. On the lateral x-ray film, the operator identifies the lowest intervertebral disk space that can be seen above the shoulders and that is wide enough for needle insertion.

The anterior part of the neck is cleansed, and several towels may be used for draping. The skin and subcutaneous fascia are infiltrated with local anesthetic adjacent to the trachea ipsilateral to the pain at the approximate level of the intended interspace. With the fingers of the left hand, the skin just lateral to the trachea and medial to the carotid sheath is compressed against the prevertebral fascia, and local anesthetic solution is infiltrated. When the tissues are thus compressed, there is only skin, platysma, and fascia for the electrode to pass through before entering the intervertebral disk.

The 18-gauge lumbar puncture needle is inserted into the intended intervertebral disk, which can be identified by palpation, at approximately the midline to a depth of 5 to 8 mm, just deep enough to hold the tip of the needle in the disk.

AP and lateral roentgenograms are taken to verify the position of the needle within the interspace.

Since it is not possible to visualize the trajectory on either the AP or the lateral film, one must imagine a right triangle superimposed on a cross section of the neck, with the tip of the needle at the apex of the triangle and the target at the acute angle at the base (14) (Fig. 13.1). By advancing the needle along the hypotenuse, it will eventually come to the target point. Thus, if one can reconstruct the imagined right triangle and adjust the angle of insertion, the needle will be pointing to the target (Fig. 13.2). The height of the triangle can be represented by the distance from the tip of the needle to the target point, as measured by the lateral roentgenogram, and the base of the triangle can be represented by the distance from the tip of the needle to the target point on the AP film, since both have identi-

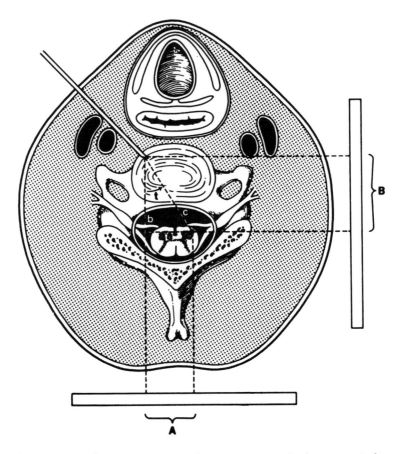

Figure 13.1 In the anterior approach to a target in the lower cervical spinal cord, the needle electrode is inserted diagonally through the intervertebral disk.

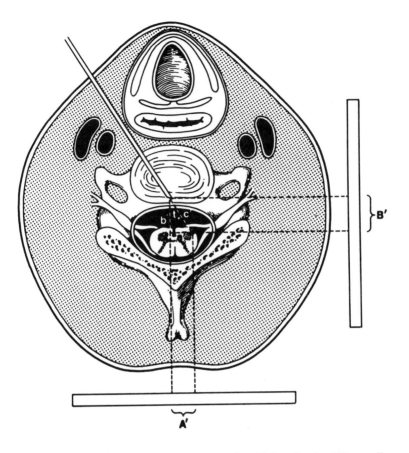

Figure 13.2   The first measurements are made with just the tip of the needle in the disk. The distance from the tip of the needle to the target point on both the AP and lateral films defines a right triangle, the hypotenuse of which indicates the proper direction of insertion.

cal magnification. The proportions remain the same and, therefore, an equivalent triangle can be drawn which has the desired angle of insertion at the apex.

A right triangle is drawn on a piece of paper with a height equivalent to the needle-target distance on the lateral film and the base equivalent to the needle-target distance on the AP film. The diagram can be held at the patient's chin, and the needle aligned with the hypotenuse to obtain the proper angle of insertion. Alternatively, one may use a mechanical device to simulate the proper angle (15).

The needle is advanced until its tip is held firmly in the posterior part of the disk (Fig. 13.2). AP and lateral films are taken and the same procedure is performed to draw another right triangle. If the needle is advancing accurately to the target point, the two right triangles will be equivalent, and the needle will still be aligned with the hypotenuse of the second right triangle.

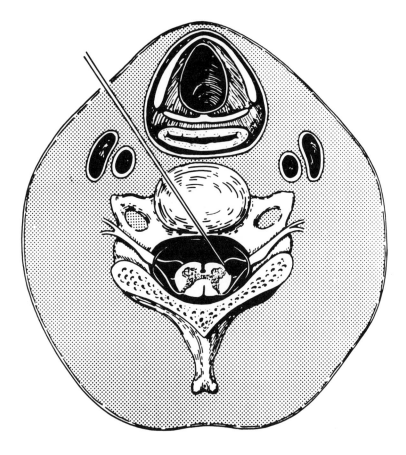

Figure 13.3 The second measurements are made with the tip of the needle at the posterior part of the disk, at which point the trajectory of the needle is fixed.

If the needle is not advancing properly, it must be withdrawn almost completely from the disk and a correction made. Rotating the needle so the bevel is in the proper direction to facilitate correction of the angle is necessary, particularly if only a small correction is to be made.

If the needle lies along the proper trajectory, it is advanced through the disk and through the dura into the subarachnoid space. Again, it is important to see the flow of cerebrospinal fluid, since subdural placement of the electrode will not result in a permanent lesion. If the arachnoid or dura mater is not readily penetrated, the insertion of a sharpened stylet through the needle may facilitate penetration.

The needle is advanced until it barely touches the spinal cord with the bevel directed medially. With the obturator removed, the needle is advanced until cessation of flow of cerebrospinal fluid indicates that the opening of the bevel lies against the cord. AP and lateral films are again taken to verify the proper position of the electrode before penetration of the spinal cord.

When it has been ascertained that the needle is in the proper position, the stylet is inserted through the needle and into the anterolateral quadrant of the spinal cord (Fig. 13.3). It is necessary to insert the stylet with a sharp thrust to penetrate the pia, since extrapial placement also will result in an incomplete lesion.

The parameters for lesion production are identical to those used for C2 cordotomy. The patient is tested for analgesia immediately on insertion of the electrode. If an area of analgesia is detected, it serves as an excellent indicator of the position of the electrode. If not, a 15-second test lesion is made, and the patient again tested for analgesia. If the patient develops analgesia in the proper area, a 30- to 60-second lesion is made to assure permanence of fiber interruption. One must warn the patient that application of the current will be painful, perhaps somewhat more so at lower cervical levels than at C2, because of stimulation of the closest nerve root. Following application of current, the patient's motor function is tested, with particular attention to hand function, since the lesion is adjacent to emerging segmental motor fibers, and excessive longitudinal spread of the lesion can cause impairment of hand strength. Even though motor weakness is seen initially in 15% to 30% of cases, it is permanent in less than 5%, but still constitutes the greatest risk of this procedure.

If the test lesion demonstrates that the electrode is either too medial or too far lateral, it must be adjusted to the proper position. It is not possible to change the trajectory of the needle after it has been inserted through the disk. Small corrections of angle are quite difficult, since the needle tends to go through the prior hole in the disk, but they can be made by substituting a second stylet with the tip slightly angled. Thus, the bent stylet can produce a lesion 1 mm more medial or more lateral, as required. A larger correction is rarely necessary.

If the patient has no detectable analgesia after the test lesion, additional AP and lateral films should be obtained to verify the position of the electrode. One must bear in mind, however, that the spinal cord can be moved slightly by the electrode, and the electrode may lie just outside the spinal cord even though the coordinates are correct by measurement. In that case, the stylet is withdrawn and reinserted sharply through the pia. If the stylet glances off the surface of the cord, the use of a curved stylet may help penetrate the pia. The use of a stylet with a sharpened point may also be helpful to penetrate the pia, which is quite tough in some patients.

The patient should be observed postoperatively for hypotension, delayed development of weakness, respiratory depression, or urinary retention. Vital signs should be recorded regularly through the first night.

CARE AFTER THE PROCEDURE

The optimal schedule to withdraw patients from analgesics varies from patient to patient. Those patients who have been taking large doses of narcotics suffer withdrawal symptoms if the narcotics are discontinued abruptly, and those symptoms may sometimes take the form of increased pain perception with the appearance of an unsuccessful result. Patients may become extremely agitated, restless, or have severe diarrhea during the withdrawal period. A program that prevents withdrawal symptoms provides the patient with scheduled administration of narcotics rather than on demand, decreasing that dose daily by 15% of the preoperative dose, so narcotics are discontinued at the end of the first week.

If patients have pain in areas not rendered analgesic by cordotomy, their narcotic requirement may remain until further treatment is provided.

Whether the C2 or lower cervical approach is used, the procedure generally takes between 30 and 60 minutes. If the desired result is not immediately apparent, however, or if there is difficulty finding the target point or penetrating the spinal cord, additional time may be required. Calm patience on the part of the operating team is required to maintain the patient in a cooperative state. As a general rule, it is best to discontinue the attempt if success has not been achieved within 90 minutes. An occasional patient with incomplete analgesia at the end of that time will have excellent pain relief, and possibly the development of more dense analgesia within the subsequent 24 hours.

There have been few, if any, complications during the procedure. Blood pressure changes may be seen at the time of lesion production or secondary to the patient's apprehension. Pneumothorax or carotid artery injury have not been reported but are possible complications.

RESULTS

Most of the large series concerning the results of percutaneous cervical cordotomy intermingle patients with cancer pain with those having pain of benign origin (1,4–6). Even so, initial relief can be expected in 80% of patients at the lower cervical level and slightly more at upper cervical levels. Long-term follow-up, however, is less optimistic, with only two-thirds of the patients with benign pain maintaining satisfactory pain relief after six months. One can anticipate adequate, lasting pain relief for the duration of the patient's life in 75% to 80% of patients with cancer, a figure comparable to surgical cordotomy.

Complications (3,4) involve hemiparesis in 5% to 10% of patients, usually resolving within two to three weeks, with similar incidence in the C2 group and the lower cervical group. Monoparesis of the ipsilateral upper extremity may occur in up to 15% of patients following the lower cervical approach, but remains permanent in only 5%.

As with any other cordotomy, there are patients who develop difficulty with urinary control following the procedure. A close look at those patients in the author's series reveals that all are patients with pelvic carcinoma who had at least some symptoms of difficulty with urinary control prior to cordotomy, so that cordotomy impaired their bladder compensation, rather than caused a neurogenic bladder per se. The risk of decompensation increases after bilateral procedures.

One complaint, similar to that after surgical cordotomy, is that the knee on the side of the lesion may occasionally buckle. This appears to be a lapse of proprioceptive control, rather than weakness, because there is good strength on testing, and the problem arises only occasionally. Nevertheless, it can be distressing to the patient and may be severe enough to cause the patient to fall.

Another complication after high cervical cordotomy is sleep-induced apnea, which may occur after production of a lesion in the anterolateral quadrant of the spinal cord above the C4 level. Sleep-induced apnea, as its name implies, is a condition wherein the patient appears normal while awake, but may stop breathing when he falls asleep, and may be found dead in bed shortly after retiring. Even though breathing normally while awake, the patient may complain of a vague feeling of apprehension. Ordinary pulmonary function studies may be normal, but the patient may have mild or moderate impairment of ventilation. The normal hyperventilation response to breathing carbon dioxide is impaired, however, suggesting that the problem is not one of interruption of motor fibers or upper motor neurons controlling the phrenic nerve, but is a failure of response to hypercapnia. Since it may also occur after a unilateral lesion contralateral to the side of a pneumonectomy, it may be concluded that the receptors must be in the lung. One must be cautious postoperatively with patients who are at high risk for sleep-induced apnea, since occasionally the problem may not become apparent until the second night after surgery.

Patients who are at high risk should have apnea monitoring, and should be in a location where they can be closely observed for at least the first two nights after cordotomy. If they become apneic upon falling asleep, they should be immediately aroused and, if necessary, ventilated manually. Once such an episode has occurred, pulmonary function studies, including response to carbon dioxide inhalation, should be performed to monitor the evolution of the problem. It may be necessary to intubate the patient and ventilate manually in order to assure that fatal apnea does not occur.

Sleep-induced apnea usually is self-limiting and may reverse itself after a few days. If not, the patient may require long-term pulmonary assistance.

It must be recognized, however, that sleep-induced apnea can be completely avoided by patient selection. Bilateral procedures should not be done at high cervical levels, nor should a unilateral lesion be made on the side opposite a significantly impaired lung. If patients require a cordotomy under those circumstances, only lower cervical cordotomy should be considered.

SUMMARY

Percutaneous cervical cordotomy has become an accepted procedure, and, indeed, should be used in preference to surgical cordotomy in most patients who meet the criteria for a cordotomy. It allows a similar result without the trauma of general anesthesia and major surgery, an important consideration in debilitated cancer patients, who are the most likely candidates for this procedure.

REFERENCES

1. Gildenberg PL: Percutaneous cervical cordotomy for relief of intractable pain. Cleve Clin Q 1969;36:183–188.
2. Gildenberg PL: Percutaneous cervical cordotomy. Appl Neurophysiol 1981;44: 233–243.
3. Wepsic JG: Complications of percutaneous surgery for pain. Clin Neurosurg 1976; 23:454–464.
4. Gildenberg PL: Percutaneous cervical cordotomy. Clin Neurosurg 1974;21:246–255.
5. Lin PM, Gildenberg PL, Polakoff PP: An anterior approach to percutaneous lower cervical cordotomy. J Neurosurg 1966;25:553–560.
6. Rosomoff HL, Brown CJ, Sheptak P: Percutaneous radiofrequency cervical cordotomy. Technique. J Neurosurg 1965;23:620–627.
7. Rosomoff HL: Bilateral percutaneous cervical radiofrequency cordotomy. J Neurosurg 1969;31:41–46.
8. Rosomoff HL, Driger AJ, Kupman AS: Effects of percutaneous cervical cordotomy on pulmonary function. J Neurosurg 1969;31:620–627.
9. Belmusto L, Brown E, Owens G: Clinical observations on respiratory and vasomotor disturbances as related to cervical cordotomies. J Neurosurg 1963;20:225–232.
10. Mullan S, Hekmatpanah J, Dobbin G, et al.: Percutaneous intramedullary cordotomy utilizing the unipolar anodal electrolytic lesion. J Neurosurg 1965;22:548–553.
11. Fox JL: Experimental relationship of radiofrequency electrical current and lesion size for application to percutaneous cordotomy. J Neurosurg 1970;33:415–421.
12. Tasker RR, Organ LW: Percutaneous cordotomy. Physiological identification of target site. Confin Neurol 1973;35:110–117.
13. Tasker RR, Organ LW, Smith KC: Physiological guidelines for the localization of lesions by percutaneous cordotomy. Acta neurochir (Wien) 1974;210:111–117.
14. Gildenberg PL, Lin PM, Polakoff PP, II, et al.: Anterior percutaneous cervical cordotomy. Determination of target point and calculation of angle of insertion. Technical note. J Neurosurg 1968;28:173–177.
15. Gildenberg PL: Angle meter to indicate the proper angle of insertion in anterior percutaneous cervical cordotomy. Technical note. J Neurosurg 1971;34:244–247.

CHAPTER 14

Stereotactic Surgery

Philip L. Gildenberg

Stereotactic surgery is a technique wherein a specialized apparatus is used to direct an electrode accurately to a target within a structure deep within the brain with minimal damage to overlying tissues. It is based on the cartesian principle that a point may be defined in space by its relationship to three planes intersecting at right angles to each other, and that those planes may be based on anatomic landmarks.

Stereotactic techniques have been used in animals since 1908, when Horsley and Clarke (1) designed a system based on measurements from three planes in relationship to an animal's skull. This was not accurate enough for humans, however, because of the great variability between the position of deep cerebral structures and the landmarks on the skull. It was not until Spiegel and colleagues (2), in 1947, established a system based on intracerebral landmarks that stereotactic surgery became clinically applicable. Since then the field has expanded tremendously.

At present, the most commonly used internal landmarks are established by intraoperative ventriculography to demonstrate the anterior and posterior commissures as they encroach on the third ventricle. The midsagittal plane is readily discernible as the midline of the third ventricle. The horizontal plane extends at right angles to this plane and passes through both the anterior and posterior commissures. The third plane is established at right angles to the other two and passes through the posterior commissure.

To relate a given anatomic structure to the reference planes, it is necessary to consult an atlas, of which many are presently available (3–9). One must take into account the variability between human brains, which can be ascertained by consulting tables in each atlas. Consequently, it is necessary to verify physiologically that the electrode or probe is in the proper anatomic target, which usually can be done by stimulation or recording.

Stereotactic surgery may be used for the treatment of movement disorders, pain, psychosurgery, or occasionally the treatment of epilepsy.

MOVEMENT DISORDERS

A variety of movement disorders can be treated by stereotactic surgery. Generally, one of the two interlocking extrapyramidal circuits that regulate movement is interrupted.

One circuit concerns the basal ganglia and the thalamus. Fibers from the putamen enter the globus pallidus, from which neurons lead into the ventral anterior nucleus of the thalamus by several pathways. The lenticular fasciculus, located above the subthalamic nucleus, and the ansa lenticularis, below the subthalamic nucleus, join together in Forel's field H. These two pathways ascend together as the thalamic fasciculus (H1) to the ventral anterior nucleus of the thalamus. Since almost the entire outflow from the pallidum to the thalamus forms a compact bundle as it traverses Forel's field H, the maximum number of fibers can be interrupted there with the smallest lesion, which is one preferred target point for stereotactic surgery for movement disorders (Fig. 14.1). From the thalamus there are connections to the supplementary motor cortex. Connections within the cortex project to the caudate nucleus, which in turn projects back to the putamen to complete the circuit from putamen to globus, pallidus to thalamus (ventral anterior) to cortex to caudate and back to putamen.

The second interlocking circuit links the cerebellum to the basal ganglia. The major outflow from the cerebellum is through the dentate nucleus, which projects to the red nucleus. Some fibers synapse in the red nucleus, and others pass through it to project to the ventrolateral nucleus of the thalamus adjacent to the area that receives fibers from the globus pallidus. This area of the ventrolateral nucleus of the thalamus is the most commonly employed target point in the treatment of movement disorders (see Fig. 14.1). Fibers from this area extend to the primary and secondary motor cortex, from which efferent fibers descend through the internal capsule to end in the pontine nuclei. Neurons from those nuclei project to the cerebellar cortex. The outflow from the cerebellar cortex passes to the dentate nucleus, completing the cerebellum-dentate-ruber-thalamus (ventrolateral)-cortex-pontine nuclei-cerebellum motor control circuit.

Regardless of the movement disorder, the general targets for stereotactic surgery are most often the ventrolateral nucleus of the thalamus or Forel's field. Within the ventrolateral nucleus, target points for rigidity and tremor are not quite identical, the target point for tremor being slightly dorsolateral to the ideal target point for rigidity.

Parkinson's disease is the most common movement disorder for which stereotactic surgery has been used. During the first decade following the introduction of stereotactic surgery, medical management of Parkinson's disease was poor, so that stereotactic surgery became the major treatment. As L-dopa therapy provided more satisfactory relief for bradykinesia and rigidity (the symptoms most likely to be disabling), the number of patients considered good candidates for stereotactic surgery diminished.

Tremor responds best to stereotactic surgery and bradykinesia responds least, which contrasts to the pattern of response to L-dopa. Consequently, patients

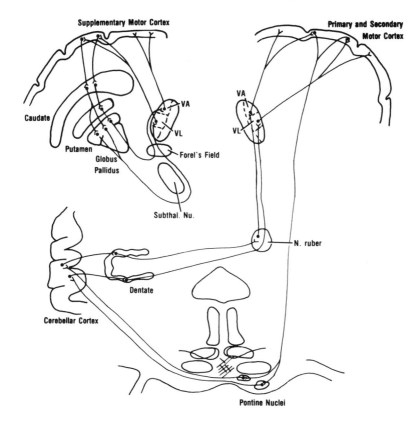

Figure 14.1 The two adjacent circuits that are part of the extrapyramidal tracts of interest in stereotactic surgery. The most common targets for movement disorders are Forel's field and the ventrolateral nucleus of the thalamus (*VL*), *VA*; ventral anterior nucleus.

who are disabled by tremor despite L-dopa therapy are candidates for stereotactic surgery; however, the tremor of Parkinson's disease is not often disabling, since it is a tremor at rest and diminishes when voluntary activity is initiated. As patients are treated with L-dopa for three to five years, many become resistant to the medication, or the progression of symptoms makes response to medical therapy inadequate (10,11). That group of patients may be considered for stereotactic surgery. There is also a group of patients who develop involuntary movements of dyskinesia from L-dopa, and stereotactic surgery may control the dyskinesia so the patient may tolerate medical management at optimal doses (11–13).

In general, the following recommendations may be made for the use of stereotactic surgery in Parkinson's disease (14).

1.   If bradykinesia is the major problem, a course of medical management is indicated.

2.   If the patient is intolerant to the medication or does not respond, stereotactic surgery may be considered, particularly if tremor is a significant symptom.
3.   If the patient still has significant bradykinesia after stereotactic surgery, L-dopa management should be tried once again, since the combination of surgery plus medical management may prove more effective than either alone.
4.   If tremor is the major problem, only a brief course of medical management should be tried, and if the patient does not respond, stereotactic surgery should be considered.
5.   If tremor persists after stereotactic surgery, a medical program should be tried once again.
6.   If the patient's symptoms are symmetrical and bilateral, the dominant side might be operated on first in order to provide the maximum rehabilitation from a unilateral procedure.
7.   Bilateral procedures should be avoided if at all possible, but if necessary, a minimum of 6 to 12 weeks should elapse before the second side is operated.
8.   If surgery is done bilaterally, every attempt should be made to make asymmetrical lesions to minimize the risk of side effects affecting mentation or speech. Bilateral lesions in Forel's fields (campotomy) should not be done because of the risk of mutism.

The risk of untoward side effects of a neurologic nature following stereotactic surgery increases after the age of 60 years, and even more so after the age of 65, so that surgery should be undertaken cautiously in elderly patients.

In well-selected patients, relief of tremor can be anticipated in 85% to 93% and some improvement in bradykinesia in up to 50%. Neurologic side effects, such as weakness or difficulty with speech or mentation, may occur in 2% to 4% (13,15,16).

Essential or familial tremor may be very disabling, since it is a tremor of intention. It becomes worse on attempting voluntary movement and may be severe enough to interfere with such activities of daily living as eating or dressing. It may be present at any age, or may become progressive in adulthood or middle years. There is no medical program to which it consistently responds. Stereotactic lesions in the ventrolateral nucleus of the thalamus or in Forel's field may produce dramatic and excellent results.

There are other causes of tremor that are amenable to stereotactic surgery. Although stroke or head trauma may produce tremor, the nervous system is no longer intact, so the response to stereotactic surgery is less predictable. Nevertheless, if the patient is sufficiently disabled by the tremor and recognizes that the outcome is uncertain, stereotactic surgery can be considered.

The involuntary movements that occur with Huntington's chorea may be amenable to stereotactic treatment. Huntington's chorea, however, is a familial disease marked by progressive mental deterioration as well as the choreiform movements associated with degeneration of the caudate nucleus. It is important to consider whether the patient's disability is due to the dementia or to the movement disorder. If mentation is good, significant improvement in involuntary movements may result from stereotactic surgery with a lesion in Forel's field or the ventrolateral nucleus.

Hemiballism may occur after vascular or surgical injury to the subthalamic nucleus and consists of involuntary hurling and irregular, frequently violent movements of the shoulder and proximal arm. Hemiballism may resolve spontaneously, and stereotactic surgery should not be contemplated unless the symptoms continue for at least two to three months. Lesions can be made in either Forel's field or the ventrolateral nucleus of the thalamus.

Dystonia musculorum deformans (torsion spasm) is a progressive condition in which disability may result from torsion of the trunk muscles with asymmetrical spasm or spasticity. There may be dystonic contractures of the extremities. Response to stereotactic thalamotomy is somewhat unpredictable, but 50% of patients may have dramatic improvement. It is necessary to make large lesions, and frequently bilateral surgery is required. The disease is progressive, however, so symptoms may recur as the disease overtakes improvement (17). A lesion in Forel's field (18) may improve symptoms, but bilateral Forel's field lesions should be avoided. Large lesions may be required in the ventrolateral nucleus (17). If necessary, lesions may be repeated and enlarged at three-month intervals provided there is some improvement.

There have been reports of the use of stereotactic surgery for spasmodic torticollis (19), but the results are unpredictable (20), or improvement may occur only after considerable delay (21). Results are so uncertain that stereotactic surgery generally is not the therapy of choice.

Certain patients with cerebral palsy may be candidates for stereotactic surgery, although the enthusiasm for this procedure has waned during the last decade. Stereotactic thalamotomy sometimes is employed for the management of cerebral palsy (22). In general, tremor responds well to thalamotomy or campotomy. Choreoathetosis may appear the same after surgery in that the involuntary movements continue, but often there is an improvement in voluntary control and the ability to perform daily activities. Spasticity responds least well. It is of interest that often the effects of surgery do not manifest themselves for some weeks after the operation, and then only with physical therapy, since a considerable amount of training is required when involuntary movements become less overwhelming. The surgery must often be done under general anesthesia because of the involuntary movements and age of the patient. A number of reports have suggested that production of a lesion in the dentate nucleus might help spastic cerebral palsy (23–25) with a 30% improvement in spasticity and perhaps facilitation of nursing care in 50% (26). The operation, which is relatively direct, involves coordinates taken from visualization of the fourth ventricle on x-ray, and has been shown to be reasonably safe. Unfortunately, the effects were unpredictable and appear to decrease with time, so that dentatomy is no longer often performed for cerebral palsy. Thalamotomy or campotomy may help choreiform movements in up to 78% of patients (27).

PAIN

There are several ways that stereotactic surgery is employed in the management of pain. Although some spnial cord techniques are referred to as "stereotactic," the present discussion is confined to stereotactic procedures involving the brain. Some of these procedures involve interrupting pathways concerned with the perception of pain, and others concern stimulation of pain inhibition centers.

Before considering any procedure that concerns management of pain, it is necessary to define the type of pain or situation in which a given procedure may be indicated. Pain can be divided generally into acute pain, cancer pain, and chronic pain of benign origin.

Acute pain is generally managed by treatment of the underlying etiology. Analgesics may be given until the pathologic process begins to abate, and stereotactic surgery is never indicated.

Cancer pain is usually managed in an aggressive fashion with analgesics, including narcotics administered in increasing dosage as tolerance develops or the pathologic process extends. When it is no longer possible to manage the pain with analgesics or noninvasive procedures, ablative procedures are indicated. Although cordotomy is the most frequently employed procedure for cancer pain, it can only be employed for pain affecting the trunk or extremities, particularly the lower body. Pain that is widespread and involves the shoulders, arms or head, or pain that involves the entire body may require stereotactic interruption of pain pathways within the brain.

The management of pain of benign origin generally involves withholding or withdrawing analgesic medication, especially narcotics, treatment of depression and regression, possibly behavior modification or other psychological techniques, resocialization and remobilization, and techniques that involve stimulation of the sensory system. It is rare that an ablative procedure is indicated, except for pain of every specific etiology, which usually involves pathology of the nervous system, such as sympathectomy for the causalgia of reflex sympathetic dystrophy. Although the initial results of interrupting a pain pathway might be encouraging, almost all studies that have included long-term follow-up reveal that there is no ablative procedure that alleviates chronic pain on a long-term basis. Stereotactic insertion of deep brain-stimulating electrodes or dorsal column stimulation may be indicated in a small number of selected patients with pain of known etiology that continues despite maximum benefit from a comprehensive pain management program.

Pain Pathways

Because pain is a complex sensation, pathways concerned with the perception of pain are multiple. Pain can be modified by numerous factors, such as mental activity and emotional tone. In addition to the pathways carrying pain perception from the body to the areas of the brain that provide consciousness, there are other pathways concerned with the modulation of pain perception. The ascending pathways are those that might be interrupted to treat cancer pain, and the descending pain modulating or inhibiting pathways are those that may be stimulated for selective management of pain of benign origin, or occasionally also widespread cancer pain.

The neospinothalamic tract, or lateral spinothalamic tract, is the best known of the ascending pain pathways and is the most clearly defined anatomically. Cells of origin lie in the posterior horn just anterior to the substantia gelatinosa, cross the midline in the anterior white commissure within a few segments of the sensory input, and ascend in the contralateral anterolateral quadrant of the spinal cord. In the brain stem, this pathway is referred to as the medial lemniscus, which sends collaterals to the pontine and mesencephalic reticular formation before ending in the ventral posterolateral nucleus of the thalamus. This is the pathway that is interrupted in cordotomy. It can also be interrupted stereotactically at midbrain levels or just as the fibers enter the thalamus.

The paleospinothalamic tract originates with the same fibers as the lateral spinothalamic tract, but concerns the collateral pathway through the pons and midbrain reticular formation. The multisynaptic ascending pathway ascends to the intralaminar nuclei of the thalamus, the centrum medianum, the parafascicular nuclei, and to the hypothalamus and those areas concerned with emotion, such as the limbic lobe, including the cingulate gyrus, the hippocampus, and amygdala (28). Distribution is not somatotopic and is bilateral, so a lesion on one side may affect pain on either or both sides of the body. Interruption of this pathway provides no detectable analgesia by usual methods of testing, in contrast to the neospinothalamic pathway, but may provide the patient with relief of cancer pain. The paleospinothalamic pathway in the brain stem is often referred to as the *extralemniscal pathway* to distinguish it from the neospinothalamic lateral spinothalamic tract, which ascends as the medial lemniscus.

It is necessary to include the limbic system in a discussion of ablation of pain pathways for cancer pain. Not only is this system concerned with emotions, but interruption of certain areas, particularly the cingulate gyrus, may be of help in managing certain types of pain, particularly cancer pain that is accompanied by a great deal of emotional distress. After interruption of this system, the patient may still perceive that pain is present but not be distressed by it.

Stereotactic Pain Procedures

Pain involving the entire head and body or pain involving the face or neck may be managed by interrupting the spinothalamic tract stereotactically at midbrain levels, a procedure known as *mesencephalotomy* (29). An electrode is inserted in a trajectory approximately in line with the brain stem. The lesion is located for maximum safety, depending on the response to stimulation at the time of surgery (30,31). If the electrode is too low or medial, stimulation may produce abrupt deviation of the eye and pupillary constriction, a sign that the electrode is too close to the oculomotor fibers. If the electrode is too far lateral or anterior, stimulation at low frequency may cause movement of the contralateral extremities, indicating that the electrode is too close to the pyramidal tract.

Interruption of the lateral spinothalamic tract alone is often unsuccessful in obtaining pain relief. This finding has led to development of procedures that also interrupt the fibers of the paleospinothalamic system. Coincidentally, attempts to produce the lesion above the level of the mesencephalon to minimize undesirable side effects, such as diplopia or hemiparesis, have been explored. Lesions in or near the thalamus are referred to as *thalamotomy*, and there are several types used for pain relief. The convergence of the various pathways that relate to the different aspects of pain makes it possible to tailor the lesion to the needs of the individual patient (see Fig. 14.2); however, since pain is intermingled with other sensations in the ventral posterior nuclei of the thalamus, it is desirable to interrupt either the extralemniscal or lemniscal fibers as they ascend to the medial portion of the thalamus, or a combination of both. This has led to nomenclature describing several types of thalamotomy for pain relief.

Basal thalamotomy involves the production of a lesion interrupting only the extralemniscal fibers as they ascend toward the intralaminar nuclei, the centrum medianum, and the parafascicular nucleus. The lesion in basal thalamotomy may be extended to interrupt the lemniscal fibers as well. In medial thalamotomy, a somewhat larger lesion is made to interrupt the extralemniscal system at its termination in the intralaminar nuclei and centrum medianum. In dorsomedian thalamotomy, a lesion is produced in the dorsomedial nucleus to interrupt the fibers that project to the frontal lobe, the same lesion that is used for affective disorders. Curiously, one may obtain pain relief with any of these three types of thalamotomy without the production of demonstrable analgesia, as long as the lemniscal fibers are avoided.

It is also possible to treat pain, particularly cancer pain, by lesions in the cingulate gyrus, that is, cingulotomy, which is used in psychosurgery. This may be helpful to alleviate the depression and emotional distress accompanying a terminal illness as well as the stresses of narcotic addiction. Even though the patient may appear more comfortable and require no analgesic medications, he may report that the pain is still there, but is no longer distressing.

The optimal procedure must be tailored to the needs of each patient. With pain from bone metastases or with a large somatic component, basal thalamotomy or mesencephalotomy with interruption of the lemniscal system may be desirable. If the patient has a great deal of emotional distress, narcotic addiction, or a large component of visceral pain, the lesion should primarily concern the extralemniscal system, as with intralaminar thalamotomy. If the emotional component is extensive, the intralaminar lesion may be extended to include dorsomedian thalamotomy, a cingulotomy may be done preferentially.

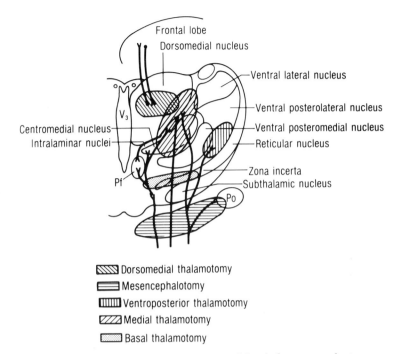

Dorsomedial thalamotomy
Mesencephalotomy
Ventroposterior thalamotomy
Medial thalamotomy
Basal thalamotomy

Figure 14.2 Pain pathways in various parts of the thalamus may be interrupted to provide relief of pain. Mesencephalotomy and basal thalamotomy interrupt the lemniscal or neospinothalamic tracts. Basal thalamotomy also interrupts the diffuse pain pathway, as does medial thalamotomy. Dorsomedial thalamotomy interrupts pathways concerned with emotion, which project to the frontal lobe. (Reprinted by permission from Gildenberg PL: Functional neurosurgery, in HH Schmidek, M.D., F.A.C.S., and WH Sweet, M.D., F.A.C.S. Operative neurosurgical techniques, vol. II. New York: Grune & Stratton, 1982.)

Deep Brain Stimulation

Descending inhibitory pain pathways were first discovered when it was observed in rats that stimulation of the area around the aqueduct at midbrain levels produced analgesia so the rats did not respond to noxious stimulation, so-called stimulation-produced analgesia (SPA) (32,33). It was later verified in patients that stimulation of the area in the posterior wall of the third ventricle and periaqueductal gray matter may lead to relief from chronic pain or cancer pain, even without the production of analgesia as tested by pin stick (34–36).

A system has been devised by which an electrode may be implanted in the brain to provide stimulation of such areas. The electrode is implanted stereotactically and is connected through subcutaneous leads to a small radio receiver that usually is located subcutaneously below the clavicle. The implanted system is passive, that is, contains no power of its own. It is activated by power transmitted from a small radio transmitter, slightly larger than a pack of cigarettes, that can be controlled by the patient and is coupled to the internalized system through an antenna secured on the chest overlying the radio receiver.

A number of sites have been found to produce analgesia when stimulated. In humans, the most effective areas are in the ventrolateral periaqueductal gray matter (37) and the gray matter just lateral to the third ventricle, near the posterior commissure (36,38). Deep brain-stimulating electrodes are inserted stereotactically. Pain relief may exceed the period of stimulation by many hours (36,39). It is curious to note that stimulation of the periaqueductal gray is amplitude dependent, that is, if the voltage for pain relief is exceeded, stimulation may make the pain worse or may cause the patient extreme distress.

Pain caused by denervation, such as phantom limb pain, can often be managed successfully with chronic deep brain stimulation of the somatosensory system. Electrodes may be inserted either into the ventral posterior nucleus of the thalamus or the posterior limb of the internal capsule, theoretically substituting sensation from electrical stimulation for the absent sensory input (34,38).

Electrodes are inserted under local anesthesia so the patient may be tested intraoperatively with stimulation for accurate placement. On stimulation of the somatosensory system, it is important that the patient have sensation projected to that area of the body concerned with pain. In deep brain stimulation of the descending pain inhibitory system, it is encouraging if the patient has abrupt relief of pain on stimulation of the inserted electrode, but reports of pain relief may be inconclusive or inaccurate during the stress and sedation of surgery. Intraoperative stimulation is nevertheless important to assure that the electrodes are not in adjacent areas of important neurologic function, such as the pyramidal tracts or near the oculomotor fibers. Even though the procedure may take three to four hours, most patients tolerate the stress sufficiently to report sensation on stimulation, but assessment for pain relief may require stimulation during the less stressful postoperative period.

PSYCHOSURGERY

Present-day psychosurgical procedures generally involve stereotactic techniques. The old prefrontal lobotomy and extensive undercutting of the frontal lobes have been supplanted by safer and more accurate techniques that are far less likely to cause deterioration of mentation or alertness and are more likely to provide the desired beneficial result. Although some surgeons still prefer an open operation based on discrete landmarks (40), most prefer the control and simplicity afforded by sterotactic surgery.

Indeed, it was the inexactness of the classic prefrontal lobotomy (41,42) that motivated Spiegel and co-workers (2,18) to develop the techniques for human stereotactic surgery. The first patients were treated for affective disorders. The indications for psychosurgery, however, have been markedly restricted since the development of tranquilizers. Despite recent political attention directed at psychosurgery, a national commission to evaluate allegations against the procedure gathered evidence demonstrating that psychosurgery is both reasonably safe and effective (43) but should not be used if nonsurgical means are effective. Conditions that are indications for psychosurgery are those characterized by stereotyped and excessive emotional response (44), that is, depression (44–47), chronic anxiety or tension state (44), obsessive-compulsive state (48), and perhaps the depressive component of manic-depressive disorders (44). There is considerable controversy as to whether psychosurgery should be used for aggressive disorders, and such conditions presently are not usually considered for psychosurgery.

Most authors use the same target point for obsessive-compulsive neurosis, anxiety, and depression. The most popular target is the cingulate gyrus, so that cingulotomy is the procedure most likely done in all three conditions (49), although some surgeons prefer to make lesions in the anterior portion of the internal capsule to interrupt the fibers radiating to the frontal lobe (50–52).

Since there is no immediate identifiable result of the production of such lesions nor accurate means for physiologic control, and because patients for psychosurgery may have difficulty cooperating with a long procedure under local anesthesia, cingulotomy or dorsomedial thalamotomy is often performed under general anesthesia.

Because of the lack of physiologic restraints, any acceptable neuroanesthetic technique may be employed; however, one should use an agent that allows the patient to awaken promptly at the conclusion of surgery. This permits evaluation for undesirable side effects, such as edema, bleeding, or interference with cerebral blood vessels. Because the patient may remain drowsy and may exhibit considerable anergia during the first seven to ten days postoperatively, with lack of contact with surroundings and lack of initiation of conversation (53,54), evaluation of the patient may be difficult during the initial postoperative period. This early condition is usually only temporary and bears no relationship to the final clinical result. In fact, during the second and third week, the patient may show increased irritability and verbal aggressiveness, and it is not until the fourth to sixth week that the ultimate clinical result becomes evident.

EPILEPSY

Stereotactic surgery can be used to treat epilepsy not otherwise amenable to surgery (see Chapter 12). Since reports of long-term follow-up in patients with partial seizures secondary to temporal lobe foci indicate that patients treated with stereotactic surgery do not generally do as well as patients treated with classic temporal lobe resection, the latter technique is the procedure of choice. There is a group of patients, however, with unilateral foci or predominantly unilateral epilepsy whose foci may not be in a resectable area of the temporal cortex (55). Such patients may benefit from the production of a stereotactic lesion in the amygdaloid nucleus (26,27) or even the same pathway leading from the globus pallidus or Forel's field as is used for treatment of movement disorders (56).

ANESTHETIC CONSIDERATIONS

Types of Apparatus

There are three types of stereotactic apparatus (Fig. 14.3), the design of which has implications for anesthesia. The apparatus should be constructed in such a way that there is free access to the patient's face to care for the airway, especially if vomiting occurs. It should be constructed so the patient's head may be quickly removed in the event of a catastrophe that may require assisted ventilation and/or intubation. Ideally, it should be possible to change the patient's position even

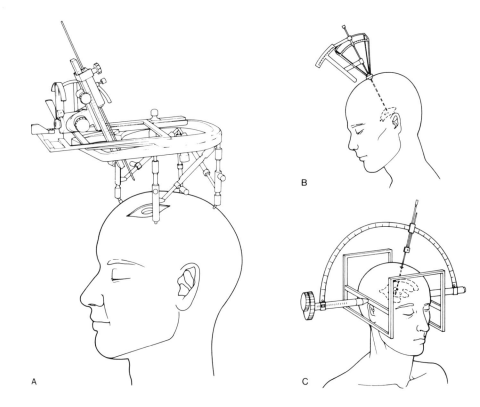

Figure 14.3 The three types of stereotactic devices; *A*, rectilinear type; *B*, aiming device; and *C*, arc type.

while in the apparatus, so that the head can be lowered in the event of hypotension or air embolism. The apparatus should be electrically safe, especially since both electronic lesion-making apparatus and monitoring devices are attached to the patient simultaneously. The stereotactic apparatus should fix firmly to the patient's skull in a manner to assure that the patient is comfortable, so it is not necessary to oversedate the patient to prevent movements of the head in relationship to the apparatus. There are many stereotactic apparatus representing each of three types that meet these requirements.

The most commonly employed type of apparatus is the arc type, which interrelates two or more arcs (Fig. 14.3C). The mechanical target point lies at the center of an arc along which an electrode holder can be adjusted. No matter at which angle the electrode is inserted, it is always directed to the mechanical target point. The patient's head is adjusted within the apparatus or the arc is adjusted to bring the desired anatomic structure to the center of the arc. In some designs using the arc principle, the arc is attached to a frame secured to the patient's head, as with the Leksell apparatus (Fig. 14.3C) (57), which has particular advantages. There is free access to the patient's face, the patient may be moved with the stereotactic apparatus in place, and the frame can be rapidly disassembled in an emergency. The Reichert (58) apparatus has a basal ring to which the patient's head is secured, and a second arc that is attached to the basal ring and adjusted according to the coordinates of the target point. This apparatus is heavy and is attached to the operating table or a pedestal, so it is not possible to change the patient's position while in the apparatus. The ring to which the patient's head is attached may provide some difficulties for access to the patient's face in an emergency, but routine care can be handled expeditiously. The most commonly employed apparatus in the United States (59) is the Todd-Wells apparatus, which works in a reciprocal fashion. The several interlocking arcs are built into the apparatus, and the patient's head is moved to bring the target point to the proper position. Again, this apparatus is attached to the operating table or to a pedestal, so the patient must remain prone or supine. The ring securing the patient's head can be rapidly removed from the apparatus or completely disassembled in event of emergency.

The rectilinear type of stereotactic apparatus is based on the same principle as the original Horsley-Clarke system, and is illustrated by the Spiegel-Wycis device (2) (Fig. 14.3A). The frame is attached to the patient's skull and bears a plate that can be moved longitudinally or transversely. The electrode holder allows controlled advance of the electrode to provide for adjustment in the third plane. Angular adjustments are included so the electrode can be inserted along the most desirable trajectory, as with the arc-type systems. The advantage of this type of system, from the viewpoint of the anesthesiologist, is total access to the patient's face and chest. The patient can be moved to any position with the apparatus in place, since the apparatus is quite light. Some systems employing the rectilinear arrangement, however, may involve a head holder that partially occludes the face (Spiegel-Wycis Model VI) or may require attachment to the operating table, which restricts the patient's mobility (5).

The third type of system is a simple aiming device (Fig. 14.3B). A burr hole is made and a ball-and-socket joint is screwed into the burr hole. The universal joint allows the apparatus to be adjusted so the electrode points to the target. Because of the difficulties of attaching the apparatus securely to the bone and the inaccuracies of fine angular adjustments, this type of apparatus is not as precise as the other two. It has been used recently in conjunction with computed tomographic (CT) scanning, since accuracy is not as critical and can be verified by repeated scans during the procedure, and the entire apparatus lies outside the scanning plane. This type of apparatus provides completely free access to the patient's head and the patient can be moved easily, but care must be taken not to dislodge or move it.

Choice of Anesthetic

Because of the necessity to test the patient physiologically during functional surgical procedures to assure accuracy of electrode placement in the anatomic target, procedures are done under local anesthesia unless the patient is too young, too confused, or too agitated to lie quietly during the procedure, or has such severe involuntary movements that general anesthesia is essential. Even patients undergoing stereotactic biopsy for tumor or aspiration of abscesses probably should have the procedure performed under local anesthesia, if feasible, to avoid potential risks of anesthesia in a patient with intracranial hypertension. Also, if intracranial bleeding were to occur, it might be identified by the appearance of a progressive neurologic deficit or decreasing level of consciousness and treated more promptly.

If local anesthesia is employed, the duration of the procedure may suggest the most appropriate agent. Most procedures are less than four hours so that 1% lidocaine with 1:100,000 epinephrine usually is adequate. If it is anticipated that the procedure will last more than four hours, it is recommended to combine 1% lidocaine containing 1:100,000 epinephrine with an equal volume of 0.5% bupivacaine, to make a final concentration of 0.5% lidocaine, 0.25% bupivacaine, and 1:200,000 epinephrine.

If general anesthesia is used, the choice of agent depends on whether the patient has intracranial hypertension and/or whether intraoperative electrical recordings are planned. If the patient has intracranial hypertension, as for stereotactic biopsy of a brain tumor, the usual precautions should be used. Because of the further increase in intracranial pressure accompanying an increase in arterial carbon dioxide tension ($PaCO_2$), the patient should be hyperventilated, ideally to maintain the $PaCO_2$ between 25 and 28 mm Hg. Agents such as ketamine that increase intracranial pressure should be avoided. The use of low-dose isoflurane, barbiturates and/or narcotics, that may decrease intracranial pressure, combined with hyperventilation, may be helpful. Animal studies with cryogenic lesions have indicated greater postoperative development of cerebral edema following use of any of the three halogenated inhalation agents. Therefore, if such a means of lesion production is to be used, a balanced anesthetic technique is, at least theoretically, preferable.

It would seem that the requirements of sedation for stereotactic surgery are sufficiently well defined that some common practices should have developed to guide the anesthesiologist new to this field. An unpublished survey of anesthesiologists and neurosurgeons (Gildenberg and Frost 1977), however, revealed that there was virtually no consensus as to the appropriate sedative or anesthetic agent used with stereotactic surgery. Some practitioners appear to be unaware of the requirements of the procedure and were using agents that should have been contraindicated for considerations discussed herein, and there appeared to be little communication about this subject, since there were few reports in the literature, and since at some centers the anesthesiologist and neurosurgeon appeared to be unaware of each other's actions and requirements.

If electrical recording is desired during the procedure, agents that affect electrical activity of the brain should be avoided. Diazepam, in particular, may cause a change in electrical activity concerned with epilepsy. Barbiturates also may cause suppression of normal activity and the production of a sleeplike electroencephalographic (EEG) state, but without normal sleep spindles. Ketamine may cause profound alterations in the EEG with alternating high-amplitude delta complexes and periods of fast activity (60) and may promote frank seizures in susceptible patients (61).

The use of a 70:30 nitrous oxide/oxygen mixture has minimal effect on electrical activity of the cortex or subcortex (62) and may be used to supplement local anesthesia unless air is used as a contrast agent.

Phenothiazines should be avoided in patients with movement disorders, since they may alter the involuntary movements used as an indication of the adequacy of lesion production.

Intravenous droperidol and fentanyl can be used if sedation is required (63) since this combination has minimal effects on the EEG (64), but care must be taken that the patient not become oversedated for those parts of the procedure that require the patient's cooperation or require demonstration of the patient's involuntary movements. A recent article has summarized the requirements for neuroleptic analgesia (65).

Antihistimines should be avoided since in some patients they cause excitement and hyperventilation rather than sedation (66). Ideally, no sedation at all should be used for patients with movement disorders, since even the calming effect of the sedation may cause sufficient suppression of the symptoms under study that adequacy of lesion production cannot be accurately determined.

Air Embolism

If the procedure is done in the sitting position, there is a potential risk of venous air embolism and appropriate precautions must be taken. Even with a burr hole, there may be sufficient settling of the brain to cause traction on the surface veins, especially as they enter the sagittal sinus, which is at subatmospheric pressure in the sitting position, and air entering the subdural space may be aspirated into the sagittal sinus. In preparation for using the sitting position, an atrial catheter should be placed prior to the procedure. A Doppler precordial monitor should be used throughout the procedure (67,68). If the Doppler monitor indicates air in the vascular system, nitrous oxide should be discontinued and other appropriate therapeutic measures adopted.

Some surgeons may perform pneumoencephalography to visualize the landmarks about the third ventricle. Usually this is done the day prior to surgery or in the operating room immediately before surgery. Patients may complain of severe headache and may require analgesics, possibly narcotics, in order to remain still after the pneumoencephalogram. There is an increased risk of air embolism after pneumoencephalography, particularly in elderly patients who may have sufficient atrophy to cause traction on the surface veins, especially in the sitting position. If an air ventriculogram is used, it may be necessary to instill the air under controlled pressure to vsualize the posterior commissure, which theoretically may increase the risk of venous air embolism. Whenever air is employed as a contrast agent, the use of nitrous oxide is contraindicated, since its differential absorption may cause a large increase in the volume of intracranial gas.

Preparation and Diagnostic Studies

The patient is placed in either the supine or sitting position on the operating table, depending on the type of apparatus to be used. The head is shaved and the scalp cleansed. It may be advantageous to mark the reference planes, or at least the midsagittal plane, or the scalp. The sites for fixation of the contact points are marked and infiltrated early with local anesthetic, depending on the type of apparatus and anticipated duration of the procedure. When the apparatus is secured to the patient's head, a burr hole is made and a ventricular cannula inserted to instill contrast material.

Perhaps the most distressing part of the procedure is the noise that the patient hears during production of the burr hole. Consequently, power instruments should be avoided. A burr, such as the D'Errico burr, that can be used with a Hudson brace to produce a hole in a single step is preferable.

Conray or Pantopaque may be used for the ventriculogram with appropriate precautions. If Pantopaque is used, it is necessary to manipulate the patient's head to visualize both the anterior and posterior commissures, since the hyperbaric contrast material settles in the most dependent area. This necessitates a sitting position, with the risk of air embolism.

Iothalamate meglumine (Conray) is the agent most usually used for ventriculography during stereotactic surgery. The most frequently occurring adverse reactions with Conray ventriculography are nausea and vomiting, which occur almost invariably if the agent leaks out of the ventricular system into the subarachnoid space, which is not uncommon with the doses required. Vomiting may be a particular problem in that the patient's head is secured in the stereotactic apparatus. Suction and emesis basin should be available. When vomiting occurs, it is usually of short duration, but the patient requires considerable reassurance during that time. In general, phenothiazines should be avoided, but diazepam may be helpful to calm the patient, with care being taken to avoid oversedation.

Conray, like other water-soluble contrast agents, has other potential complications. It has been associated with fatal anaphylactic reactions. In these cases there is usually a history of allergy to such agents or iodine. The anesthesiologist should be prepared to deal with these reactions with cardiovascular support, high doses of steroids, epinephrine, vasopressors, and airway maintenance.

Water-soluble contrast agents may cause seizures. If it is anticipated that they will be used, anticonvulsant medication should not be discontinued. Should a seizure occur, intravenous diazepam, sodium thiopental, or phenobarbital is recommended. If the contrast agent may enter the subarachnoid space, anticonvulsant medication should be considered prophylactically. Drugs that lower the seizure threshold, especially phenothiazine derivatives, should not be used, nor should monoamine oxidase inhibitors, tricyclic antidepressants, or psychoactive drugs.

THE PROCEDURE

Following ventriculography, anteroposterior and lateral roentgenograms are obtained. The midline of the third ventricle is indicated on the anteroposterior film and its relationship to the coordinate system of the apparatus noted. On the lateral films, the anterior and posterior commissures are identified and a line drawn between the two. The coordinates of the intended target point are determined from an atlas and indicated by measurement on the anteroposterior and lateral films, taking x-ray magnification into account.

The apparatus is adjusted by a series of progressive approximations, that is, the apparatus is adjusted to the target point as indicated on the anteroposterior and lateral films, and another pair of films is obtained; any inaccuracies are corrected and the procedure is repeated. With each correction, the errors should decrease until accuracy is achieved.

When the apparatus is adjusted so that the proper coordinates are at the center or target point of the apparatus, final films are made with the electrode probe secured in the apparatus with the tip of the electrode on the scalp. The trajectory is indicated on the anteroposterior and lateral films by drawing a line through the image of the electrode and beyond, which should pass through the target point in both views.

If adjustment is accurate, the electrode or probe is temporarily removed and the scalp incision and burr hole are made where the electrode contacted the scalp. The dura is coagulated and opened, and the electrode is replaced and advanced to the target point. Final anteroposterior and lateral films are made with the electrode in position to verify accuracy before stimulation, lesion production, or aspiration is attempted.

Even though the electrode may lie at the proper coordinates, it is necessary to use physiologic verification to assure that the tip of the electrode is in the intended anatomic structure and avoids nearby areas of vital brain function. If both stimulation and recording are to be done, recording is performed first, since stimulation may affect spontaneous activity. The parameters of recording and whether stimulation is used to evoke electrical activity depend on the specific target. The frequency of stimulation depends on the observations to be made, and may vary between 50 and 120 Hz. It is usually necessary that the patient be awake during testing to obtain maximum information from the procedure.

After it has been verified that the electrode is in the proper position, the lesion is made. The three most common methods of lesion production are radiofrequency current, application of cold, or leukotome. When electrical current is applied at a rapidly alternating frequency, usually between 500 kHz and 2 MHz (frequencies usually employed in radio transmission), the ionic oscillation of the surrounding tissues is vigorous enough to cause those tissues to heat. If a temperature of 45 °C is exceeded, a permanent lesion will result. The usual temperature employed in stereotactic surgery is 80 °C, usually maintained for 1 to 2 minutes. Most radiofrequency generators are calibrated to provide that temperature, or a thermistor is incorporated into the electrode to monitor the temperature during the lesion production.

In the use of cold, an insulated probe is inserted stereotactically. As liquid nitrogen circulates through the probe, the uninsulated tip cools to sufficiently low temperatures to cause the surrounding brain tissue to freeze, producing a permanent lesion. In the usual system, the temperature at the tip of the probe is monitored, and this information is fed back to a valve system to regulate the flow of liquid nitrogen and attain the desired temperature for the necessary duration, ordinarily − 40 °C to −100 °C for three minutes. Disadvantages of the cold probe are that electrical stimluation or recording are not possible with the same instrument, and the probes tend to be larger than radiofrequency electrodes. In animal studies, creation of a cryogenic lesion during the use of inhalation agents has been associated with increases in intracranial pressure. One theoretical advantage is that the narrow area surrounding the probe shows temporary alteration in activity as the temperature decreases, so that a test may be employed prior to the production of a permanent lesion.

A leukotome is an instrument with a small wire loop that can be extended from the side near the tip. The leukotome is inserted with the wire loop retracted, which can then be extended and the instrument rotated, usually one quadrant at a time, to cut the surrounding tissue and produce a lesion. The sole advantage of the system is its simplicity, since expensive apparatus is not required. Disadvantages include the inability to perform recordings or stimulate through the leukotome at the area to be incorporated within the lesion and the risk to surrounding blood vessels, which may cause intracerebral bleeding. The leukotome presently is used by only a few stereotactic neurosurgeons (59).

Following lesion production, the electrode or probe is withdrawn and the small scalp incision sutured. The patient should be observed closely for the development of complications, particularly intracranial bleeding. Even though the incision is small, production of a lesion causes a major disruption in neurophysiologic regulation and the patient should be afforded the same care that one would give any postoperative craniotomy patient.

STEREOTACTIC SURGERY GUIDED BY
COMPUTED TOMOGRAPHY

Perhaps the most important new development in the field of stereotaxis is the combination of computed tomographic (CT) scanning with stereotactic surgery—a significant advance in both fields. Although these procedures are just beginning to be used clinically, it becomes possible to introduce a probe, biopsy forceps, or aspiration needle into any lesion that can be seen on CT scans (69).

Most techniques involve the use of specialized stereotactic apparatus that is attached to or incorporated into a CT scanner (70–76). Other techniques involve calculation of coordinates from the CT scan (77) or attachment of a head frame during the scanning procedure (72), with the actual surgery being done in the operating room.

The advantages of performing the surgery in the CT scanner are increased accuracy and the ability to monitor the progress of tissue removal or aspiration intraoperatively. The disadvantages, however, are numerous, especially for the anesthesiologist. Most CT rooms are not equipped for anesthesia or surgery and may compromise sterility or availability of necessary gases, suction, and emergency facilities. The anesthesiologist is removed from the operating area where personnel and equipment are available to handle any emergency. The CT apparatus itself may restrict access to the patient's face and/or chest, depending on the system used and whether the stereotactic apparatus is in place (Chapter 5).

In general, it is preferable to do most procedures under local anesthesia, which affords an additional degree of safety, since the major complication is bleeding from a biopsy site, which can be detected promptly if the patient is awake. Since many patients have increased intracranial pressure from tumor, abscess, or hematoma at the time the procedure is done, the usual cautions concerning anesthesia for patients with intracranial hypertension should be taken.

REFERENCES

1. Horsley V, Clarke RH: The structure and function of the cerebellum examined by a new method. Brain 1908;31:45–124.
2. Spiegel EA, Wycis HT, Marks M, et al.: Stereotactic apparatus for operations on the human brain. Science 1947;106:349–350.
3. Spiegel EA, Wycis HT: Stereoencephalotomy. Part I. New York, Grune & Stratton, 1952.
4. Shaltenbrand G, Bailey P: Introduction to stereotaxis with an atlas of the human brain. Stuttgart, Thieme, 1959.
5. Talairach J, David M, Tournoux P: Atlas d'anatomie stereotaxique. Paris, Masson, 1957.
6. Andrew J, Watkins ES: Stereotaxic atlas of the human thalamus. Baltimore, Williams & Wilkins, 1969.
7. Emmers R, Tasker RR: The human somesthetic thalamus. New York, Raven Press, 1975.

8. Van Buren JM, Buorke RC: Variations and connections of the human thalamus, vol 2, Variations of the human diencephalon. New York, Springer, 1972.

9. Afshar F, Watkins ES, Yap JC: Stereotaxic atlas of the human brainstem and cerebellar nuclei. New York, Raven Press, 1978.

10. Hoehn MM, Yahr MD: Parkinsonism: Onset, progression and mortality. Neurology 1976;17:427–442.

11. Kelly PJ, Gillingham FJ: The long-term results of stereotaxic surgery and L-dopa therapy in patients with Parkinson's disease. A 10-year follow-up study. J Neurosurg 1980;53:332–337.

12. Siegfried J: Is the neurosurgical treatment of Parkinson's disease still indicated? J Neural Transm (Suppl) 1980;16:195–198.

13. Wycis HT, Cunningham W, Kellett G, et al.: L-Dopa in the treatment of postsurgical Parkinson patients. J Neurosurg 1970;32:281.

14. Gildenberg PL: Current indications for stereotactic surgery in Parkinson's disease. Med J St Josephs Hosp (Houston) 1981;16:219–223.

15. Laitinen L: Surgical treatment, past and present, in Parkinson's disease. Acta Neurol Scand (Suppl) 1972;51:43–58.

16. Van Buren JM, Li C-L, Shapiro DY, et al.: A qualitative and quantitative evaluation of Parkinsonians three to six years following thalamotomy. Confin Neurol 1973;35: 202–235.

17. Cooper IS: Movement disorders. New York, Hoeber, 1969.

18. Spiegel EA: Guided brain operations. Basel, Karger, 1982.

19. Hassler R, Dieckman G: Stereotaxic treatment for spasmodic torticollis, in Schaltenbrand E, Walker AE (eds): Stereotaxy of the human brain. New York, Thieme-Stratton, 1982, pp 522–531.

20. Gildenberg PL: Comprehensive management of spasmodic torticollis. Appl Neurophysiol 1981;44:233–243.

21. Laitinen L: Short-term results of treatment for infantile cerebral palsy. Confin Neurol 1965;26:258–263.

22. Broggi G, Angelini L, Bono R, et al.: Stereotactic surgery of abnormal movements: Clinical results in 33 cerebral palsy patients. Appl Neurophysiol 1982;45:306–310.

23. Heimburger RF, Whitlock CC: Stereotaxic destruction of the human dentate nucleus. Confin Neurol 1965;26:346–358.

24. Siegfried J: Neurosurgical treatment of spasticity, in Rasmussen T, Marino R (eds): Functional neurosurgery. New York, Raven Press, 1979, pp 123–128.

25. Zervas N: Long-term view of dentatectomy in dystonia musculorum deformans and cerebral palsy. Acta Neurochir (Wien) (Suppl) 1977;24:49–51.

26. Narabayashi H: Stereotaxic surgery for athetosis or the spastic state of cerebral palsy. Confin Neurol 1962;22:363–367.

27. Spiegel EA, Wycis HT, Szekely EG, et al.: Campotomy in various extrapyramidal disorders. J Neurosurg 1963;20:871–881.

28. Mehler WR: Some neurological species differences—a posteriori. Ann NY Acad Sci 1969;167:424–468.

29. Spiegel EA, Wycis HT: Mesencephalotomy in the treatment of "intractable" facial pain. Arch Neurol 1953;69:1–13.

30. Nashold BS, Jr: Extensive cephalic and oral pain relieved by midbrain tractotomy. Confin Neurol 1972;34:381–388.

31. Voris HC, Whistler WW: Results of stereotaxic surgery for intractable pain. Confin Neurol 1975;37:86–96.

32. Mayer DJ, Hayes RL: Stimulation-produced analgesia: Development of tolerance and cross-tolerance to morphine. Science 1975;188:941–953.

33. Reynolds DV: Surgery in the rat during electrical analgesia induced by focal brain stimulation. Science 1969;164:445.

34. Adams JE: Technique and technical problems associated with implantation of neuroaugmentive devices. Appl Neurophysiol 1977/78;40:111–123.

35. Nashold BS Jr, Wilson WP, Boone E: Depth recordings and stimulation of the human brain: A twenty-year experience, in Rasmussen T, Marino R (eds): Functional neurosurgery. New York, Raven Press, 1979, pp 181–195.

36. Richardson DE, Akil H: Pain reduction by electrical brain stimulation in man. II. Chronic self-administration in the peri-ventricular gray matter. J Neurosurg 1979;47: 184–194.

37. Mayer DJ, Liebeskind JC: Pain reduction by focal electrical stimulation of the brain. An anatomical and behavioral analysis. Brain Res 1974;68:73–93.

38. Hosobuchi Y, Adams JE, Rutkin B: Chronic thalamic stimulation for the control of facial anesthesia dolorosa. Arch Neurol 1973;29:158–161.

39. Hosobuchi Y, Adams JE, Linchitz R: Pain relief by electrical stimulation of the central gray matter in humans and its reversal by naloxone. Science 1977;197:183–186.

40. Ballentine HT, Jr, Giriunas IE: Advances in psychiatric surgery, in Rasmussen T, Marino R: Functional neurosurgery. New York, Raven Press, 1979, pp 155–164.

41. Freeman W: Frontal lobotomy in early schizophrenia. Long-term follow-up in 415 cases, in Hitchcock E, Laitinen L, Vaernet K (eds): Psychosurgery. Springfield, Ill, Charles C Thomas, 1972, pp 311–321.

42. Freeman W: Frontal lobotomy in early schizophrenia: Long-term follow-up in 415 cases. Br J Psychiatry 1971;114:1223–1246.

43. National Commission for the Protection of Human Subjects of Biomedical and Behavioral Research: Report and recommendations. Psychosurgery. Washington, DC, DHEW, Publication No (05) 77–0001, 1977.

44. Sweet WH, Obrador S, Martin-Rodriguez JG (eds): Neurosurgical treatment in psychiatry, pain and epilepsy. Baltimore, University Park Press, 1977.

45. Bailey HE, Dowling JL, Davies E: Cingulotractotomy and related procedures for severe depressive illness (studies in depression, IV), in Sweet WH, Obrador S, Martin-Rodriguez JG (eds): Neurosurgical treatment in psychiatry, pain and epilepsy. Baltimore, University Park Press, 1977, pp 229–251.

46. Ballantine HT Jr, Cassidy WL, Bordeur J: Frontal cingulotomy for mood disturbance, in Hitchcock E, Laitinen L, Vaernet K (eds): Psychosurgery. Springfield, Ill, Charles C Thomas, 1972, pp 221–229.

47. Ballantine HT Jr, Cassidy WL, Flanagan NB: Stereotaxic anterior cingulotomy for neuropsychiatric illness and intractable pain. J Neurosurg 1967;26:488–495.

48. Orthner H, Muller D, Roeder F: Stereotaxic psychosurgery. Techniques and results since 1955, in Hitchcock E, Laitinen L, Vaernet K (eds): Psychosurgery. Springfield, Ill, Charles C Thomas, 1972, pp 37–390.

49. Sweet WH; Treatment of medically intractable mental disease by limited frontal leucotomy—justifiable? N Engl J Med 1973;189:1117–1125.

50. Crow HJ, Cooper R, Phillips DG: Controlled multifocal frontal leucotomy for psychiatric illness. J Neurol Neurosurg Psychiatry 1961;24:353–360.

51. Smith JS, Kiloh LG, Boots JA: Prospective evaluation of prefrontal leucotomy: Results at 30 months follow-up, in Sweet WH, Obrador S, Martin-Rodriguez JG (eds):

Neurosurgical treatment in psychiatry, pain and epilepsy. Baltimore, University Park Press, 1977, pp 217–224.

52. Storm-Olsen R, Carlisle S: Bifrontal stereotactic tractotomy. A follow-up study of its effects of 210 patients. Br J Psychiatry 1971;118:141–154.

53. Lopez-Ibor JJ, Lopez-Ibor A: Selection criteria for patients who should undergo psychiatric surgery, in Sweet WH, Obrador S, Martin-Rodriguez JG (eds): Neurosurgical treatment of psychiatry, pain and epilepsy. Baltimore, University Park Press, 1977, pp 151–162.

54. Bailey HR, Dowling JL, Davies E: Studies in depression, III: The control of affective illness by cingulotractotomy. A review of 150 cases. Med J Aust 1973;2:366–371.

55. Sypert GW: New concepts in the management of epilepsy. Medical and surgical. Clin Neurosurg 1977;24:600–641.

56. Yoshii N: Follow-up study of epileptic patients following Forel-H-totomy. Appl Neurophysiol 1977/78;40:1–12.

57. Leksell L: Stereotaxis and radiosurgery. An operative system. Springfield, Ill, Charles C Thomas, 1971.

58. Reichert T: Stereotactic brain operations. Bern, Hans Huber, 1980.

59. Gildenberg PL: Survey of stereotactic and functional neurosurgery in the United States and Canada. Appl Neurophysiol 1975;38:31–37.

60. Rosen I, Hagerdal M: Electroencephalographic study of children during ketamine anesthesia. Acta Anaesthesiol Scand 1976;20:32–39.

61. Bennett DR, Madsten JA, Jordan WS, et al.: Ketamine anesthesia in brain damaged epileptics. Electroencephalographic and clinical observations. Neurology 1973;23:449–460.

62. Babb TL, Ferrer-Brechner T, Brechner VL, et al.: Limbic neuronal firing rates in man during administration of nitrous oxide-oxygen or sodium thiopental. Anesthesiology 1975;43:402–409.

63. Gilbert RGB, Brindle GF, Galindo A: Anesthesia for neurosurgery. Boston, Little Brown & Co, 1966, pp 132–137.

64. Nilsson EE, Ingvar DH: EEG findings in neuroleptanalgesia. Acta Anaesthesiol Scand 1967;11:121–127.

65. Zukic A, Kelly PJ: Neuroleptic analgesia for stereotactic surgery. Affl Neurophysiol 1883;46:172–174.

66. Melville KI: Antihistamine drugs, in Schacter M (ed): Histamines and antihistamines. Section 74, International encyclopedia of pharmacology and therapeutics. Oxford, Pergamon, 1973, pp 127–171.

67. Adornato D, Gildenberg PL, Ferrario CM, et al.: Pathophysiology of intravenous air embolism in dogs. Anesthesiology 1978;49:120–127.

68. Gildenberg PL, O'Brien RP, Britt WJ, et al.: The efficacy of Doppler monitoring for the detection of venous air embolism. J Neurosurg 1981;54:75–78.

69. Gildenberg PL, Kaufman HH, Murthy KSK: Calculation of stereotactic coordinates from the computed tomographic scan. Neurosurgery 1982;10:580–586.

70. Bergstrom M, Boethius J, Eriksson L: Head fixation device for reproducible position alignment in transmission CT and positron emission tomography. Technical note. J Comput Assist Tomogr 1981;5:136–141.

71. Brown R: A computerized tomography-computer graphics approach to stereotaxic localization. J Neurosurg 1979;50:715–720.

72. Greitz T, Bergstrom M: Stereotactic procedures in computer tomography, in Newton TH, Potts DG (eds): Radiology of the skull and brain. Technical aspects of Computer Tomography. St. Louis, CV Mosby, 1981, pp 4286–4296.

73. Jacques S, Shelden CH, McCann GD: Computerized three-dimensional stereotaxic removal of small central nervous system lesions in patients. J Neurosurg 1980;53: 816–820.

74. Koslow M, Abele MG, Griffith RC: Stereotactic surgical system controlled by computed tomography. Neurosurgery 1981;8:72–82.

75. Rosenbaum A, Lunsford LD, Perry J: Computerized tomography guided stereotaxis. A new approach. Appl Neurophysiol 1980;43:172–173.

76. Rushworth RG: Stereotactic guided biopsy in the computerized tomographic scanner. Surg Neurol 1980;14:451–454.

77. Kaufman HH, Gildenberg PL: New head positioning system for use with computer tomographic scanning. Neurosurgery 1980;7:147–149.

PART III

Central Nervous System Trauma

CHAPTER 15

The Management of Head Injury
Kamran Tabaddor and
Elizabeth A.M. Frost

Head injuries constitute not only major medical emergencies but also serious socioeconomic problems. Optimal outcome depends on a team approach, involving, among others, the anesthesiologist, the neurosurgeon, and the emergency room physician. Rational therapy depends on a full understanding of the pathophysiology of this trauma.

EPIDEMIOLOGY

Information on the occurrence of head trauma is important to formulate health care policies, plan treatment and rehabilitation facilities, and efficiently allocate resources. Few, if any, national and local statistics providing this data are kept; hence, estimates are made from special national sample surveys or from intensive study of local communities. Estimates of the annual incidence of head injury in the entire United States range from 673 per 100,000 (1) to 204 per 100,000 (2). This discrepancy is due to methodologic variations in the definition of a "case" and in the sampling design. In regional communities, the annual incidence rate of head injury ranges from 180 per 100,000 in Olmstead County, Minnesota (3), to 249 per 100,000 in the Bronx, New York (4), to 295 per 100,000 per year in San Diego County, California (5). These regional differences may be due to real urban-rural differences in the occurrence of head trauma or to methodologic differences in the study design.

Several studies (6,7) have observed that most head injuries occur and present to the emergency room between the hours of 4 PM and midnight. Moreover, the frequency of head injury is highest between Friday and Sunday. Seasonal variation of head injuries has been apparent in most studies, but no consistent patterns have been observed (2–6).

Populations at special risk for head trauma have been identified through community surveys and case series. These data identify groups for the most efficient targeting of preventive strategies. Studies of head injury consistently show that males are at a two to four times higher risk than are females (3–5). The age distribution of head injury in the Bronx is shown in Figure 15.1 (4). Increased

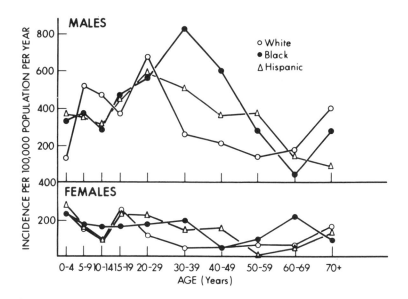

Figure 15.1 The age distribution of head injury in the Bronx indicates the highest frequency in blacks at age 30 years and in whites and Hispanics at age 20 years. (From Cooper KD, Tabaddor K, Hauser WA et al.: The epidemiology of head injury in the Bronx. Neuroepidemiology, in press. Reprinted by permission.)

rates of head injury are consistently found in young males and in the elderly and probably are due to violence (4) and traffic accidents (2,3,5) in the young and falls in the elderly.

In most communities studied, traffic accidents are the cause of over 50% of head injuries (3,5); however, several studies in urban communities (4,8,9) have found that violence accounted for a substantial proportion of head trauma. These differences may be due to the low socioeconomic status and the fewer available highways and the more frequent use of public transportation in urban areas.

Among the factors most prominently associated with traumatic injury in general and head trauma in particular is alcohol consumption, which has been indicated in over 50% of fatal motor vehicle accidents in the United States (10). Two studies (11,12) found that approximately 50% of emergency room patients with head injury had detectable blood alcohol levels. Recently, many states have increased the legal age for alcohol consumption in an effort to reduce traffic accident mortality and morbidity.

Unpublished data from the Health Interview Survey (13) suggest that only 25% of all "head injuries" involve skull fractures or intracranial injuries. That only a small fraction of head injuries are moderate to severe was supported by a one-month study of all emergency room contacts in a large teaching hospital (7). Only 15% of the total head injury population in this study was admitted to the hospital and only 9.6% of those admitted had moderate or severe injuries as defined by a Glasgow Coma Score between 3 and 11 (14).

The annual mortality rate from head injuries in the United States is unknown. Mortality data published by the National Center for Health Statistics catalog death from external causes rather than death from the site of insult.

A recent study of head injury in three urban counties indicates that the mortality rates were similar for Bronx County, New York, San Diego County, California, and Harris County, Texas, despite differences in the socioeconomic structures of these counties (15). The annual mortality rate from head injuries averaged 29 per 100,000 and varied among the counties from 27 to 32 per 100,000. Since over 60% of head trauma mortalities occur prior to hospital admission and admission to specialized neurosurgical units, these authors suggest that primary prevention may be the key component in any program geared to reduce head trauma mortality.

EMERGENCY CARE

Head injury constitutes a dynamic process and has a variable course, depending both on the initial injury and on secondary brain damage. The initial brain damage resulting from the impact is not amenable to treatment. Therefore, the goals of management are to prevent secondary brain damage resulting from the development of intracranial or extracranial complications and to provide the brain with the optimal physiologic environment to maximize the potential for recovery. The ability to talk after head trauma implies that since the initial impact was not fatal, death may then be related to subsequent deterioration. Hence, by the prevention of secondary brain injury, death might be avoided (16). In a group of patients known to have talked before dying from head injury, hypoxia and shock were the most common extracranial causes of death (17). Misdiagnosis or delay in diagnosis of hematomas, as intracranial complications, contributed most to fatal outcome. Therefore, in the emergency room, every effort should be made to diagnose promptly intracranial complications and establish an optimal level of cerebral oxygenation and perfusion.

Respiratory Care

The oxygen requirement of the injured brain is higher than that of the normal brain. A borderline hypoxia, commonly tolerated in the normal brain, can produce hypoxic damage in the acutely insulted brain. Thus, adequate cerebral oxygenation must be a priority. Early recognition and prompt aggressive treatment of respiratory dysfunction are of major importance in the initial care of the head-injured patient. It is far preferable to intubate the trachea of a patient who has marginal difficulty but who can soon maintain his respiration adequately rather than risk a delay that can have catastrophic consequences. Endotracheal intubation must be considered if both a patent airway and adequate spontaneous ventilation cannot be maintained. Arterial blood gases are the best determinant of the ventilatory function. An arterial oxygen partial pressure (PaO_2) of less than 70 mm Hg on room air or arterial carbon dioxide tension ($PaCO_2$) of greater than 45 mm Hg are indications for ventilatory assistance. The methods of securing the airway are of paramount importance. Attempting to intubate the trachea of an otherwise healthy, young, muscular semicomatose male may precipitate extreme struggling and enormous rises in intracranial pressure (ICP), with potential risk for tentorial herniation (Fig. 15.2). Administration of small doses of sodium thiopental and succinylcholine allows securing the airway under less traumatic circumstances (Fig. 15.3). These principles also apply to patients in whom a concomitant cervical fracture is suspected. Prior to intubation, which must again be done as atraumatically as possible, the cervical vertebrae should be distracted by applying cervical traction or by simply pulling on the hair. It is not advisable to administer succinylcholine prior to stabilization of the neck since the unstable bony fragments may be maintained in their position only by muscular spasm. Cervical fractures are rare, however, especially in young children, as compared with the frequent occurrence of hypoxia in patients with traumatic coma. Therefore, the need for establishing an airway should take precedence over the concern for potential cervical instability.

Stomach distention, a common finding after severe head injury, can compromise respiration by limiting diaphragmatic excursion. But passing a nasogastric tube may stimulate the gag reflex, causing regurgitation and aspiration. This procedure, therefore, should be done only after endotracheal intubation.

In addition to airway obstruction and pulmonary contusion, respiration may be compromised by primary central nervous system (CNS) dysfunction. Neurogenic respiratory difficulties may be due to trauma and/or intoxication.

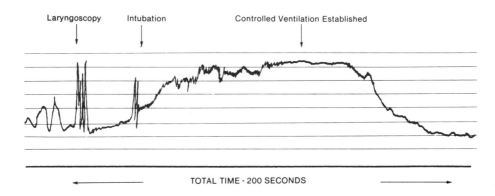

Figure 15.2 Intracranial pressure may rise precipitously during uncontrolled intubation. (From Frost EAM: Head trauma and the anesthesiologist. Weekly Anesthesiology Update, vol 10, lesson 2, 1979. Reprinted by permission.)

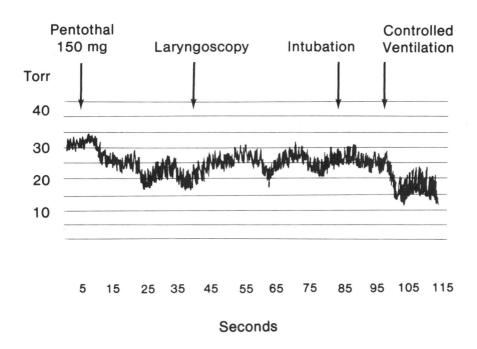

Figure 15.3   Intubation may be achieved more safely in the head-injured patient by prior administration of pentothal.

The respiratory pattern varies with the level of brain or brain-stem injury and may present as Cheyne-Stokes, neurogenic hyperventilation, apneustic, or ataxic respiration (18). Cheyne-Stokes respiration has also been observed after upper respiratory tract obstruction and is not diagnostic of cerebral dysfunction. Neurogenic hyperventilation is referred to as deep rapid respiration of over 35 cycles per minute (19). Several studies have shown that periodic respiration or central neurogenic hyperventilation is consistently associated with poor outcome (20,21). Neurogenic pulmonary edema may result from hypothalamic damage, which causes release of a massive sympathetic discharge. Regardless of their origin, these respiratory difficulties are associated with hypoxemia and necessitate assisted or controlled ventilation. When clinical doubt exists regarding the effectiveness of ventilation, prompt intubation is indicated (22). Controlled respiration not only improves oxygenation, but it allows the regulation of $PaCO_2$, which plays an important role in the control of intracranial hypertension.

Hypoxia secondary to neurogenic pulmonary shunting is a common finding in severe head injury and usually responds to affiliation of positive end-expiratory pressure (PEEP). Although it has been suggested that PEEP may increase ICP, reduced thoracic compliance (due to alimentation in the lung vasculature) and head elevation may prevent direct transmission of pressure (19,23,24). Improvement in arterial oxygenation and intracranial compliance outweighs potential deleterious effects. If increased pulmonary shunting is secondary to fluid overload, it can be corrected with a loop diuretic such as furosemide. Osmotic diuretics such as mannitol should be avoided in this situation.

Hypotension

The next step in emergency care is to ensure adequate cerebral perfusion. Sustained posttraumatic hypotension in adults frequently points to extracranial sources, but transient hypotension after head injury is not an infrequent occurrence (25). In infants, intracranial hemorrhage, particularly if associated with subgaleal hemorrhage, can lead to hypovolemia. In adults, intracranial hematomas do not reach a volume sufficient to cause hypovolemic shock. Therefore, sustained hypotension in adults is due to either other systemic injuries or brain-stem failure. The latter condition commonly is a terminal event.

Concomitant spinal cord injury may cause shock secondary to the loss of sympathetic innervation of vascular smooth muscle. This vasoparalysis results in a sudden increase in the vascular bed and pooling of a large portion of blood volume into the lower extremities. Elevating the legs above the heart level or using mast trousers is the management of choice for this condition.

All external bleeding, including scalp lacerations, must be controlled and if no other causes for hypotension are readily apparent, it must be treated symptomatically by rapid infusion of blood or crystalloids. Blood transfusion is preferred because it increases the oxygen-carrying capacity. This function of the blood, even in the absence of systemic hypotension, may have a significant impact on brain oxygenation.

Neurologic Assessment

Once cardiopulmonary resuscitation is completed, neurologic examination can be performed. The initial assessment can estimate the extent of primary cerebral damage while subsequent examinations can evaluate the level of recovery or the emergence of complications. The initial evaluation should include information as to the time, location, and mechanism of injury. This information can be obtained from paramedical personnel, relatives, or other witnesses.

In order to compare initial findings with those on subsequent examinations (which may be given by different observers), the neurologic examination must be succinct and reproducible. Assessment of level of consciousness, examination of the eye, and assessment of brain-stem function are of special importance. The level of consciousness is the sentinel point in evaluating the extent of injury. Popular expressions used to describe the patient's level of consciousness, such as "stuporous," "semicomatose," or "obtunded" have different meanings to different examiners, and thus are imprecise. Evaluating and quantifying the patient's level of response to different intensities of external stimuli is a more objective measure, and correlating this quantitative measure of neurologic function with outcome is desirable for both clinical and research needs. This purpose appears to be served by the Glasgow Coma Scale (GCS), which consists of three components: eye opening, motor response, and verbal response (26–28) (Table 15.1). Motor response appears to be the most sensitive component, and it correlates best with both the extent and outcome of severe injury (28,29). In particular, this correlation is highest in severe injuries, indicated by a motor score of 4 or less. Such patients commonly score only two additional points and obtain a total GCS of 6 or below.

For GCS scores greater than 6, other circumstances may confound the score. For example, patients who are in shock, hypoxic, intoxicated, or postictal may have a GCS that does not accurately reflect the degree of brain damage. In addition, associated injuries, such as bilateral orbital trauma or cervical cord damage, may interfere with application of the scale. In the agitated, uncooperative, dysphasic, or intubated patient, accurate scoring may be impossible (30). The GCS cannot be applied to the preverbal children. Furthermore, since the motor score is obtained from the side with the best response, it fails to reflect unilateral deterioration. For example, the coma score in a patient who can localize the stimulus bilaterally and then become unilaterally decerebrate remains the same. This misrepresentation can be avoided by recording the motor response of both sides. Hence, GCS must be regarded as a crude quantitative measure of consciousness and not a substitute for a detailed neurologic assessment.

Table 15.1 The Glasgow Coma Scale

Best verbal response	
None	1
Incomprehensible sound	2
Inappropriate words	3
Confused	4
Oriented	5
Eyes open	
None	1
To pain	2
To speech	3
Spontaneously	4
Best motor response	
None	1
Abnormal extensor	2
Abnormal flexion	3
Withdraws	4
Localizes	5
Obeys	6
Total coma scale	15–3

Nontraumatic causes of brain dysfunction, such as alcohol or drug inges-tion, should not be held responsible for a depressed level of consciousness unless organic causes have been ruled out. Galbraith (31) has pointed out that misdiagnosis or delay in diagnosis of secondary complications often is the result of failure to recognize the organic basis of the depressed sensorium, and hence findings have been erroneously attributed to alcohol or cerebrovascular accident. Under these conditions, the correct diagnosis may not be made until signs of brain-stem compression become apparent. For example, in a patient who was driving a motor vehicle prior to the accident and who presents with a GCS of 13 or less, the neurologic condition should not be attributed to intoxication. This level of mental function is incompatible with driving. Likewise, epileptics may sustain head trauma resulting in an intracranial hemorrhage with minimal exter-nal evidence of injury. Intracranial hematoma should be suspected whenever postictal focal deficit, focal seizures, or status epilepticus are observed in an epileptic without a previous history of such seizure patterns (32).

A complete neurologic examination can be performed only in alert and cooperative patients. Only a limited objective examination is available when the level of consciousness is depressed. Under these circumstances, the eye examina-tion acquires prime importance. The eye position, movement, shape, size, and the reaction of pupils should be noted and recorded.

Spontaneous eye movements in coma usually are roving and may be con-jugate or dysconjugate. As coma deepens, spontaneous eye movements cease. Horizontal roving eye movement indicates only that midbrain and pontine tegmentum are intact. This form of eye movement, however, does not require an intact occipital or frontal cerebral cortex (33). In addition, this phenomenon can be observed despite complete destruction of supratentorial cerebral tissues. In deeper coma, the integrity of the brain-stem function can be tested with the oculovestibular or the oculocephalic reflex, but the latter should not be done until the stability of the spine has been determined. The oculocephalic phenomenon re-quires integrity of proprioceptive fibers from the neck muscle, and this reflex is particularly brisk in certain types of metabolic coma, especially hypoglycemic and hepatic encephalopathy (34). As coma deepens, the oculocephalic reflex usually disappears first, followed by the oculovestibular reflex (cold caloric), which is a much stronger stimulus.

Pupillary light reflex is an important diagnostic test in comatose patients. Traumatic damages of the brain that are strong enough to render patients comatose usually are associated with abnormal pupillary light reflex, whereas metabolic diseases that result in deep coma spare this reaction (34). Abnormal pupillary light reaction may be valuable in localizing the injury. Small, reactive pupils are seen in diencephalic injury and/or metabolic disorders. Pinpoint pupils generally occur with pontine hemorrhages and are believed to result from simultaneous sym-pathetic interruption and parasympathetic irritation. Midbrain damage may pro-duce midposition, nonreactive pupils with spontaneous fluctuation of size (hippus) (18). A unilaterally dilated and fixed pupil usually indicates a supratentorial ex-panding mass with a midline shift and uncal herniation. Occasionally, small but reactive pupils may be observed during early phases of cerebral herniation. At this stage, patients usually are responding appropriately to painful stimuli, but as the coma deepens, the pupils become fixed and dilated. This phenomenon has been explained by hypothalamic compression in early stages of herniation with resultant bilateral Horner's syndrome (33,34). If the process of herniation is not reversed by decompression of the expanding mass, the brain stem will be irreversibly damaged. Rare instances of uncal herniation with third nerve palsy may occur in an awake patient. The third nerve is occasionally damaged directly by orbital trauma, but in such circumstances, this is commonly associated with fourth and sixth nerve injuries. In the presence of a fixed dilated pupil, optic nerve injury must also be excluded. This can be done by attempting to elicit the consensual light reflex. Although bilaterally fixed, dilated pupils following head trauma has been considered a sign of fatal cerebral injury, this sign can also be observed in the early postictal state (35). Rarely, a unilaterally dilated pupil also occurs after a seizure. Becker and associates (36) have noted that the absence of the oculocephalic reflex in posttraumatic coma is associated with a higher mortality rate (63%) than when the oculocephalic reflex is intact. Likewise, an absent light reflex is associated with an 85% chance of poor outcome, while an intact pupillary light reaction is associated with only a 28% chance of poor outcome. Similar correlations have been reported in other adult and pediatric case series (29, 35, 37).

Other neurologic findings, such as hemiparesis and dysphasia, are evidence of hemispheric lesions, and their progression may reflect an expanding mass lesion. Hemiplegia is seen commonly in the contralateral side, whereas third nerve palsy occurs on the side of the lesion. Occasionally, hemiplegia and third nerve palsy are seen on the same side. The ipsilateral weakness is the result of rapid shift of the brain stem by the hippocampus, causing compression of the contralateral corticospinal tract against the opposite tentorial edge (Kernohan's notch). Unilateral impairment of the third nerve almost always occurs on the same side as the lesion, however. Therefore, the side of the third nerve palsy is a more reliable indicator than hemiparesis in determining the side of pathology. Localization by these means is even more important when there is rapid deterioration, as in acute epidural hematomas, which mandate surgical exploration without diagnostic studies. Other clinical findings that have localizing value include postictal hemiparesis (Todd's paralysis) and posttraumatic focal seizures. Ataxia and nystagmus should draw attention to the posterior fossa as the site of pathology.

Abnormal reflex posture may be associated with increased tone in the extensor or flexor muscles, commonly referred to as decerebrate or decorticate posturing, respectively. Distinction between the two forms of reflex posture is not always possible. Decorticate posture commonly refers to triple flexion of the upper extremities and hyperextension of the lower extremities. Decerebrate posture is characterized clinically as hyperextension of the upper and lower extremities. Patients may demonstrate decerebrate posture on one side of the body and decorticate response on the other side (combined decerebrate rigidity). Decortication and decerebration may also alternately occur on the same side. The Sherringtonian implication of these terms has been loosely transferred to humans to imply brain-stem damage (38, 39). Recent pathologic studies, however, indicate that the correlation between decerebrate posturing and structural brain-stem damage does not always exist (40).

The other form of reflex posture has been called *mixed decerebrate rigidity* and is clinically recognized by the hyperextension of upper extremities and flexor posture of the lower extremities (18). This reaction is commonly elicited by noxious stimuli but can also occur spontaneously. Bricolo et al. (40) reported fatal outcome in every head trauma patient who manifested this form of posturing. These authors have also noted 55% and 70% mortality in patients with combined decerebrate rigidity and alternate decerebrate and decorticate rigidity, respectively.

Diagnostic Studies

After the stability of the cervical spine is determined, the patient can be positioned for radiographic studies. The importance of skull films in the early management of head injury is debatable. Lateralized neurologic findings are markedly better for locating the side of a lesion in a comatose patient than is the demonstration of a skull fracture. Nevertheless, the recognition of a linear skull fracture is significant in a patient who, after a lucid interval, suffers neurologic deterioration; it may suggest an ipsilateral epidural hematoma. The fracture line can be used as a landmark for placing the exploratory burr hole.

In the patient with minimal neurologic impairment, skull fractures may indicate significant head injury and should alert the physician to a higher probability of posttraumatic complications (41). Certain linear fractures, including fractures crossing the middle meaningeal artery, major venous sinuses, and those extending to the base of the skull, carry higher risks for intracranial hematoma and cerebrospinal fluid (CSF) leak. Fractures through air sinuses with opacification or an air-fluid level should be considered compound fractures.

A shift of a calcified pineal-habenular commissure beyond the range of technical error (1 to 2 mm) is unequivocal evidence of a space-occupying lesion. A midline pineal, however, does not exclude the presence of lesions such as bilateral hematomas or frontally located lesions.

Computerized tomographic (CT) scanning has revolutionized the management of head injury by providing a noninvasive technique for identifying and demonstrating the location, nature, and effects of an intracranial lesion. Unlike any other diagnostic study, the CT scan is capable of differentiating between cerebral edema, contusion, and hematoma.

Between 30% and 40% of patients with severe head injuries have normal CT scans initially (42,43). Early negative CT scan, corollary of the clinically known lucid interval, may sometimes give a false sense of security to the clinician, who attributes subsequent deterioration to causes other than intracranial hematomas. Thus any patient whose neurologic condition worsens or who fails to achieve expected improvement should have a repeat CT scan (44–48). This will not only rule out operative pathology, but frequently it will provide a plausible explanation (e.g., edema, hemorrhagic infarct, etc.) for an unsatisfactory recovery.

All patients with a GCS of less than 12 should be studied by CT scan. Exception can be made for patients who present with the classic symptoms and signs of rapidly expanding epidural hematomas. In this situation time is of the essence, and the patient can be operated upon without the benefit of preoperative scanning.

Presently, the role of angiography in the evaluation of acute head injury is limited to those penetrating injuries where the possiblility of vascular involvement exists. Angiography can also provide information on vasospasm and circulation time, but this information rarely contributes to the patient's management (49,50).

INJURY TO THE BRAIN COVERINGS

Examination of the head can provide invaluable information. Scalp contusions and lacerations not only provide proof of head trauma, but also indicate the probable side of the lesion. Scalp lacerations are commonly handled in emergency rooms by the general surgical staff. Thus, valuable information concerning the depth of the wound and the extent of bony involvement may get buried under the sutures. Since hair and dirt usually are driven into the wound, liberal irrigation and thorough débridement of devitalized tissue are necessary. Hemostasis can be accomplished temporarily by digital pressure on the wound margins and ultimately by galeal sutures. Before repairing the scalp laceration, hair should be shaved at least 2.5 cm on both sides of the wound. Small scalp avulsions may be repaired primarily by undermining the galea, but larger avulsions commonly require rotation of the scalp flap.

Depressed skull fractures under lacerations should be considered compound and require early surgical repair. In fact, over 75% of depressed skull fractures in adults are compound (51). It has been shown that the rate of infection increases in patients operated on later than 24 hours after injury (52,53). The diagnosis of depressed skull fracture should always be confirmed by appropriate radiographic views since the accumulation of a subperiosteal hematoma may sometimes appear erroneously as a depressed bone to palpation. The purposes of surgery are to débride the devitalized tissue, elevate the depressed bone, and evaluate the dura and underlying brain. Care must be taken not to manipulate any bony fragment in the emergency room. A bony fragment may be tamponading a lacerated vessel or a dural sinus, and its removal may result in uncontrollable intracranial hemorrhage.

The same principles apply to penetrating objects that are still in place. The offending object must be protected from any movement during transportation of the patient from the emergency room to the radiology department and to the operating room (Fig. 15.4). Radiographic views of the object within the skull are helpful in planning the surgical exposure. Furthermore, if the impaling object is lying close to a large vessel, angiography may be advisable prior to dislodging the object. Tangential high-velocity scalp wounds may not penetrate the skull or

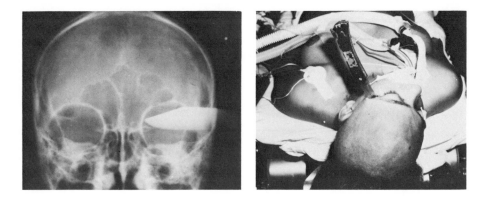

Figure 15.4   Penetrating objects should be left in place until the patient's cardiorespiratory status is stabilized under operating conditions. This patient sustained a major knife injury behind the orbit.

cause early neurologic disorders; however, delayed surgical complications such as subdural, extradural, or cortical hematomas may occur (54). Hemotympanum, ecchymosis over the mastoid area (Battle's sign), or lid ecchymosis without extension to the eyebrows (raccoon eyes) often indicate a basal skull fracture. In these conditions there is a high risk of complications, such as meningitis and CSF rhinorrhea.

The incidence of meningitis is untreated cases of basilar skull fracture is about 25% (55). CSF rhinorrhea usually appears in the first 48 hours after injury. If the patient complains of fluid dripping from his nostril after mild frontal injury, it is important to determine the nature of the fluid in the emergency room. In order to confirm the diagnosis of CSF rhinorrhea, the fluid accumulated from the nose must contain more than 30 mg/dl of glucose. Dextrostix may give a positive reaction with as little as 5 mg/dl of glucose and is positive in 75% of patients with normal nasal secretions. A negative reaction can reliably rule out the presence of CSF. In our experience, the CSF otorrhea or rhinorrhea following gunshot wounds does not heal spontaneously and virtually always leads to an intracranial infection if not surgically repaired in the first 24 hours. Delayed forms of CSF rhinorrhea may also occur several days to months later, suggesting that the tract has been temporarily sealed by a blood clot or that damaged brain tissue has herniated into the dural and bony defect. Lysis of the clot or resolution of necrotic brain tissue reinstitutes a pathway for CSF. It is, therefore, important for the emergency room examiner to alert the patient with basal skull fractures to possible complications should the patient be discharged.

PENETRATING INJURIES OF BRAIN

Most of the neurosurgical experience in cerebral missile injuries comes from military sources. Significant reductions of the morbidity and mortality rates in more recent wars have been attributed to the progress in technology and the methods of delivering early medical care in the combat field. The judicious use of antibiotics has been most effective in improving outcome.

Civilian gunshot wounds differ from military missile injuries in that the civilian population has rapid access to well-equipped neurosurgical facilities. In addition, the ballistics of the missile differ. Most civilian injuries are caused by low-velocity bullets, whereas the shell fragments, other penetrating objects from explosions, and high-velocity bullets are common in military wounds. The destructive power of a bullet depends on its kinetic energy as well as its size and shape (kinetic energy is a function of the mass of the bullet and the square of its velocity: $E = 1/2\,mV^2$) (56). In penetrating the tissue, bullets with higher kinetic energy produce proportionately more tissue damage. Butler et al. (57) have demonstrated that the bursting fracture of the skull results from a high-pressure wave transmitted from the brain itself (Fig. 15.5). Experimental studies reveal that this sort of fracture does not occur when the missile strikes an empty skull. Kocher, in 1874, demonstrated that when a bullet passes through an empty can, it leaves only entrance and exit holes, but when the can is filled with water, the container bursts (58). Bone fragments as a rule do not contain high kinetic energy but soon come to rest in the brain tissue alongside the bullet tract.

Barnett reported epidural, subdural, or intracerebral hematomas in 56% of 316 consecutive cases of penetrating wounds (59). The author considered vascular laceration responsible for the high incidence of intracranial hematoma in this series. Others, however, have reported extremely low incidence rates of intracranial hematomas following penetrating injuries (60). In the absence of a hematoma, devitalized brain tissue may often act as a mass lesion and may be responsible for increased ICP and poor outcome. Crockard has identified three categories of high, normal, and low ICP patterns in the early hours following injury; in all of these patterns, the ICP rose to extremely high levels within the ensuing few hours (61).

Diagnostic Studies

Routine radiographic views of the skull, including a base view, are usually sufficient to determine the trajectory of the bullet and evaluate the position of penetrated bony fragments.

CT scanning can delineate further the indriven bony fragments, evaluate the extent of brain injury, and identify intracranial hematomas. Intracranial hematomas are commonly associated with tangential bullet wounds of the skull and also occur when the bullet ricochets from the inner table of the skull (62). This latter phenomenon may result in rupture of a cortical vessel, causing a subdural hematoma.

Cerebral angiography is performed only if major vascular injury is expected. Occurrence of a delayed intracranial hemorrhage is also an indication for angiography, since it is commonly related to rupture of a traumatic aneurysm.

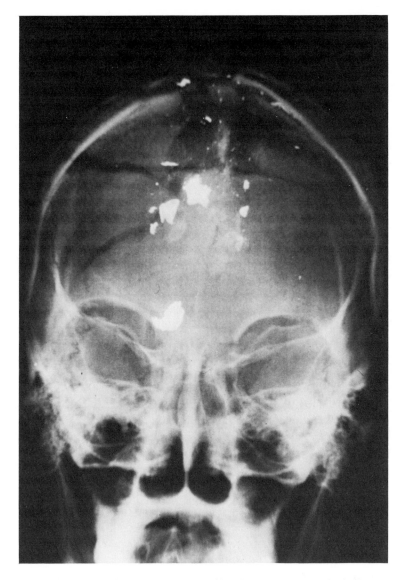

Figure 15.5 Missile injuries, especially those imparting high kinetic energy, exert a bursting type of injury.

Treatment

The general management of an acute head injury should also be employed in resuscitation of a patient with gunshot wounds. The purpose of surgery is to débride the devitalized scalp, bone, and brain tissues around the bullet tract, and to evacuate any intracerebral or extracerebral hematomas. Bone fragments are the main source of infection, and every attempt must be made to ensure their complete removal (63,64). The bullet and metallic fragments are infrequent causes of complications, and the attempt at their removal should only be made if they are easily accessible. In order to prevent the spread of infection to brain tissue, a thorough débridement of the scalp wound and bone fragments must precede manipulation of the brain. Devitalized brain tissues are then débrided and the tract is observed. Gentle digital palpation of the brain tissue around the bullet tract is done routinely in search of hidden bone fragments. After completion of brain débridement, the bullet tract must remain open. Collapse of the tract walls and closure of the tract should raise the suspicion of a hematoma in surrounding tissues. Water-tight closure of the dural membrane provides an effective barrier to superficial infections and protects the brain from adhering to the scalp.

The rate of infection can be markedly reduced by early débridement and proper use of antibiotics. Bacteriologic studies have shown that the most common bacteria found in the devitalized scalp and bone are gram-positive cocci. Forty-five percent of indriven bones, according to Carey and colleagues (65,66), are contaminated, and the sole contaminant is *Staphylococcus*, irrespective of the type of organism cultured from the wound. It is therefore advisable to use an antistaphylococcal antibiotic preoperatively and to continue its use for five to seven days after débridement.

Prognosis

Although civilian neurosurgical facilities are better equipped and more readily available to victims of urban conflicts than those in combat zones, the mortality rate of civilian bullet injuries is reportedly higher (60,67). In military situations there is a high incidence of mortality in the early hours after severe missile injuries. This is primarily attributed to respiratory distress and does not enter into the military neurosurgical statistics.

The level of consciousness after penetrating wounds is a major predictor of mortality. Byrnes and associates (68) have reported 100% mortality in 25 deeply comatose patients and 78% mortality in those who reacted only to pain stimuli regardless of pupillary response to light. Other factors that have an adverse influence on the prognosis are the presence of high systemic blood pressure (systolic > 150 mm Hg) or hypotension (< 90 mm Hg systolic) on admission. Moreover, bullet wounds that traverse the brain side-to-side carry a higher mortality risk than if the injury is frontal-occipital (67,69).

TRAUMATIC INTRACRANIAL HEMATOMA

Traumatic intracranial hematomas may occur in different anatomic locations including the intracerebral, subdural, or epidural spaces. Since the clinical course, treatment, and prognosis vary significantly from one form to another, they are best discussed in relation to their anatomic site. Although intracranial hematomas occur predominantly in only one of the three anatomic sites, their occurrence in combination is not rare and carries a very poor prognosis (70,71).

Epidural Hematoma

Traumatic epidural hematoma (EDH) is an infrequent complication of head injury. The incidence of EDH in hospitalized cases of head trauma varies from 0.2% in Galbraith's series (72) to 3% in McKissock's (73) and 4.6% in Heiskanen's (74). These variations, however, may be related to the admission policies and referral patterns within the communities studied.

EDH is usually a result of an automobile accident, but since automobile accidents are the most common cause of head injury, their association with EDH may be a reflection of the increased frequency. The most common cause is lacerated middle meningeal vessels and their branches, and is due to fracture of the squamous portion of temporal bone, resulting in a temporal hematoma (75). Lacerations of the frontal branch or parieto-occipital branches of the meningeal vessels are not uncommon, however, (Fig. 15.6). The incidence of EDH is greatest between the ages of 15 and 20 years. Middle meningeal vessels and their branches do not become firmly adherent to their respective bony groove until early adult life. Hence, the infrequent occurrence of this complication in childhood can be explained by a developmental factor as well as the more pliable bones of childhood. On the other hand, the incidence of EDH declines in older age groups as the dura becomes firmly adherent to the skull and is readily torn rather than separated from the bone by a linear fracture.

A venous hemorrhage in the epidural space may result from a dural sinus laceration. Smaller dural veins may also cause an epidural hematoma after the dura is dissected from the bone by the skull fracture (76). Since pressure in the epidural space usually is higher than in the venous system, it is difficult to explain the mechanism by which a venous epidural clot expands. It seems likely that the venous pressure transiently exceeds that of the epidural space during Valsalva maneuvers, and this results in stepwise expansion of the hematoma and further dissection of the dura from the bone. This slow expansion can explain the chronic clinical presentation of venous EDH (77-79).

In over 90% of cases of EDH, the presence of a skull fracture can be confirmed by surgery (71,72). Radiographic evidence of skull fracture is not as high, however. The direction of the skull fracture can provide information concerning the source of hemorrhage. Fracture lines crossing the middle meningeal groove are commonly associated with arterial bleeding, whereas fractures which transverse the major dural sinuses are likely to produce a venous hematoma. Unlike other traumatic intracranial clots that can be seen with a contralateral skull fracture, epidural hematomas are almost always associated with ipsilateral fracture. This correlation has an important clinical implication. When rapid deterioration of the patient's neurologic condition does not allow for diagnostic

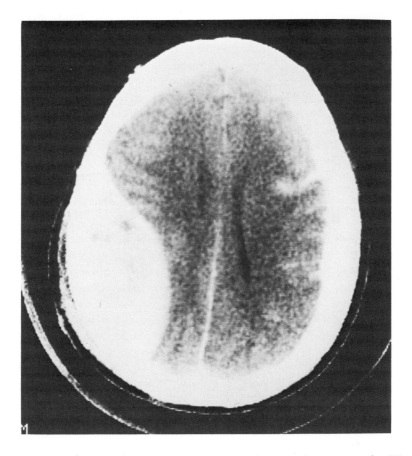

Figure 15.6   An epidural hematoma presents this typical picture on the CT scan.

studies other than skull films, the fracture line can serve as a guide to the placement of exploratory burr holes.

The clinical course of an arterial EDH consists of rapid deterioration of neurologic status following a lucid interval. In its classic form, the clinical presentation is that of a young man who experiences brief loss of consciousness after a relatively minor head injury from which he recovers only to lapse into coma a few hours later. Clinical signs of tentorial herniation with ipsilateral third cranial nerve palsy are often present at this stage and can serve to localize the side of the hematoma for cranial exploration without diagnostic measures.

This classic presentation of epidural hematoma occurs in fewer than 50% of patients (71,73,75). Absence of the lucid interval and a depressed sensorium from the outset indicate intradural pathology in addition to EDH. Jamieson and Yelland (70,80) noted that the lucid interval is not pathognomonic of EDH and, in fact, a higher rate of lucid intervals is seen in patients with intradural lesions. Venous epidural hemorrhages often are slow to develop; in contrast, the arterial form of EDH takes a rapid course and usually results in brain-stem compression within a few hours (77). Therefore, once the diagnosis is suspected, treatment should not be delayed for radiographic confirmation; however, the availability of CT scan in many trauma centers can provide more detailed information in the few minutes that it takes to prepare the operating room. If the rate of deterioration is not rapid, this valuable information may justify the few minutes' delay. If deterioration is rapid, however, exploratory burr holes must be made immediately.

The preoperative use of diuretics and limitation of fluid replacement often results in hypovolemia; however, increased ICP and brain-stem compression are associated with a rise in systemic blood pressure (Cushing reaction). This neurogenic systemic hypertension may, therefore, mask the hypovolemic hypotension and result in normal blood pressure values. When ICP is rapidly reduced by surgical decompression, the driving force behind the hypertension is precipitously removed and hypovolemic hypotension becomes apparent. If this systemic hypotension is not anticipated and prevented, the brain may sustain an additional ischemic insult. Therefore, when preoperative intracranial hypertension is suspected, intraoperative systemic hypotension can be avoided by monitoring central pressures and by empirically expanding the circulating volume by infusion of blood or crystalloids during anesthesia.

The outcome of EDH relates directly to the preoperative extent of intradural pathology and the brain-stem compression. Postoperative management is similar to the general guidelines used in patients with closed head injury.

Subdural Hematoma

A subdural hematoma (SDH) is a collection of blood between the dura and arachnoid membrane. The most common cause of SDH is trauma, but it also occurs spontaneously, in various coagulopathies, cerebral aneurysms, arteriovenous malformations, and in certain neoplasms. SDH is considered acute when it becomes clinically symptomatic within 72 hours after injury, subacute when it manifests between 3 and 15 days, and chronic when the hematoma is more than two weeks old. The pathophysiology, clinical course, and outcome vary between the acute form and the subacute and chronic forms.

Acute Subdural Hematoma

Acute SDH (ASDH) is the most common intracranial hematoma of traumatic origin to require surgical attention. The incidence of this complication varies from 1% to 13% in various case series (70,81,82). This wide variation is due to the diversity of referral patterns and admission policies of hospitals. The occurrence of ASDH in patients with traumatic coma varies from 22% in Richmond, Virginia

(83), to 17% in San Diego, California (84), and 29% in a multicenter study reported by Gennarelli et al. (85).

Venous ASDH results from rupture of the bridging veins to the sagittal sinus during the acceleration-deceleration movement of the brain following impact. This hematoma may therefore be associated with a variety of underlying brain damage; ASDH without associated parenchymal damage or brain laceration is an uncommon event. In the series of Jamieson and Yelland, however, 45% of the patients with ASDH had no associated brain damage and the mortality rate was 22% (70).

The other common causes of ASDH, frequently associated with contrecoup injuries, are brain lacerations, cerebral contusions, and intracerebral hematomas that bleed into the subdural space (70). Recently, it has been shown that some ASDHs may be arterial in origin. These comprise most of the hematomas that overlie the cortical contusion (86,87).

Bilateral ASDH varies in occurrence from 8% to 33% (88,89). These lesions commonly are associated with a high mortality rate (90).

The association of cerebral contusion and ASDH was noted in 43% of patients studied by CT scanning (91). CT findings in these patients usually demonstrate a disproportionately greater midline shift than the thickness of subdural clot. This is due to associated cerebral contusion and/or swelling, which are seen infrequently in epidural hematomas. Since the subdural space does not exert resistance against spread of hematoma, this lesion commonly covers the entire hemisphere, and although it is not often as thick as epidural, it can assume a large volume and reduce intracranial compliance.

Clinical Presentation.   Clinically, ASDH presents as primary brain damage with a secondary elevation of ICP. Those patients who are comatose from the outset and remain in coma have sustained significant brain damage. Outcome in these patients directly depends on the extent of brain damage.

The lucid interval, which commonly is considered pathognomonic of EDH, is not infrequent in ASDH. McLaurin and Tutor (92) in reviewing 90 SDHs noted that the lucid interval, characterized by unconsciousness followed by a period of relative improvement and subsequent deterioration, was present in 18% of the patients. They noted mortality in this group (6%) was lower compared to those who remained in coma (77%). In the large group of SDHs reported by Jamieson and Yelland (80) there was a classic lucid interval in 13%, and this group showed a lower mortality rate. The rate of lucid intervals in this group was comparable to that in patients with EDHs (12%) and in those with intracerebral hematomas (19%) (93).

The presence of a lucid interval has been attributed to the time it takes for the hematoma to expand, but pathologic documentation of expanding hematoma is not often possible. The use of the CT scan permits accurate estimation of the size of the hematoma, and scans repeated at short time intervals may document its expansion. Some patients, therefore, may undergo diagnostic studies during the lucid interval. The absence of a surgically treatable lesion should not result in a false sense of security and delay in diagnosis, especially if the patient's condition deteriorates several hours later (Fig. 15.7).

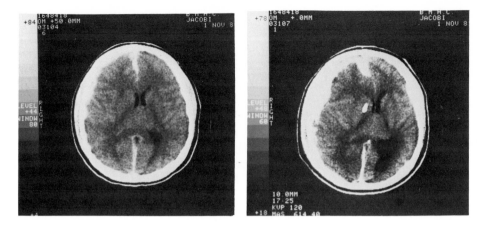

Figure 15.7 Rapid expansion of a subdural hematoma may occur over a one-hour period, as seen in these two CT scans.

Surgical evacuation of ASDH is achieved either by multiple burr holes or by craniotomy. McKissock, Richardson, and Bloom (89) found no difference in the outcome of patients treated by either method. They noted, however, that in several cases an intracerebral hematoma or some portion of the SDH was not evacuated by multiple burr holes. In the past decade most investigators have preferred a large craniotomy for treatment of ASDH (83,90,94). This approach allows complete evacuation of the clot, securing of all bleeding points, and removal of necrotic tissue.

The timing of surgery is considered an important factor in determining the outcome. Early evacuation, that is, within four to six hours after injury, is noted to result in a more favorable outcome (83,95,96). Other prognostic factors such as age, pupillary reactivity, and state of consciousness also affect outcome, as they do in other traumatic injuries of the brain (97).

Subacute and Chronic Subdural Hematoma

Subacute and chronic SDHs are most frequently observed in patients over 50 years old. The annual age-specific incidence rate for chronic SDH in the United States in the third decade of life is approximately 0.13 per 100,000, and it is approximately 7.4 per 100,000 for patients over 70 years of age.

In chronic alcoholics, epileptics, and individuals over 50 years of age, a considerable amount of brain atrophy results in an increased extraparenchymal volume. This extra volume can be occupied by a slowly expanding hematoma without any rise in ICP. The gradual expansion of the clot allows the brain to adjust itself to the new situation by compressing the venous channels and providing further space for the hematoma to expand.

The mechanism by which the hematoma expands remains controversial. The osmotic theory of Gardner (98), popularized in the 1930s, postulated that the hyperosmolar state of the subdural fluid will attract CSF across the subdural membrane, which will result in expansion of the mass. He demonstrated that by dialysing SDH fluid in a cellophane bag against CSF, the volume of hematoma fluid will increase; however, expansion of the hematoma did not occur when the subdural membrane was utilized as the dialysing membrane. Gitlin (99) later challenged this theory by demonstrating the effusion of albumin from serum into the subdural fluid. This argument was further supported by Rabe, Flyn, and Dodge (100), who recovered intravenously injected ^{131}I-tagged albumin in the subdural fluid. The effusion of albumin may be due either to the partial permeability of the capillary endothelium or recurrent hemorrhages from the thin-walled vessels of the subdural membrane.

Rebleeding in the SDH cavity may be frequent and usually results from minor head injuries or other mechanisms that lead to transient elevation of venous pressure. This frequent rebleeding was demonstrated by Ito, Komai, and Yamamoto (101), who injected ^{51}Cr-labeled red cells into the peripheral circulation and recovered them in the SDH shortly thereafter. They postulated that frequent rehemorrhage is enhanced by the presence of fibrinolytic enzymes in the hematoma membrane. In 18 patients studied with ^{51}Cr-labeled red blood cells, a rebleeding rate that averaged 10% of the hematoma volume was noted.

The subdural membrane functions to absorb its contents (100). Clinical demonstration of spontaneous resolution of SDH has been attributed to the presence of this absorptive ability of the subdural capsule (102). Both absorption and effusion are directly related to the surface area of the membrane, while rebleeding is often the result of minor trauma and fibrinolytic activity of the membrane and its contents (103). As long as there is a balance between the expanding and absorptive forces, the size of the hematoma remains constant and the patient is asymptomatic. If the overall volume of the bleeding becomes greater than the absorptive system can handle, the hematoma will expand. If factors encouraging the bleeding can be eliminated, the absorption may exceed the expansion and the patient may return to his presymptomatic condition.

The outer membrane of subdural capsule that forms on the dural side of the clot gradually becomes thicker. The inner layer of the membrane is very thin. Both layers are pathologically distinct within seven to ten days.

A history of head trauma is often absent. Clinical presentation of chronic and subacute SDH may vary from focal signs of brain dysfunction to a depressed level of consciousness to the development of an organic mental syndrome. This clinical presentation can often mimic that of a stroke or brain tumor. The presence of a white matter lesion, such as a visual field defect or dysphasia, does not negate the presence of chronic SDH. Subacute SDH generally presents signs of elevated ICP, such as decreased levels of consciousness and headaches, while chronic forms of hematomas usually resemble the clinical presentation of stroke.

The diagnosis of subacute or chronic SDH is readily made by a CT scan. The density of the SDH is higher than that of normal brain tissue during the acute state. It gradually becomes isodense about two weeks later, and becomes hypodense in the chronic phase. The diagnosis may be missed during the isodense period. Indirect evidence, such as unilateral ventricular compression or a midline shift without the presence of an intracerebral lesion, should raise the suspicion of an isodense SDH. In this situation, double-dose contrast enhancement can be used to visualize the cortical blush or subdural membrane.

Treatment. Treatment of chronic SDH has undergone a significant change during the past several decades. Removal of the membrane surrounding the hematoma was once thought to be required, but this is presently deemed unnecessary (104). Adequate drainage of the liquid portion of the hematoma by twist drill and needle aspiration generally produces good results, and craniotomy can be reserved for those instances in which the SDH reaccumulates, when there is a solid clot, or when the brain fails to reexpand and the patient remains symptomatic (105–108). This procedure, as a definitive method of treatment, was first described by Tabaddor and Shulman (105) and is commonly performed at the bedside under local anesthesia (Fig. 15.8). The use of local anesthetic with appropriate monitoring is beneficial since most of the patients are old and are at considerable risk for complications of general anesthesia.

Postevacuation CT scans show that the brain does not ordinarily reexpand to obliterate the space until about 40 days later (108). This slow reexpansion is inconsequential and does not require treatment.

Intracerebral Hematoma

The diagnosis of intracerebral hematoma has become more frequent since the advent of CT scanning. Before this, angiography could not visualize the hematoma in certain areas of the brain and was unable to differentiate hematoma from contusion; the diagnosis was routinely made in the operating room while the brain was being explored for traumatic intracerebral mass lesions or during postmortem examinations. Jamieson and Yelland (93) reported 63 surgically verified intracerebral hematomas in a series of 11,100 head trauma patients, an incidence of 0.6%. Lin et al. (109) reported an incidence of 0.3% of surgically significant intracerebral hematomas. More recent studies with CT scanning report an incidence of 6.3% for intracerebral hematomas as compared with 21.3% for cerebral contusions (110).

The two most common mechanisms of cerebral contusion and intracerebral hematomas are coup and contrecoup injuries (111–113). Coup lesions are referred to as the parenchymal damage that occurs beneath the point of cranial impact and is caused by the inbending bone slapping the brain surface. They are also caused by a transient depression of a linear skull fracture to produce cortical laceration. Contrecoup injuries are cerebral contusions distant from the point of impact. These lesions are the result of a blow delivered to the unsupported head. During this motion the skull moves in the direction of force before the kinetic energy is transmitted to the brain. This delay produces a high-pressure wave in

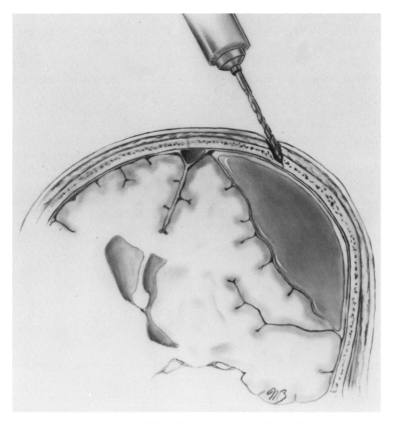

Figure 15.8 A chronic subdural hematoma may be safely aspirated by twist drill under local anesthesia.

the brain beneath the point of impact and a negative pressure at the antipole, which causes cavitation in the brain tissue. When the skull motion comes to a sudden halt, the brain, which lags behind, strikes the opposite part of the skull. Actual contrecoup injury is more complex, however, since the inner surface of the skull is not smooth but contains several ridges that are divided by falx and tentorium, contrecoup injuries have predilection for certain locations. Following frontal or occipital impacts, contrecoup lesions frequently involve the orbital surface of the frontal lobe and the basal and lateral surfaces of the temporal lobe. A posterior parietal blow may be associated with a lateral temporal contrecoup contusion. Contrecoup lesions of the occipital lobe are rare. A cephalocaudal acceleration-deceleration movement results in transient crowding of supratentorial tissues in the tentorial hiatus and cerebellar tonsils in the foramen magnum. The result is a high or low brain-stem injury. In this instance, the diaphragm sellae may also tear or damage the pituitary stalk, leading to development of diabetes insipidus. Diffuse axonal injury is most likely to occur with lateral acceleration-deceleration head motion (114). Ommaya, Grubb, and Naumann (115) have shown that, irrespective of the site of impact, over 90% of cerebral contusions develop in the temporofrontal region.

The developmental mechanism of intracerebral hematomas is unclear. Their delayed appearance often is correlated with deterioration of neurologic state (110). Baratham and Dennyson (116) described 21 of 7866 head injuries where the initial recovery was followed by a deterioration in neurologic function owing to the delayed development of an intracerebral hematoma. These delayed hematomas are clinically indistinguishable from EDHs or SDHs (93,109). Several theories have been offered to explain the delayed development. Evans and Scheinker (117) postulated that local reduction of pH produced vasodilation with subsequent perivascular petechiae coalescing to form the hematoma. Brain softening, especially when it involves a vessel wall, after trauma may also produce a hematoma. The final factor contributing to the development of intracerebral hematomas is the increased blood flow around the contused brain, which is exacerbated by hypoxia, hypercapnia, and elevated venous pressure. These three factors can precipitate or expand a hematoma (116). The evolution of intracerebral hematomas has been documented by serial CT scanning (110).

The development of delayed intracerebral hematoma correlates with poor prognosis. Cooper and colleagues (110) suggested that the outcome could not be altered by surgical intervention, while Levinthal and Stern (118) found that further improvement can be achieved by evacuating the clot. The discrepancy in their results may be due to the different methods of patient selection and differences in the patients' neurologic conditions at the time treatment was rendered. It is also our experience that when a delayed hematoma is associated with clinical deterioration, evacuation of the clot often produces neurologic improvement. The development of intracerebral hematomas sometimes can be detected by ICP monitoring in early stages before the neurologic findings are elicited.

MANAGEMENT OF INTRACRANIAL HYPERTENSION

Although more than half of all deaths from head trauma are associated with intracranial hypertension, the causal role of various degrees of ICP elevation in the outcome of head trauma remains unclear (21,119–122). Significant intracranial hypertension, however, may reduce the perfusion pressure below the critical level (60 mm Hg) required to maintain normal cerebral metabolism and thus be responsible for some form of secondary brain damage. In order to prevent secondary brain damage, intracranial hypertension must be detected and controlled early. In appropriate cases, this may be done soon after the patient is resuscitated and diagnostic studies are completed. Neurologic deterioration secondary to marked ICP elevation occurs after ICP has been elevated for some time. This makes clinical evaluation an inappropriate method for early detection of increased ICP. Most clinicians consider any ICP level above normal (10–15 mm Hg) to be detrimental, although the actual level at which ICP elevation becomes harmful remains controversial. There is no direct relationship between ICP elevation and neurologic impairment. For example, the marked intracranial hypertension seen in conditions such as pseudotumor cerebri is associated with minimal neurologic dysfunction, while the moderate ICP elevation in severe head injury may be associated with a fatal outcome. Hence, ICP values can provide useful information only when used in conjunction with other clinical data.

Experience with ICP monitoring in head trauma patients has led to the isolation of several factors critical in the management of intracranial hypertension (123). Elevated ICP in the presence of a unilateral mass lesion is associated with higher morbidity. This probably is due to the structural displacement and, ultimately, to the brain-stem compression resulting from the pressure gradient between compartments of the intracranial space. These midline structural shifts are related also to the location of lesions within the cranium. Frontal lobe masses, for example, are commonly associated with marked elevation of ICP before manifesting clinical signs of brain-stem compression. ICP monitoring in these patients can provide a margin of safety before brain-stem compression occurs. On the other hand, temporal lobe lesions can result in brain-stem compression before ICP becomes markedly elevated. The safety margin is therefore quite narrow, and any elevation of ICP requires vigorous medical or surgical treatment (124).

Since intracranial volume is constant, the introduction of additional volume, such as a hematoma or edema, needs to be compensated for by displacement of an equal volume out of the cranium. This volume compensation is accomplished by a reduction in venous blood volume and/or intracranial CSF. When these two compensatory mechanisms are exhausted, any additional volume results in a sharp rise of ICP. The status of these compensatory mechanisms is measured by the intracranial compliance, a parameter that can be estimated from the pressure/volume curve. The biomechanics and pathophysiology of ICP have been discussed in Chapter 3.

In patients with basilar skull fractures and leakage of CSF, ICP does not accurately reflect the influence of an expanding lesion (25). As the volume of the mass increases, the CSF is forced out of the cranium without a significant rise in ICP. The determination of intracranial compliance is no longer valid because the cranial cavity loses the property of a closed box. Under these circumstances, a normal ICP value should not militate against the surgical treatment of a focal intracranial mass lesion. Intracranial hypertension should be treated along several lines.

Hyperventilation

Although most clinicians commonly use "edema" and "swelling" interchangeably, these terms can be more precisely applied to two distinct and temporal processes that occur after head injury (125). The pathophysiologic distinction between cerebral edema and swelling after head injury has led to a logical approach to their management. Brain swelling is defined as an increase in the cerebral blood volume.

It is postulated to result from cerebral vasoparalysis with resulting hyperemia and may last from several hours to several days. Prolonged hyperemia of the brain may lead to vasogenic edema and possibly to increased ICP with brain herniation. The CT scan characteristics of cerebral hyperemia show slightly increased brain density and compressed ventricles. This increased density can be enhanced further by use of intravenous contrast infusion (126).

Brain edema, on the other hand, is defined as increased water content of the extravascular spaces of the brain. The white matter density of edematous brain is less than that of normal brain on CT scanning. Water content, which can be quantitatively determined by tissue density, is higher in edematous than in normal brain. Brain edema, usually focal or unilateral, does not develop shortly after trauma, while hyperemia occurs early.

The influence of hyperventilation on ICP is related to the lower carbon dioxide level, which can be achieved in brain tissue in a short period of time. Extracellular alkalosis in the brain produced by hypocapnia directly affects vascular muscles and causes constriction of cerebral resistance arterioles. Consequently, systemic blood pressure transmitted to thin-walled cerebral vessels is decreased, and this results in the reduction of cerebral blood volume. The effect of hyperventilation on ICP begins in less than one minute and usually stabilizes within five minutes.

Early after injury, the increased cerebral blood flow (CBF) and cerebral blood volume may gradually lead to ICP elevation. In a later stage, sustained intracranial hypertension is accompanied commonly by cerebral edema and may compromise the CBF; in extreme situations, this leads to complete cessation of flow. It is in the hyperemic phase that hyperventilation is expected to be most effective. In patients with normal or reduced blood flow, the pressure response might rapidly become adapted to hyperventilation.

During continued hyperventilation, ICP slowly rises and becomes stable after three to five hours, usually at a level lower than the original pressure. This is due to an adaptive mechanism. Cerebral vascular response to hypocapnia is markedly reduced or abolished in the presence of hypoxia. Therefore, the shallow rapid respiration of neurogenic hyperventilation, which is accompanied commonly by hypoxia caused by shift of the oxygen dissociation curve to the left, is ineffective in lowering ICP. Some authors have cautioned against prolonged and severe hyperventilation for fear of producing tissue hypoxia with all its side effects (18). A patient who is spontaneously hyperventilating is apt to develop fatigue, increased body metabolism, and hyperthermia, which in turn raise the cerebral metabolic demand. Under these circumstances it is best to sedate the patient and mechanically control the respiration.

Hyperventilation to reduce the $PaCO_2$ below 20 mm Hg may compromise oxygenation. When rapid temporary reduction of ICP is desired, hypocapnia of 25 mm Hg can be effective. For long-term treatment of ICP, $PaCO_2$ levels of 30 to 35 mm Hg may be as effective as lower levels. Since acute head injury is associated with cerebral hyperemia, the treatment of raised ICP can best be controlled by lowering the $PaCO_2$. By the same token, hypercapnia can rapidly lead to a marked ICP elevation and cerebral herniation. In the emergency room this process may occur during a difficult intubation with a combination of hypoxia and hypercapnia. Figure 15.2 illustrates a critical ICP rise during intubation. This event can be avoided or minimized by adequate mask ventilation before any attempt at intubation is made.

Steroid Therapy

Controversies over the purported beneficial effects of steroids in head injury are not surprising (127–131). The brain's reaction to the impact is complex and at different times may consist of various combinations of swelling, vasogenic edema, and cytotoxic edema. Swelling is defined as an increased cerebral blood volume owing to either vasoparalysis or venous outflow obstruction, and it may be transient or minor. When massive, however, swelling may lead to vasogenic cerebral edema. The cerebral swelling typically observed in hypercapnia is unresponsive to steroid therapy.

Vasogenic edema is characterized by increased permeability of brain capillary endothelial cells. Cerebral white matter is particularly vulnerable to this form of edema. Vasogenic edema is commonly observed in the periphery of metastatic tumors, in abscesses, and in experimental cryogenic lesions in animals (132,133). There is ample clinical and experimental evidence to support the effectiveness of steroid therapy in vasogenic edema (133–136), but the importance of this form of edema in the traumatized brain is unknown.

Cytotoxic edema is defined as engorgement of cellular elements of brain with concomitant reduction of the extracellular fluid space. The clinical conditions commonly associated with cytotoxic edema include hypoxia and water intoxication. This form of edema is shown to be unresponsive to steroid therapy. Since most severe head injuries are associated with some degree of focal or generalized cerebral hypoxia, the occurrence of cytotoxic edema is a frequent pathologic finding. The assessment of the effectiveness of steroid therapy after head trauma by means of randomized clinical trails is difficult because of the occurrence of these different forms of edema. Moreover, those injuries that produce extreme tissue disruption and hemorrhage probably would not respond favorably to any form of treatment. Therefore, bias in the selection of patients often invalidates the results of clinical trials.

Dehydration

ICP can be lowered by a variety of hypertonic solutions and diuretics. The most extensively used osmotic diuretic is mannitol, which lowers ICP, improves intracranial compliance, scavenges free radicals, and improves CBF. Since mannitol is not metabolized and does not disrupt the normal blood-brain barrier, it seems unlikely that the agent has a direct effect on cerebral metabolism. It does have an indirect effect, however, increasing CBF and decreasing preexisting cerebral ischemia. The mechanism by which mannitol reduces ICP is based on a rapid rise of serum osmolarity, which creates an osmotic gradient between blood and brain and favors the passage of water from the brain, thus producing an increase in brain volume and ICP. The parts of the brain most likely to shrink are areas with normal permeability of the capillary endothelial bed. In the presence of vasogenic edema, mannitol shrinks the normal areas of the brain and does not affect the edematous region. This mechanism raises the potential risk of an increased midline dislocation when mannitol is used in unilateral cerebral disorders. The occurrence of this phenomenon, however, has not been demonstrated in clinical studies. After a rapid infusion over a period of 15 minutes, serum osmolarity reaches the peak level within 30 minutes; diuresis begins within 45 minutes, followed by a blood-brain osmolarity equilibrium a few hours later. The ICP reduction occurs within 10 to 20 minutes. Once equilibrium has been reached, mannitol no longer lowers the ICP; hence, continuous infusion becomes rapidly ineffective. With the exception of clinical emergencies, mannitol should not be used without monitoring of ICP and serum osmolarity. In patients with impending heart failure, mannitol should be used with extreme caution (137). A nonosmotic diuretic such as furosemide is the drug of choice in this condition as well as when serum osmolarity is 20 to 30 mOsm above normal. ICP monitoring permits careful adjustment of diuretic dose to minimize the fluid and electrolyte imbalance.

ANESTHETIC MANAGEMENT

Premedication

Preoperative sedation is best avoided in head-injured patients. Pain usually is not a major complaint of these patients, and therefore the use of narcotics is not justified. Moreover, even 25 mg of meperidine can cause significant increase in $PaCO_2$, which may be extremely hazardous if intracranial compliance is reduced. Diazepam has a half-life of about 12 hours and, especially in older patients, may cause sufficient CNS depression to interfere with neurologic assessment.

Phenobarbital, which is frequently used for seizure control, has a marked sedative effect and a long duration of action. Phenytoin causes less sedation and is the initial drug of choice. Side effects (hypotension, cardiac arrhythmias, and CNS depression) are minimized if the drug is given at an intravenous rate no faster than 50 mg/min.

The routine use of belladonna alkaloids is not recommended because the cardiac effects of these drugs may obscure changes in intracranial dynamics.

Monitoring

Appropriate intraoperative monitoring includes continuous electrocardiography with the capability of strip recording. Arterial cannulation should be performed to provide a port for frequent blood gas analyses and continuous systemic arterial blood pressure monitoring. Trend recordings with the availability of a final hard copy of systolic, diastolic, and mean arterial pressures provide indications of continued adequate cerebral perfusion during the administration of anesthesia.

Blood loss and prior administration of diuretic agents complicate the maintenance of fluid balance. Patients are frequently hypovolemic, hypokalemic, and hypochloremic. This state may not cause hypotension initially because the victims generally have a healthy vasculature that can compensate and because intracranial damage often causes arterial hypertension. Hence, the true state of hydration may be realized for the first time following induction of anesthesia, when catastrophic hypotension may occur. Rational fluid replacement involves monitoring of central venous pressure. Placement of a flow-directed balloon flotation catheter is indicated especially in elderly patients with heart disease, in whom administration of large volumes of hyperosmolar solutions (e.g., mannitol) and large volume fluid replacement may precipitate pulmonary edema. Cardiopulmonary function should also be monitored in all patients in whom the development of neurogenic pulmonary edema is suspected.

Urinary output must be carefully monitored for the potential development of diabetes insipidus.

Continuous temperature recording is indicated, as meningeal irritation by blood and hypothalamic injuries may cause hyperthermia.

When operation is performed in a head-up position or if the injury involved a venous sinus, Doppler monitoring and prior placement of a right atrial catheter are recommended (see Chapter 7).

Anesthetic Technique

Intubation frequently has been performed prior to the patient's arrival in the operating room. If not, this maneuver must be accomplished as atraumatically and expeditiously as possible using small incremental doses of sodium thiopental, succinylcholine, and lidocaine. This last drug is administered both intravenously (1 mg/kg) and topically (4 ml of 4% laryngotracheal spray).

Considerable controversy has continued over what constitutes the best anesthetic technique for patients with head injury. An intravenous or balanced anesthetic technique involves incremental administration or continuous infusion of drugs such as barbiturates, narcotics, tranquilizers, and muscle relaxants (in combination with nitrous oxide). The timing of injection and the dosage are guided mainly by the vital signs. Proponents of this regimen have claimed that the decrease in CBF and metabolic rate afforded by narcotic and barbiturate drugs is essential to care safely for patients with decreased brain reserves. Furthermore, in the severely injured patient, appropriate postoperative management includes continued control of ventilation in order to attenuate intracranial hypertension. Therefore, the delayed sedative effect that may occur following a multipharmacologic technique may be desirable. The potential increase in seizure activity that occurs with administration of higher doses of enflurane, especially when the patient is hypocapnic, is of serious concern and would mandate against its use (138). Moreover, both halothane and enflurane increase CBF significantly. Although increased CBF may lead to an ICP elevation, this side effect can be minimized or even prevented by sodium thiopental and hyperventilation. The beneficial effect of higher CBF rate is an excess of blood flow in relation to metabolic demand (139,140). Anesthetic concentrations of inhalation agents above minimum alveolar concentration (MAC) usually abolish autoregulation, although hypocapnia and hypercapnia may potentiate or antagonize MAC, respectively (141).

The inhalation technique affords ease of administration (especially in children), rapid reversal of anesthetic effect at the end of the procedure, and a decreased risk of adverse pharmacologic interaction since fewer drugs are used. If an intravenous technique is used, emergence from anesthesia may be prolonged and arterial hypertension is less easily controlled intraoperatively. Should air embolism occur, necessitating the discontinuation of nitrous oxide, anesthetic depth becomes difficult to control.

Isoflurane provides adequate depth of anesthesia for intracranial procedures without myocardial depression or increase in intracranial pressure (142). Prior establishment of hypocapnia is not necessary to prevent an increase in CBF (143). Autoregulation and vascular reactivity to carbon dioxide are preserved up to at least 1 to 5 MAC. Therefore, should sudden decrease in ICP be desirable, this may still be achieved by hyperventilation. Isoflurane causes a dose-related decrease in cerebral oxygen consumption as neuronal function decreases until an isoelectric electroencephalographic tracing occurs. This effect is produced in humans at clinical concentrations (2 MAC) that do not cause adverse cardiovascular effects (144). Although isoflurane is an isomer of enflurane, it does not produce seizure activity even in the presence of hypocapnia (145).,

In our study of 132 patients, significant improvement in outcome was demonstrated in those anesthetized with inhalation agents rather than with intravenous drugs following blunt trauma (146). This study was flawed in that grouping was only by preoperative condition and not by pathology. In all groups, however, patients who received nitrous oxide alone fared significantly worse. This finding may be explained by animal studies in which nitrous oxide was demonstrated to increase cerebral metabolism out of proportion to increases in CBF (147). Clinical reports have also documented ICP elevation in neurosurgical patients associated with the use of nitrous oxide anesthesia (Fig. 15.9) (148,149). Nevertheless, in injuries characterized by diffuse vasodilation (immediately after injury or gunshot wounds), barbiturate and narcotic drugs probably constitute the preferred technique.

Emergence from Anesthesia

If the patient were conscious and breathing spontaneously preoperatively, the same state should be realized within minutes of the end of surgery.

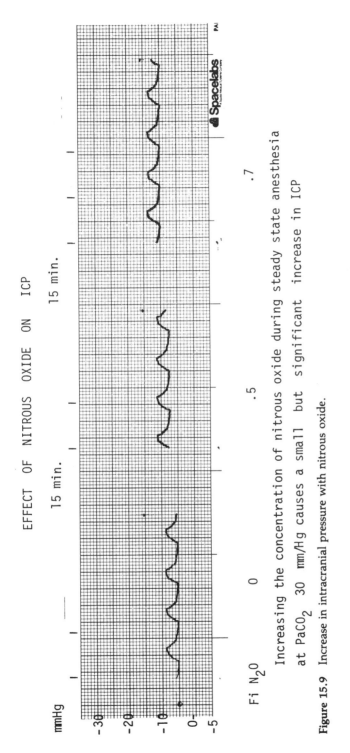

Figure 15.9 Increase in intracranial pressure with nitrous oxide.

With the release of an intracranial mass lesion, many patients regain consciousness promptly. As soon as the patient is able to follow commands and respiratory status is stable, early extubation can decrease the likelihood of developing pneumonic complications and can improve the ability to cough. Note, however, that patients in whom considerable cerebral edema was demonstrated preoperatively must be carefully observed for the development of hypercapnia and alteration in the sensorium and further increase in ICP. Should any of these conditions occur, reintubation and assisted ventilation must be performed immediately.

ACKNOWLEDGMENT

The authors wish to acknowledge the invaluable assistance of Ms. Pam R. Factor, M.S., M. Phil., in the preparation of this chapter.

Vascular Injuries Associated with Head Trauma

Michael E. Miner and
Steven J. Allen

Because of the extreme vascularity of the head, trauma frequently involves major vessels. Special consideration should be given to identification, therapy, and possible complications in these situations.

Although the incidence of major vascular injury following head injury is not high, when these "associated" vascular injuries do develop, they frequently become the overwhelming issue in the patient's management. Such lesions may cause quite dramatic physical findings, but more frequently they require a high index of suspicion and experience for the clinician to make a timely diagnosis (150). Computerized brain imaging has greatly improved our diagnostic ability in head injury, but it has also diminished the use of angiography. Since most of the vascular lesions associated with head trauma require angiography for proper evaluation, there is a need to reestablish the indications for angiography in the head-injured patient. This is especially true because many of these vascular lesions are recoverable if diagnosed and treated early. Vascular lesions in the neck also are occasionally associated with head injury with little or no evidence of neck injury. Such injuries are particularly treacherous diagnostic problems. To treat these patients properly there must be an ongoing, coordinated effort between the anesthesiologist, radiologist, surgeon, and the trauma team.

MECHANISMS OF VASCULAR INJURY FOLLOWING HEAD INJURY

Simple linear fractures of the calvarium are rarely the source of vascular injuries. We have seen one case of dural arteriovenous fistula that apparently resulted from a linear skull fracture. On the other hand, fractures at the base of the skull can result in sudden occlusion of the carotid or vertebral arteries with major acute neurologic deficit. Traumatic false aneurysms of the carotid artery can be caused by fractures through the foramen lacerum or the lesser wing of the sphenoid with

This work was supported in part by NIH Grant #N01NS92314.

local weakening of the vessel wall (151). Similarly, carotid-cavernous fistula can be caused by basilar skull fractures when both the carotid artery and the cavernous sinus are lacerated (152). Depressed calvarial fractures are not commonly associated with vascular injuries except when they occur over the major venous sinuses. The patient often is not in severe neurologic straits, and the fracture may appear quite benign until the bony fragment is removed (153). Such sinus injuries can also result in thrombosis, but massive hemorrhage is more commonly seen by the surgeon and anesthesiologist.

Missile wounds to the brain may result in direct vascular injuries but may cause linear, basilar, or depressed skull fractures that can also yield secondary vascular injuries. Bullet wounds more commonly result in vascular injury because of the "shock" effect of the bullet. This effect is related to the velocity, yawl, and size of the bullet, as well as the bullet tract. Therefore, thrombosis, hemorrhage, arteriovenous fistula, and aneurysm formation may result either within or outside the direct tract.

Nonpenetrating head injuries not associated with skull fractures can also result in vascular injuries, but the mechanism is often conjectural (154). Severe vascular spasm may occur with such injuries, presumably related to subarachnoid hemorrhage (155). Vascular thrombosis, apparently caused by either intimal injuries or hemorrhage into the media, have been frequently described. False aneurysms and arteriovenous fistula following nonpenetrating injuries are rare in the absence of basilar skull fractures.

Just as spinal cord injuries can result from primary head trauma, so may injury to the cervical vessels (150). These injuries presumably occur because of acute stretching of the vessels. Intimal tears of the carotid artery are particularly likely to occur with primary injury to the head. Such injuries may result in acute or progressive vessel occlusion, emboli to the cerebral circulation, dissection of the intima, or aneurysm formation (154). Carotid artery injuries may cause progressive, unexplained neurologic deterioration, even in the absence of direct neck trauma, and obviously require a high index of suspicion to diagnose. Unrecognized blunt trauma to the neck can also occur in association with head injury, resulting in a clinical problem that is primarily the result of cervical vascular injury. The vertebral artery can be injured secondary to cervical spine fractures or distraction injuries to the vertebrae, or with injuries to the region of the occipital condyles.

MANAGEMENT OF SPECIFIC VASCULAR INJURIES

Carotid-Cavernous Fistula

Head trauma is a common cause of carotid-cavernous fistula (156) (Fig. 15.10). These fistulas are most frequently associated with major fractures of the base of the skull, but occasionally result from penetrating wounds. Clinical abnormalities arise because of a change in the direction of blood flow in the venous side with distention of the orbital vascular channels, mass effect behind the eye, or the

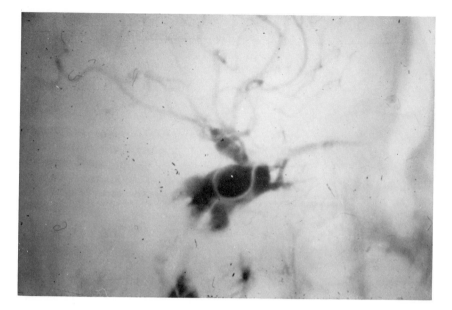

Figure 15.10 Lateral view of a subtracted carotid angiogram in a 37-year-old man who developed a carotid-cavernous fistula after a severe closed head injury and basilar skull fracture. The full symptoms did not develop until five days after the injury. There is minimal intracranial flow owing to almost complete emptying of the carotid blood flow into the cavernous sinus.

shunting of blood away from the eye and brain. The resultant ischemia and hypoxia cause the visual disturbances and unilateral neurologic signs. Ocular signs include exophthalmos, orbital bruit, ocular pulsations, headache, chemosis, extraocular palsies, and visual failure (157–159). Characteristically, the globe is displaced downward and laterally because the dilated ophthalmic veins are located superiorly and medially in the orbit. The exophthalmos may be so severe as to result in exposure keratitis. The bruit is frequently the most disturbing problem to the patient. It may be present constantly and increase when the patient is reclining, making sleep difficult. Of the extraocular nerves, the abducens is affected twice as often as the ocular motor or trochlear. Impaired vision occurs in approximately 90% of cases and may be quite severe (157). Occasionally there can be bilateral ocular signs with a unilateral fistula. There is frequently an associated subtle hemiparesis, which may develop into a profound hemiplegia.

Although CT and skull roentgenograms are useful, angiography is the definitive diagnostic procedure for carotid-cavernous fistulas. Characteristically, angiography demonstrates early opacification and enlargement of the cavernous sinus and ophthalmic and other veins that normally drain into the cavernous sinus (see Fig. 15.8). This often is associated with decreased filling of the cerebral circulation (151).

Although 5% to 10% of patients spontaneously improve, life-threatening intracranial hemorrhage occurs in approximately 3%. Epistaxis and severe orbital bleeding are rare, but when they do occur the hemorrhage is dramatic (160). The signs and symptoms are often not immediately apparent after injury and may take several months to reach their full clinical manifestation. Indications for operative intervention include intolerance to the bruit, delayed visual loss, hemorrhage, and progressive hemiparesis. Cosmetic disfiguration may also become unacceptable. Therefore, the goals of treatment are to preserve vision, eliminate the bruit, restore the appearance of the eye, and improve CBF.

A variety of surgical techniques have been used to correct carotid-cavernous fistula. The Jaeger-Hamby procedure is the most commonly employed carotid ablative procedure (152,156). In this approach the carotid artery is initially ligated intracranially proximal to the origin of the ophthalmic artery. A muscle strip is then introduced into the cervical internal carotid artery and flow-directed to the fistula. Auscultation of the eye confirms loss of the bruit, and plain X-ray films document the location of the metallic clips applied to the muscle strip (152). A double-lumen catheter has been developed that allows angiographic visualization while a balloon is placed in the fistula, thus allowing carotid blood flow to continue after the fistula is corrected. Once the balloon is appropriately positioned, it is inflated with contrast media. Parkinson (161), using adjunctive hypothermia in cardiac arrest, has been able to obliterate the fistula directly and preserve the carotid artery. This procedure is technically difficult but very innovative. The catheter technique of Serbinenko (162) uses a detachable balloon tip that can be placed directly in the orifice of the fistula. Once positioned, the balloon is filled with silicon and detached from the catheter. This technique also allows for obliteration of the fistula while preserving patency of the carotid artery. Extracranial-intracranial bypass procedures may further reduce the incidence of postocclusion neurologic deficits (163).

False Aneurysms

Traumatic false aneurysms occur predominantly in the intracavernous portion of the internal carotid artery (Fig. 15.11). These lesions may expand and become symptomatic by causing pressure on the ipsilateral optic nerve or extraocular nerves. They can also cause pulsating exophthalmos or rupture into the cavernous sinus and cause a carotid-cavernous fistula, or they may rupture into the sphenoid sinus and cause massive epistaxis (164). The findings of unilateral blindness, orbital fracture, and epistaxis after head injury require angiography for diagnosis. Trapping procedures (i.e., intracranial and cervical internal carotid artery ligation) produce satisfactory results in most patients.

Traumatic cerebral aneurysms may also occur in the peripheral cerebral arteries. The course is difficult to predict, but Asari and co-workers (165) have observed late catastrophic rupture in nearly 50% of all patients with distal traumatic cerebral aneurysms. Thus, a direct approach to obliterate the aneurysm is recommended.

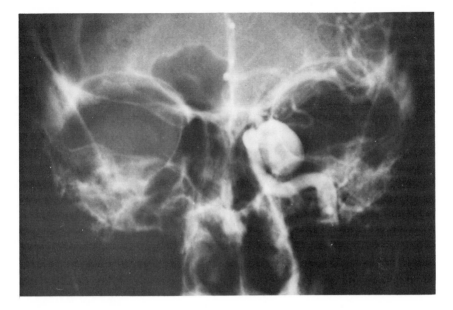

Figure 15.11   Anteroposterior view of a carotid angiogram performed in a 28-year-old man five months after head trauma. He had a LeFort 3 facial fracture and a mild brain injury from which he fully recovered within six weeks. While bowling he developed massive epistaxis, which prompted this angiogram. The false aneurysm of the infraclinoid portion of the internal carotid artery was compressing the optic nerve laterally but had ruptured into the sphenoid sinus. Intracranial ligation of the internal carotid artery just proximal to the ophthalmic artery was followed by ligation of the cervical portion of the internal carotid artery. The patient continues to have a field defect but has not had any other signs or symptoms in five years.

Dural Venous Sinus Injury

Injury to the dural venous sinuses is associated most commonly with depressed skull fractures over the major venous sinuses but can also occur as a result of direct bullet wounds. Depressed fractures over the major sinuses require angiography preoperatively unless a life-threatening mass effect is demonstrated on CT or there is active hemorrhage. A conservative approach to treatment is frequently the best course of action. Rarely, a sudden tear in a large sinus may result in venous air embolism and an air lock develops in the heart. Outcome is usually promptly fatal.

When surgical treatment is required, the team should be well aware that massive bleeding may occur. Direct ligation of the anterior half of the superior sagittal sinus is relatively safe and carries a low mortality rate. Ligation of the posterior half of the sinus has an unacceptably high mortality (153). Angiographic demonstration that the major venous drainage from the brain goes down one transverse sinus suggests that ligation of the opposite sinus may carry a low mortality; however, ligation of the transverse sinus is hazardous.

A variety of closure techniques can be used on the sinuses, including direct suturing and oversewing with a variety of agents such as small pieces of muscle and pericranial or dural patch grafts. When the sinus is destroyed over a great distance, autogenous saphenous vein grafts are extremely helpful. The use of an intravascular shunt, as described by Kapp, Gielchinsky, and Deardourff (153), with inflatable balloons at both ends allow relatively leisurely anastomosis of the saphenous vein to the dural sinus.

The key to treating these lesions is preoperative diagnosis with angiography, adequate exposure before the sinus is opened, immediate availability of blood and fluid replacement, experience with a wide variety of suture and shunt materials to stem the hemorrhage, and close cooperation between all members of the operating team.

Cervical Vasculature

Injuries to the head may themselves result in cervical carotid or vertebral artery injury by abrupt hyperextension or lateral flexion of the neck, intraoral trauma, basilar skull fracture, or fracture of the occipital condyles (166). Nonpenetrating injury to the carotid artery characteristically results in extracranial thrombosis caused by dissection of the intima or hemorrhage into the media (154,167–169). Rarely, cerebral embolism may occur after missile wounds to the neck (170,171). The resulting neurologic findings often are delayed over several hours to several days. In young people the lesion may initially be asymptomatic, but delayed embolization into the intracranial branches may result in a neurologic syndrome that is not easily differentiated from primary head injury. The distinguishing characteristics are progressive deterioration of neurologic status unexplained by brain CT findings, ipsilateral Horner's syndrome, and a cervical hematoma. Major and minor syndromes of vertebrobasilar insufficiency can be produced by head injury. The vertebral artery can also be injured by acute hyperflexion of the neck or fractures of the skull base or vertebral canal. The resultant thrombosis may also involve the anterior spinal artery with subsequent ischemia or infarction of the cervical spinal cord (172). Treatment is geared toward maintaining CBF, preventing embolization of the cerebral vasculature, and avoiding delayed rupture of weakened vessels. Extracranial-intracranial bypass surgery has not been shown to be of value in these patients.

ANGIOGRAPHY FOLLOWING HEAD INJURY

CT has been a major advance in the diagnosis and treatment of head-injured patients. It is a rapid, accurate, definitive, and cost-effective test in most patients. Hand in hand with the increased use of CT scanning has been a decrease in the use of angiography; however, angiography continues to yield information that CT does not provide. There is a need to redefine the role of angiography following head injury. Digital subtraction angiography, a technique still not widely available, may prove of considerable diagnostic value.

A clear history of trauma and a nondiagnostic CT scan still does not supply a clear understanding of the intracranial pathology. In the event of neurologic deterioration, angiography is clearly indicated. Certainly, in patients with stable vital signs who have fractures over the major dural sinuses, angiography is indicated prior to surgery. Patients with basilar skull fractures who develop either epistaxis, extraocular nerve palsies, or decreased vision deserve to be evaluated for false aneurysms. Patients who have the signs and symptoms of a carotid-cavernous fistula require angiography. Similarly, in patients who have no obvious reason for their neurologic deterioration, cervical angiography, even in the absence of evidence of neck injury, may provide valuable diagnostic information if the study is done before the patient's condition has severely deteriorated. Perhaps the most controversial group of patients are those who have prolonged coma in the face of an improving CT scan. To be categorically certain that there is not a remedial lesion, angiography is indicated. The combination of information provided by angiography and CT scanning in difficult diagnostic problems in head injury can more frequently lead to a diagnosis than either test alone.

ANESTHETIC MANAGEMENT

Preparation for anesthesia in these procedures must start with discussion of the case and its particular problems with the surgeon. It is only by clear communication that all the potential problems can be anticipated and rational provision for them made. In our experience, these patients generally are young and in good medical health.

Positioning

Most of the procedures require a supine position with unobstructed surgical access to the head. Circuit hoses, ocular protection, and esophageal tubes need to be adequately secured before the procedure begins. Occasionally, a head-up position will be needed and precautions for air embolism need to be taken, especially if opened venous sinuses are suspected.

Perhaps the main emphasis to be made about positioning in these patients is adequate padding. Any of these lesions may require several hours to repair, and peripheral nerve palsies are to be avoided.

Monitors

Massive and sudden blood loss tends to be the major intraoperative problem facing the anesthesiologist. Adequate monitoring is essential. An arterial line placed in the patient's arm or foot on the side next to the anesthesiologist has been of great benefit not only for continuous blood pressure monitoring but also for measuring hematocrit and oxygenation. A central cannula or flow-directed thermodilution catheter should be placed to help assess blood and fluid replacement. Long operating times and the infusion of large amounts of ambient temperature fluids may predispose the patient to hypothermia. Some provision for the monitoring and maintenance of body temperature should therefore be made. A bladder catheter must be placed prior to surgery.

In cases of carotid-cavernous sinus fistula, a Doppler probe often is placed over the ipsilateral eye to monitor the bruit. The anesthesiologist may be asked to monitor this sound as successful repair of the fistula results in its disappearance.

These patients generally do not have raised ICP, and ICP monitoring usually is not indicated. Communication with the surgeon will decide whether techniques to decrease brain volume are needed.

In addition to the central venous pressure catheter, one other secure, large-bore intravenous cannula should be placed. The rapidity of exsanguination that can occur with a dural venous sinus laceration probably has to be witnessed before one can fully appreciate the magnitude of the problem. Similar hemorrhage can also occur with rupture of false aneurysms and carotid-cavernous fistulas.

Technique

Since raised ICP is not usually a problem, the anesthetic induction and maintenance technique should be planned with avoidance of hypertension as a major aim. Additionally, some patients with a carotid-cavernous sinus fistula may be predisposed to intracerebral steal and subsequent cerebral ischemia if hypotension occurs. Another factor to be considered in the maintenance phase is the need to avoid exacerbating the cardiac output by the anesthetic agent if sudden, large blood loss is encountered. Conversely, there may be selected cases such as false aneurysms, where controlled hypotension may be of technical benefit to the surgeon and also reduce the amount of blood loss.

Finally, the question of iatrogenic barbiturate coma arises in the context of cerebral preservation in those patients in whom the surgery poses a risk for cerebral ischemia. The efficacy of this technique has yet to be established (see Chapter 20).

Anesthetic effect can generally be reversed and the trachea extubated at the end of the procedure to allow evaluation of the patient's neurologic status. Patients should, however, be monitored in a recovery room or intensive care setting for at least 24 hours so that acute postoperative complications such as bleeding or cerebral ischemia can be noted quickly and appropriate treatment begun.

Following head injury, perhaps more than after any other disease process, the intense monitoring that characterizes the intraoperative period must be rigidly continued into the recovery room and intensive care unit.

REFERENCES

1. Caveness WF: Incidence of craniocerebral trauma in the United States with trends from 1970 to 1975, in Thompson RA, Green JR (eds): Complications of nervous system trauma, New York, Raven Press, 1979, pp 1–3.
2. Kalsbeek WD, McLaurin RL, Harris BSH, III, et al.: The national head and spinal cord injury survey: Major findings. J Neurosurg 1980;53:S19–S31.
3. Annegers JF, Graybow JD, Kurland LT, et al.: The incidence, causes and secular trends of head trauma in Olmsted County, Minnesota, 1935–1974. 1980;30:912–919.
4. Cooper KD, Tabaddor K, Hauser WA, et al.: The epidemiology of head injury in the Bronx. Neuroepidemiology, in press.
5. Klauber MR, Barrett-Connor E, Marshall LF, et al.: Epidemiology of head injury: A prospective study of an entire community, San Diego, California. Am J Epidemiol 1981;113:500–509.
6. Klonoff H, Thompson GB: Epidemiology of head injuries in adults: A pilot study. Can Med Assoc J 1969;100:235–241.
7. Tabaddor K, Factor PR, Shapiro K, et al.: Characteristics of head trauma patients in emergency room. In preparation.
8. Barber J, Webster JC: Head injuries—review of 150 cases. J Natl Med Assoc 1974; 66:201–204.
9. Galbraith S, Murray WR, Patel AR: Head injury admissions to a teaching hospital. Scot Med J 1977;22:129–132.
10. National Safety Council: Accident facts. Chicago, National Safety Council, 1978.
11. Galbraith S, Murray WR, Patel AR, et al.: The relationship between alcohol and head injury and its effect on the conscious level. Br J Surg 1976;63:128–130.
12. Honkanen R, Visuri T: Blood alcohol levels in a series of injured patients with special reference to accident and type of injury. Ann Chir Gynaecol 1976;65:287–294.
13. U.S. Department of Health, Education and Welfare: Unpublished data from the Health Interview Survey, 1980. Cited in PR Cooper (ed): Head injury. Baltimore, Williams & Wilkins, 1982, p 1.
14. Jennett B: Assessment of the severity of head injury. J Neurol Neurosurg Psychiatry 1976;39:647–655.
15. Frankowski RF, Klauber MR, Tabaddor K, et al.: Head injury mortality: A comparison of three metropolitan counties. Am J Public Health, in press.
16. Reilly PL, Adams JH, Graham DJ, et al.: Patients with head injury who talk and die. Lancet 1975;2:375–380.
17. Rose J, Valtonen S, Jennett B: Avoidable factors contributing to death after head injury. Br Med J 1977;2:615–618.
18. Plum F, Posner JB: The diagnosis of stupor and coma, ed 2. Philadelphia, FA Davis, 1972.
19. Frost EAM: The physiopathology of respiration in neurosurgical patients. J Neurosurg 1979;50:699–714.
20. North JB, Jennett S: Abnormal breathing patterns associated with acute brain damage. Arch Neurol 1974;31:338.
21. Vapalahti M, Troup H: Prognosis for patients with severe brain injuries. Br Med J 1971;3:404–407.
22. Laner MB, Lowenstein E: Lung function following trauma in man. Clin Neurosurg 1972;19:133–174.

23. Aidinis SJ, Lafferty J, Shapiro HM: Intracranial response to PEEP. Anesthesiology 1976;45:275–286.

24. Huseby JS, Pavlin EG, Butler J: Effect of positive end-expiratory pressure on intracranial pressure in dogs. J Appl Physiol 1978;44:25–27.

25. Miller JD, Sweet RC, Narayan R, et al.: Early insults to the injured brain. JAMA 1978;240:439–442.

26. Teasdale G, Jennett B: Assessment of coma and impaired consciousness. A practical scale. Lancet 1974;2:81–84.

27. Jennett B, Teasdale G, Galbraith S, et al.: Severe head injuries in three countries. J Neurol Neurosurg Psychiatry 1973;40:291–298.

28. Teasdale G, Murray G, Parker L, et al.: Adding up the Glasgow Coma Score. Acta Neurochir [Suppl] (Wien) 1979;28:13–16.

29. Overgaard J, Hvid-Hansen O, Land A, et al.: Prognosis after head injury based on early clinical examination. Lancet 1973;2:631–635.

30. Bouzarth WF: Coma scale (letter). J Neurosurg 1978;49:477–478.

31. Galbraith S: Misdiagnosis and delayed diagnosis in traumatic intracranial hematoma. Br Med J 1976;1:1438–1439.

32. Tabaddor K, Balagura S: Acute epidural hematoma following epileptic seizures. Arch Neurol 1981;38:198–199.

33. Caronna JJ, Simon RP: The comatose patient. A diagnostic approach and treatment. Int Anesthesiol Clin 1979;17:3–18.

34. Posner JB: Clinical evaluation of unconscious patient. Clin Neurosurg 1975;22:281–301.

35. Jennett B. Prognosis after head injury. Handbook of Clinical Neurology 1976;24:669–681.

36. Becker DP, Miller JD, Ward JD, et al.: The outcome from severe head injury with early diagnosis and intensive management. J Neurosurg 1977;47:491–502.

37. Bruce DA, Schut L, Bruno LA, et al.: Outcome following severe head injury in children. J Neurosurg 1978;48:679–688.

38. Sherrington CS: Decerebrate rigidity and reflex coordination of movement. J Physiol 1898;22:319–332.

39. Busch EAV: Brain stem contusions. Differential diagnosis, therapy and prognosis. Clin Neurosurg 1963;9:18–33.

40. Bricolo A, Turazzi S, Alexandre A, et al.: Decerebrate rigidity in acute head injury. J Neurosurg 1977;47:680–698.

41. Jennett B, Teasdale G, Braakman R, et al.: Predicting outcome in individual patients after severe head injury. Lancet 1976;1:1031–1034.

42. French BN, Dublin AB: The value of computerizing tomography in the management of 1000 consecutive head injuries. Surg Neurol 1977;7:171–183.

43. Marino de Villasante J, Taveras JM: Computerized tomography (CT) in acute head trauma. Am J Roentgenol 1976;126:765–778.

44. Robertson FC, Kishor PRS, Miller JD, et al.: The value of serial computerized tomography in the management of severe head injury. Surg Neurol 1979;12:161–167.

45. Brown FD, Mullan S, Duda EE: Delayed traumatic intracerebral hematoma. J Neurosurg 1978;48:1019–1022.

46. Diaz FG, Yock DH, Larson D, et al.: Early diagnosis of delayed posttraumatic intracerebral hematomas. J Neurosurg 1979;50:217–223.

47. Baratham G, Dennyson WG: Delayed traumatic intracerebral hemorrhage. J Neurol Neurosurg Psychiatry 1972;35:698–706.

48. Sweet RC, Miller JD, Lipper M, et al.: Significance of bilateral abnormalities on the CT scan in patients with severe head injury. Neurosurgery 1978;3:16–21.

49. Bergeron RT, Rumbaugh CL: Non space-occupying sequelae of head trauma. Radiol Clin North Am 1974;12:315–331.

50. McDonald EJ, Winestock DP, Hoff JT: The value of repeat cerebral arteriography in the evaluation of trauma. Am J Roentgenol 1976;126:792–797.

51. Braakman R: Survey and follow-up of 225 consecutive patients with a depressed skull fracture. J Neurol Neurosurg Psychiatry 1971;34:106.

52. Miller JD, Jennett WB: Complications of depressed skull fracture. Lancet 1968; 2:991–995.

53. Jennett B, Miller JD: Infection after depressed fracture of skull: Implications for management of nonmissile injuries. J Neurosurg 1972;36:333–339.

54. Dodge PR, Meirowsky AM: Tangential wounds of scalp and skull. J Neurosurg 1952;9:472–483.

55. Lewin W: Cerebrospinal fluid rhinorrhea in nonmissile head injuries. Clin Neurosurg 1966;12:237–252.

56. DeMuth WE: Bullet velocity as applied to military rifle wounding capacity. J Trauma 1969;9:27–38.

57. Butler EG, Puckett WO, Harvey EN, et al.: Experiments on head wounding by high velocity missiles. J Neurosurg 1945;2:358–363.

58. Horsley V: The destructive effects of projectiles. Proceedings Royal Institution 1894–5;14:228–238.

59. Barnett JC: Hematomas associated with penetrating wounds, in Coates JB Jr (ed): Neurological surgery of trauma. Washington, DC, Office of the Surgeon General, Department of the Army, 1965, pp 131–134.

60. Hubschmann O, Shapiro K, Baden M, et al.: Craniocerebral gunshot injuries in civilian practice—prognostic criteria and surgical management: Experience with 82 cases. J Trauma 1979;19:6–12.

61. Crockard HA: Early intracranial pressure studies in gunshot wounds of the brain. J Trauma 1975;15:339–347.

62. Dodge PR, Meirowsky AM: Tangential wounds of scalp and skull. J Neurosurg 1952; 9:472–483.

63. Martin J, Campbell EH: Early complications following penetrating wounds of the skull. J Neurosurg 1946;3:58–73.

64. Hammon WM: Retained intracranial bone fragments. Analysis of 42 patients. J Neurosurg 1971;34:142–144.

65. Carey W, Young HF, Rish BL, et al.: Follow-up study of 103 American soldiers who sustained a brain wound in Vietnam. J Neurosurg 1974;41:542–549.

66. Carry ME, Young HF, Mattis JL: A bacteriological study of craniocerebral missile wounds in Vietnam. Surg Gynecol Obstet 1972;135:386–390.

67. Raimondi AJ, Samuelson GH: Craniocerebral gunshot wounds in civilian practice. J Neurosurg 1970;32:647–653.

68. Byrnes DP, Crockard HA, Gordon DS, et al.: Penetrating craniocerebral missile injuries in the civil disturbances in Northern Ireland. Br J Surg 1974;61:169–176.

69. Hernesniemi J: Penetrating craniocerebral gunshot wounds in civilians. Acta Neurochir 1979;49:199–205.

70. Jamieson KC, Yelland JDN: Surgically treated traumatic subdural hematomas. J Neurosurg 1972;37:137–149.

71. Jonker C, Oosterhuis HJ: Epidural hematoma; a retrospective study of 100 patients. Clin Neurol Neurosurg 1975;78:233–245.

72. Galbraith SL: Age distribution of extradural hemorrhage without skull fracture. Lancet 1973;1:1217–1218.

73. McKissock W, Taylor JC, Bloom WH, et al.: Extradural hematoma—observations on 125 cases. Lancet 1960;2:167–172.

74. Heiskanen O: Epidural hematoma. Surg Neurol 1975;4:23–26.

75. Hooper RS: Observations on extradural haemorrhage. Br J Surg 1959;47:71–87.

76. Ford LE, McLaurin RL: Mechanisms of extradural haematomas. J Neurosurg 1963; 20:760–769.

77. Iwakuma T, Brunngraber CV: Chronic extradural hematoma: A study of 21 cases. J Neurosurg 1973;38:488–493.

78. Jackson IS, Speakman TJ: Chronic extradural hematoma. J Neurosurg 1950;7:444–447.

79. Trowbridge WV, Porter RW, French JD: Chronic extradural hematomas. Arch Surg 1954;69:824–830.

80. Jamieson KG, Yelland JDN: Extradural haematoma report of 167 cases. J Neurosurg 1968;29:13–23.

81. Echlin FA, Sordillo SVR, Garney TQ Jr: Acute, subacute and chronic subdural hematoma. JAMA 1956;161:1345–1350.

82. Kennedy F, Wortis H: Acute subdural hematoma and acute epidural hemorrhage. A study of seventy-two cases of hematoma and seventeen cases of hemorrhage. Surg Gynecol Obstet 1936;63:732–742.

83. Seelig JM, Becker DP, Miller JD, et al.: Traumatic acute subdural hematoma, major mortality reduction in comatose patients treated within four hours. N Engl J Med 1981;304:1511–1518.

84. Marshall LF, Smith RW, Shapiro HM: The outcome with aggressive treatment in severe head injuries. Part I: The significance of intracranial pressure monitoring. J Neurosurg 1979;50:20–25.

85. Gennarelli TA, Spielman GM, Langfitt TW, et al.: Influence of the type of intra-cranial lesion on outcome from severe head injury. J Neurosurg 1982;56:26–32.

86. Shenkin HA: Acute subdural hematoma. Review of 39 consecutive cases with high incidence of cortical artery rupture. J Neurosurg 1982;57:254–257.

87. O'Brien PK, Norris JW, Tator CH: Acute subdural hematomas of arterial origin. J Neurosurg 1974;41:435–439.

88. Talalla A, Morin MA: Acute traumatic subdural hematomas. Acta Chir Scand 1964; 128:471–482.

89. McKissock W, Richardson A, Bloom WH: Subdural hematoma. A review of 389 cases. Lancet 1960;1:1365–1369.

90. Fell DA, Fitzgerald S, Moiel RH, et al.: Acute subdural hematomas. A review of 144 cases. J Neurosurg 1975;42:37–42.

91. Dolinskas CA, Zimmerman RA, Bilanink LT, et al.: Computed tomography of post traumatic extracerebral hematomas. Comparison to pathophysiology and responses to therapy. J Trauma 1979;19:163–169.

92. McLaurin RL, Tutor FT: Acute subdural hematoma. Review of ninety cases. J Neurosurg 1961;18:61–67.

93. Jamieson KG, Yelland JDN: Traumatic intracerebral hematoma. Report of 63 surgically treated cases. J Neurosurg 1972;37:528–532.

94. Ransohoff J, Benjamin MV, Gage EL Jr, et al.: Hemicraniectomy in the management of acute subdural hematoma. J Neurosurg 1971;34:70–76.
95. Cooper PR, Rovit RL, Ransohoff J: Hemicraniectomy in the treatment of acute subdural hematoma: A re-appraisal. Surg Neurol 1976;5:25–28.
96. Gutterman P, Shenkin HA: Prognostic features in recovery from traumatic decerebration. J Neurosurg 1970;32:330–335.
97. Wassertheil-Smoller S, Tabaddor K, Feiner C, et al.: Factors affecting short-term outcome of head trauma patients. Neuroepidemiology 1982;1:154–166.
98. Gardner WJ: Traumatic subdural hematoma with particular reference to the latent interval. Archives of Neurology and Psychiatry 1932;27:847–858.
99. Gitlin D: Pathogenesis of subdural collections of fluid. Pediatrics 1955;16:345–352.
100. Rabe EF, Flyn RE, Dodge PR: A study of subdural effusions in an infant, with particular reference to the mechanisms of their persistence. Neurology 1962;12:79–92.
101. Ito H, Komai T, Yamamoto S: Fibrinolytic enzyme in the lining walls of chronic subdural hematoma. J Neurosurg 1978;48:197–200.
102. Bender MB, Christoff N: Nonsurgical treatment of subdural hematoma. Arch Neurol 1974;31:73–79.
103. Weir B, Gordon P: Factors affecting coagulation. Fibrinolysis in chronic subdural fluid collections. J Neurosurg 1983;58:242–245.
104. Robinson RG: The treatment of subacute and chronic subdural hematomas. Br Med J 1955;1:21–22.
105. Tabaddor K, Shulman K: Definitive treatment of chronic subdural hematoma by twist-drill craniostomy and closed system drainage. J Neurosurg 1977;46:220–226.
106. Markwalder TM: Chronic subdural hematomas, a review. J Neurosurg 1976;45:26–31.
107. Hubschmann OR: Twist drill craniostomy in the treatment of chronic and subacute subdural hematomas in severely ill and elderly patients. Neurosurgery 1980;6:233–236.
108. Markwalder TM, Steinsiepe KF, Rohner M, et al.: The course of chronic subdural hematomas after burr hole craniostomy and closed-system drainage. J Neurosurg 1981;55:390–396.
109. Lin TH, Cook AW, Browder EJ: Intracranial hemorrhage of traumatic origin. Med Clin North Am 1958;3:603–610.
110. Cooper PR, Maravilla K, Moody S, et al.: Serial tomographic scanning and the prognosis of head injury. Neurosurgery 1979;5:566–569.
111. Lindenberg R, Freytag F: The mechanism of cerebral contusions. A pathological-anatomic study. Arch Pathol 1960;69:440–469.
112. Gurdjian ES, Gurdjian ES: Cerebral contusions: Re-evaluation of the mechanism of their development. J Trauma 1976;16:35–51.
113. Courville CB: Coup countrecoup mechanism of craniocerebral injuries. Arch Surg 1942;45:19–43.
114. Gennarelli TA, Thibault LE, Adams JH, et al.: Diffuse axonal injury and traumatic coma in primates. Ann Neurol 1982;12:564–574.
115. Ommaya AK, Grubb RL, Naumann RA: Coup and contrecoup injury: Observations on the mechanics of visible brain injuries in the rhesus monkey. J Neurosurg 1971;35:503–516.
116. Baratham G, Dennyson WG: Delayed traumatic intracerebral hemorrhage. J Neurol Neurosurg Psychiatry 1972;35:698–706.

117. Evans JP, Scheinker IM: Histologic studies of the brain following head trauma. II. Posttraumatic petechial and massive intracerebral hemorrhage. J Neurosurg 1946;3: 10–113.

118. Levinthal R, Stern WE: Traumatic intracerebral hematoma with stable neurological deficit. Surg Neurol 1977;7:269–273.

119. Mitchell DE, Adams JH: Primary focal impact damage to the brain stem in blunt head injuries. Does it exist? Lancet 1973;2:215–218.

120. Troupp H: Intraventricular pressure in patients with severe brain injuries. J Trauma 1965;5:373–378.

121. Tindall GT, Fleischer AS: Intracranial pressure (ICP) monitoring and prognosis in closed head injury, in McLaurin RL (ed): Head injuries, second Chicago symposium on neural trauma. New York, Grune & Stratton, 1976, pp 31–34.

122. Miller JD, Becker DP, Ward JD, et al.: Significance of intracranial hypertension in severe head injury. J Neurosurg 1977;47:503–516.

123. Marmarou A, Tabaddor K: Intracranial pressure: Physiology and pathophysiology, in Cooper PR, (ed): Head injury. Baltimore, Williams & Wilkins, 1982, pp 115–128.

124. Teasdale G, Galbraith S, Jennett B: Operate or observe? ICP and the management of the silent traumatic intracranial haematoma, in Shulman K, Marmarou A, Miller JD, et al. (eds): Intracranial pressure. New York: Springer-Verlag, 1980, vol IV, pp 36–38.

125. Fishman RA: Brain edema. Br Med J 1976;1:1438–1439.

126. Zimmerman RA, Bilaniuk LT, Bruce D, et al.: Computed tomography of pediatric head trauma. Acute general cerebral swelling. Radiology 1978;126:403–408.

127. Braakman R, Schouten HJA, Dishoeck MB, et al.: Megadose steroids in severe head injury. Results of a prospective double-blind clinical trial. J Neurosurg 1983;58:326–330.

128. Faupel G, Reulen HJ, Muller D, et al.: Double-blind study on the effects of steroids on severe closed head injury, in Pappius HM, Feindel W (eds): Dynamics of brain edema. New York, Springer-Verlag, 1976, pp 337–343.

129. Gobiet W, Bock WJ, Leisegang J, et al.: Treatment of acute cerebral edema with high dose dexamethasone, in Beks JWF, Bosch DA, Brock M: Intracranial pressure. New York, Springer-Verlag, 1976, vol III, pp 231–235.

130. Cooper PR, Moody S, Klark WK: Dexamethasone and severe head injury, a prospective double-blind study. J Neurosurg 1979;51:307–316.

131. Gudeman SK, Miller JD, Becker DP: Failure of high-dose steroid therapy to influence intracranial pressure in patients with severe head injury. J Neurosurg 1979;51:301–306.

132. Meining G, Aulich A, Wende S, et al.: The effect of dexamethasone and diuretics on peritumor brain edema, comparative study of tissue water content and CT, in Pappius HM, Feindel W (eds): Dynamics of brain edema. New York, Springer-Verlag, 1976, pp 301–305.

133. Galicich JH, French LA: The use of dexamethasone in the treatment of cerebral edema resulting from brain tumors and brain surgery. American Practitioner 1961; 12:169–174.

134. Garde A: Experiences with dexamethasone treatment of intracranial pressure caused by brain tumors. Acta Neurol Scand (Suppl) 1965;13:439–441.

135. Long DM, Hartman JF, French LA: The response of experimental cerebral edema to glucosteroid administration. J Neurosurg 1966;24:842–854.

136. Maxwell RE, Long DM, French LA: The effects of glucosteroids on experimental cold induced brain edema. J Neurosurg 1971;34:477–487.

137. Buckell M: Blood changes on intravenous administration of mannitol or urea for reduction of intracranial pressure in neurosurgical patients. Clin Sci 1964;27:223–227.

138. Neigh JL, Gorman JK, Harp JR: The electroencephalographic pattern during anesthesia with Ethrane. Anesthesiology 1971;35:472–87.

139. Sakabe T, Kuramoto T, Kumagal S, et al.: Cerebral responses to the addition of nitrous oxide to halothane in man. Br J Anaesth 1976;48:957–962.

140. Smith AL: Effect of anesthetic and oxygen deprivation on brain blood flow and metabolism. Surg Clinics North Am 1975;55:819–836.

141. Miletich DJ, Ivankovitch AD, Albrecht RF, et al.: Absence of autoregulation of cerebral blood flow during halothane and enflurane anesthesia. Anesth Analg (Cleve) 1976;55:100–109.

142. Murphy FL Jr, Kennel EM, Johnstone RE, et al.: The effects of enflurane, isoflurane and halothane on cerebral blood flow and metabolism in man, abstracted. Annual Meeting Amer Soc Anesth, 1974, p 61.

143. Adams RW, Cucchiera RF, Gronert GA, et al.: Isoflurane and cerebrospinal fluid pressure in neurosurgical patients. Anesthesiology 1981;54:97–99.

144. Stockard J, Bickford R: The neurophysiology of anesthesia, in Gordon E (ed): A basis and practice of neuroanesthesia. Amsterdam, Excerpta Medica, 1975, pp 3–46.

145. Eger EI, II, Stevens WC, Cromwell TH: The electroencephalogram in man anesthetized with Forane. Anesthesiology 1971;35:504–508.

146. Frost EAM, Kim B, Thiagarajah S, et al.: Anesthesia and outcome in severe head injury. Br J Anaesth 1981;53:310.

147. Sakabe T, Kuramoto T, Inoue S, et al.: Cerebral effects of nitrous oxide in the dog. Anesthesiology 1978;48:195–200.

148. Laitinen LV, Johansson GG, Tarkkanen L: The effect of nitrous oxide in pulsatile cerebral impedance and cerebral blood flow. Br J Anaesth 1967;39:781–785.

149. Merricksen HT, Jorgensen PB: The effect of nitrous oxide on intracranial pressure in patients with intracranial disorders. Br J Anaesth 1973;45:486–492.

150. Schneider RC, Gosch HH, Taren JA, et al.: Blood vessel trauma following head and neck injuries. Clin Neurosurg 1972;19:312–354.

151. Pool JL, Potts DG: Aneurysms and arteriovenous anomalies of the brain; diagnosis and treatment. New York, Harper & Row, 1965.

152. Morley TP: Appraisal of various forms of management in 41 cases of carotid cavernous fistula, in Morley TP (ed): Current controversies in neurosurgery. Philadelphia, WB Saunders 1976, pp 223–236.

153. Kapp JP, Gielchinsky I, Deardourff SL: Operative techniques for management of lesions involving the dural venous sinuses. Surg Neurol 1977;7:339–342.

154. Fields WS: Non-penetrating trauma of the cervical arteries. Seminars in Neurology 1981;1:284–290.

155. Ecker AD: Spasm of the internal carotid artery. J Neurosurg 1945;2:479–84.

156. Hamby WB: Carotid cavernous fistulae. Springfield, Ill, Charles C Thomas, 1966.

157. De Schweinitz GE, Holloway TB: Pulsating exophthalmos. Philadelphia, WB Saunders, 1908.

158. Locke CE Jr: Internal carotid arteriovenous aneurysm, or pulsating exophthalmos. Ann Surg 1924;80:1–24,285.

159. Martin JD Jr, Mabon RF: Pulsating exophthalmos: Review of all reported cases. JAMA 1943;121:330–334.
160. Lee SH, Burton CV, Chan GH: Post-traumatic ophthalmic vein arterialization. Surg Neurol 1974;4:483–484.
161. Parkinson D: Carotid-cavernous fistula: direct repair with preservation of the carotid artery. J Neurosurg 1973;38:99–106.
162. Serbinenko FA: Balloon catheterization and occlusion of major cerebral vessels. J Neurosurg 1974;41:125–145.
163. Guegan Y, Javalet A, Eon JY, et al.: Extra-intracranial anastomosis preliminary to treatment of carotid artery-cavernous sinus fistula. Surg Neurol 1978;10:85–88.
164. Handa J, Handa H: Severe epistaxis caused by traumatic aneurysm of cavernous carotid artery. Surg Neurol 1976;5:241–243.
165. Asari S, Nakamura S, Yamada O, et al.: Traumatic aneurysm of peripheral cerebral arteries. Report of two cases. J Neurosurg 1977;46:795–803.
166. Yamada S, Kindt GW, Youmans JR: Carotid artery occlusion due to nonpenetrating injury. J Trauma 1967;7:333–342.
167. Crissey MM, Bernstein EF: Delayed presentation of carotid intimal tear following blunt craniocervical trauma. Surgery 1974;75:543–549.
168. Gleave JRW: Thrombosis of the carotid artery in the neck in association with head injury, in Third international congress of neurological surgery: Excerpta Medica, International Congress Series 110. Amsterdam, Excerpta Medica, 1966, pp 200–206.
169. Gurdjian ES, Audet B, Sibayan RW, et al.: Spasm of the extracranial internal carotid artery resulting from blunt trauma demonstrated by angiography. J Neurosurg 1971; 35:742–747.
170. Fletcher R, Woodward J, Royle J, et al.: Cerebral embolism following blunt extra-cranial vascular trauma: A report of two cases. Aust NZ J Surg 1974;44:269–272.
171. Miner ME, Handel S: Traumatic embolization of the intracranial internal carotid artery. J Neuroradiol 1978;15:141–143.
172. Schneider RC, Crosby EC: Vascular insufficiency of brainstem and spinal cord in spinal trauma. Neurology 1959;9:643–656.

CHAPTER 16

Cardiovascular Effects of Severe Head Injury
Michael E. Miner and
Steven J. Allen

Abnormalities of cardiovascular and pulmonary function are the rule rather than the exception following severe head injury; however, because pulmonary gas exchange is inherently linked to cardiovascular performance, it is often difficult to evaluate the independent function of these two systems. Over the past few years it has become increasingly apparent that treatment geared toward the head injury must be seen as only a part, albeit a major part, of the total treatment of brain-injured patients.

At the beginning of the twentieth century, Cushing described the combination of hypertension and bradycardia caused by extremely high intracranial pressures (1). This observation was very important because it focused attention on the systemic response to increased intracranial pressure (ICP). Unfortunately, it is rarely applicable to the human condition, because by the time the ICP reaches diastolic blood pressure levels, most patients are brain dead. Over the ensuing years it has become clear that in the therapy of head-injured patients, assessment of cardiovascular function is important. Unfortunately, most studies to date have not been conclusive as to what abnormalities to treat or if treatment of specific cardiovascular abnormalities should be different in this group of patients. Moreover, both the anesthesiologist and the neurosurgeon should be alerted to cardiovascular changes in the head-injured patient and be able to attribute them either to the disease process, to secondary complications, or to preexistent pathology.

This chapter reviews the literature, presents our own experience with head-injured patients, and describes a rational protocol for treatment interventions. We propose that there is a hyperdynamic cardiovascular state associated with severe head injuries, mediated by catecholamines, that is responsible for the cardiovascular sequelae observed in these patients (Fig. 16.1).

This work was supported in part by NIH Grant #N01NS92314.

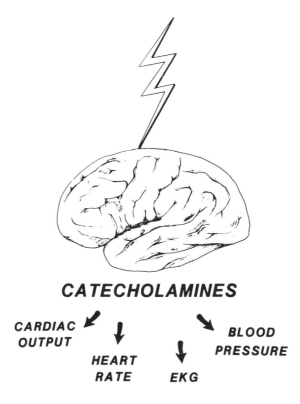

Figure 16.1   Severe brain injury causes activation of the autonomic nervous system. In most patients this results in a hyperdynamic cardiovascular response caused by the systemic release of catecholamines. In the majority of patients this is evidenced by tachycardia, systemic hypertension, an increase in cardiac output, and electrocardiographic changes suggesting diffuse myocardial ischemia.

THE ELECTROCARDIOGRAM

The electrocardiogram (ECG) in head-injured patients may show a variety of changes. Hersch examined the ECG of 164 patients with head injuries, 100 patients with injuries other than of the head, and 164 normal patients (2). He found that P waves of increased amplitude and prolonged corrected QT intervals (QTc) were almost entirely confined to those who had suffered head injury, while in patients with head injury and in those with other types of severe trauma, there was an increased incidence of prolonged QRS interval, elevated ST segments, inverted T waves, large U waves, and sinus arrhythmias with either fixed or wandering pacemakers. Vander Ark correlated mortality with ECG abnormalities in patients with subdural hematomas and found that any abnormality of the ECG was associated with an increased mortality rate (3).

The most common ECG abnormalities found in patients with subarachnoid hemorrhage can be explained by increased sympathetic tone, that is, tachycardia, prolonged QTc interval, large U waves, and T- and ST-wave changes (4). Cruickshank, Neil-Dwyer, and Brice (5) noted that the occurrence of peaked P waves, long PR intervals, prolonged QTc intervals, and U waves indicated a poor prognosis.

We reviewed 88 consecutive patients with severe head injury. Ninety-one percent showed some change in their ECG pattern. The most common abnormality was a prolonged QT interval, but a wide variety of changes were observed. Major ventricular extrasystoles and heart blocks rarely were seen; however, fatal arrhythmias have been reported in young head-injured patients who have no pre-existing cardiac abnormalities (2). Table 16.1 lists the ECG changes observed in our head-injured patients.

Studies indicate that the ECG abnormalities observed early after head injury are due primarily to the combination of activation of the autonomic nervous system and hypoxia. There is evidence that both the parasympathetic and sympathetic nervous systems are involved in the autonomic effect. Therapeutic regimens to correct hypoxia and excess vagal tone are well delineated, and clinical experience with the use of sympathetic pharmacologic blockade in head-injured patients is encouraging (6).

Prolongation of the QTc has been correlated with increased levels of epinephrine, and there is evidence that a sudden surge of epinephrine, independent of norepinephrine, occurs following brain injury (4,7). We noted a correlation between outcome and prolongation of the QTc interval. In those patients in whom the QTc was moderately prolonged, 440 to 490 msec, the mortality rate

Table 16.1   Abnormal ECG Findings in Head-Injured Patients

Finding	% (N = 88)
Bradycardia (⁵60)	9
Tachycardia (⁶100)	45
PR interval prolonged	5
QRS interval prolonged	17
Peaked T waves	7
ST segment	
Depressed	23
Elevated	15
Large U waves	17
QTc (>440 msec)	62
Ventricular extrasystoles	2
Heart block	9

NOTE: Electrocardiograms of 88 consecutive patients with severe brain injury were analyzed. All ECGs were obtained within two hours of injury, after hypotension or hypoxia was corrected.

was double that observed in patients with a normal QTc. The mortality rate more than tripled in patients with extremely prolonged QTc intervals. The QTc interval is a reflection of the depolarization-repolarization time and can be caused by increased systemic sympathetic discharge. Since this effect may be deleterious, treatment protocols geared toward its reversal (i.e., β-adrenergic blockade) may be of value.

SYSTEMIC BLOOD PRESSURE AND HEART RATE

Normovolemic hypotension after closed head trauma, in the absence of other injuries, is very unusual in the patient who survives transport to the hospital. A brain-stem injury severe enough to destroy the vasomotor center in the medulla is incompatible with life (8). Hypotension in these patients almost always is due to some other factor, such as blood loss from a scalp laceration, facial fractures, or thoracic and/or abdominal trauma. Should severe hypotension occur without evidence of other injury, it usually is immediately preterminal.

Hypertension and tachycardia are the most frequently observed hemodynamic disorders that follow head injury. Heart rates exceeding 120 beats per minute have been reported in over one-third and systolic blood pressures above 160 mm Hg in one-fourth of head-injured patients upon admission to hospital (9).

Hypertension is a common hemodynamic abnormality requiring treatment in both the acute and convalescent head-injured patient, although treatment is based more on inferential grounds than on direct evidence. Cerebral vasomotor paralysis or impaired autoregulation, either regional or global, occurs frequently in head-injured patients (10,11). Hypertension, especially in the face of these abnormalities, results in an increase in cerebral edema and ICP, which causes further compromise of the already injured brain. Therefore, systemic arterial pressure more than 30% above normal mean values should be treated. It is prudent, however, to measure ICP concurrently to ensure maintenance of cerebral perfusion pressure above 70 mm Hg.

The choices for antihypertensive therapy are between systemic vasodilators and adrenergic blockade. The adverse effect of sodium nitroprusside on ICP is well known (12). Less discussed is the similar adverse effect of hydralazine (13). Cerebral blood flow might be expected to decrease as cerebral perfusion pressure is reduced. With the use of vasodilators, however, as cerebrovascular resistance decreases, cerebral blood flow may actually rise, with a concomitant increase in cerebral blood volume and ICP. It would appear that vasodilators are poorly suited to the patient in whom the cranium is closed and rising ICP is a concern.

As pointed out by Clifton, Ziegler, and Grossman (14), a hyperactive sympathetic nervous system exists in the head-injured patient. Therefore, an attempt at pharmacologic blockade would seem to attack the problem directly. We have used propranolol successfully to control hypertension and have had no adverse reactions. We infuse propranolol at a rate of 1 mg every 15 minutes until the systolic blood pressure is less than 160 mm Hg and diastolic pressure is below 90 mm Hg or until the heart rate is under 70 beats per minute. ICP has not been noted to rise with this regimen. Careful monitoring is required to prevent deleterious effects of hypotension. Results have been more satisfactory than with vasodilator therapy.

CARDIAC OUTPUT

The data concerning cardiac output in head-injured patients are conflicting. Schulte am Esch, Murday, and Pfeifer (15) documented a moderate elevation in cardiac output with decreased peripheral vascular resistance. Clifton, Ziegler, and Grossman (14) recently reported similar findings. On the other hand, Brown et al. (9) and Popp and associates (16) have documented decreased cardiac output. Our findings indicate that patients with both mild and severe head injuries have an increased cardiac output and cardiac index. This is of even greater significance because these patients usually are hyperventilated, and resultant hypocapnia has been shown to further decrease cardiac output (17,18). The outcome in young patients with a decreased cardiac output is generally poor.

We have found it of value to monitor cardiac output routinely in severely injured patients because unexpected systemic hemorrhage, induced intravascular volume depletion, and antihypertensive drugs all exert potentially reversible effects on cardiac output. Calculation of fluid therapy is made by measuring right heart pressures (central venous, pulmonary artery, and wedge pressures) and cardiac output. We have not specifically tried to lower an elevated cardiac output by fluid restriction or by diuretic administration. Nevertheless, treatment with β-adrenergic blocking agents may be beneficial by preventing myocardial damage.

The effects of aggressive hyperventilation and continued diuretic therapy on these variables, especially cardiac output and oxygen delivery to the brain, are unknown. It is possible that cerebral hypoperfusion not completely represented by the blood pressure occurs, and the clinician should attempt to determine if therapy is protecting the brain or contributing to the disease process. Further investigation in this area is necessary before significant improvement in the care of these patients can be realized. The use of ICP monitoring is of real assistance in deciding whether to attempt to decrease an elevated cardiac output. Measurement of oxygen and other substrate utilization by the injured brain will provide invaluable information in guiding therapy. With the development of nuclear magnetic resonance techniques, this monitoring may become practical in the near future.

Few data on pulmonary artery and pulmonary capillary wedge pressures in the acutely head-injured patient are available. Reports and our experience indicate that these parameters are either within normal range or only modestly elevated (15,16).

CARDIAC PATHOLOGY

Several investigators have described myocardial lesions in patients with lethal head injuries. Clifton, Ziegler, and Grossman (14) noted that 50% of these patients had diffuse subendocardial hemorrhagic necrosis. The ECG would support the notion of a diffuse myocardiopathy rather than large vessel infarcts. Indeed, the evidence suggests that the necrotic lesions are initiated at the myoneural junction in the heart. Hackenberry and co-workers (19) reported elevated levels of the creatine kinase myocardial isoenzyme as confirmatory evidence of myocardial cell death in severely injured patients. The degree to which these lesions impair myocardial energetics either acutely or at later times is unknown; however, treatment aimed at minimizing or preventing these lesions, including adrenergic blockade, control of cerebral perfusion pressure, and adequate oxygenation, is appropriate (20).

POST-HEAD-INJURY DICF SYNDROME

A systemic coagulopathy is associated with severe brain injury. Disseminated intravascular coagulopathy and fibrinolysis (DICF) syndrome is initiated by the outpouring of tissue thromboplastin from the injured brain. This results in a consumptive coagulopathy with both hemorrhagic and thrombotic components. At one extreme, the patient exsanguinates, although most patients have a less dramatic but still important coagulopathy. Our data indicate that the postinjury DICF syndrome occurs immediately after head injury, is a reflection of continuing brain injury if the coagulation profile does not return to normal, and has a significant influence on outcome. We found that the mortality rate from head injury tripled in patients who had laboratory evidence of DICF compared with those with similar pathology and neurologic status but with normal coagulation profiles (21). This represents a treatable secondary effect of head injury that can diminish morbidity and mortality if the syndrome is recognized early. Treatment consists of fresh-frozen plasma, cryoprecipitate and, if needed, fresh-frozen platelet packs. We do not insert ventricular catheters in the face of laboratory evidence of DICF, but rather rely on the subdural hollow bolt technique of ICP monitoring (22).

SUMMARY

Severe head injury results in a hyperdynamic cardiovascular state as evidenced by systemic hypertension, elevated cardiac index, and tachycardia. Such patients are also in a hypermetabolic and hyperthermic state. The available data strongly suggest that these responses are caused by catecholamine excretion and may initially be protective to the injured patient but may also contribute to the cerebral pathology.

Treatment must be individualized. Frequently, a compromise must be reached, as the treatment of one organ system may prove deleterious to optimal function of another system. Appropriate therapy requires invasive monitoring of cardiovascular variables. Our protocol requires placement of indwelling catheters in the pulmonary artery and a peripheral artery so that pulmonary artery and wedge pressures, right atrial pressure, systemic arterial pressure, and mixed venous gases can be continuously monitored; cardiac index can be measured episodically; and peripheral and pulmonary vascular resistance, cardiac index, stroke volume, and stroke work can be calculated. The ECG is continuously monitored. Trend recordings of all measurements are invaluable.

Hypotension is treated wth infusion of colloid solutions and packed red blood cells. Although use of vasopressors is occasionally beneficial, patients who do not respond to fluid replacement have a high mortality rate. Hypertension above 160 mm Hg is evaluated and treated according to the past medical history. The respirator settings are recorded frequently.

Reliance is on β -adrenergic blocking agents rather than vasodilators. Central venous pressure should be maintained between 5 and 10 mm Hg. Although osmotic diuretics frequently are used to control intracranial hypertension, significant depletion of intravascular volume should be avoided. Major bradycardias and arrhythmias are treated appropriately (atropine, lidocaine, etc.). Although at present we continuously monitor ICP, the more precise monitoring of intracranial metabolism and flow is preferable and may shortly become a reality.

REFERENCES

1. Cushing H: Concerning a definite regulatory mechanism of the vaso-motor centre which controls blood pressure during cerebral compression. Johns Hopkins Hosp Bull 1901;12:290–292.

2. Hersch C: Electrocardiographic changes in head injuries. Circulation 1961;23:853–860.

3. Vander Ark GD: Cardiovascular changes with acute subdural hematoma. Surg Neurol 1975;3:305–308.

4. Boddin M, Van Bogaert A, Dierick W: Catecholamines in blood and myocardial tissue in experimental subarachnoidal hemorrhage. Cardiology 1973;58:229–237.

5. Cruickshank JM, Neil-Dwyer G, Brice J: Electrocardiographic changes, their prognostic significance in subarachnoid haemorrhage. J Neurol Neurosurg Psychiatry 1974;37:755–759.

6. Feibel JH, Baldwin CA, Joynt RJ: Catecholamine associated refractory hypertension following acute intracranial hemorrhage: Control with propranolol. Ann Neurol 1981;9:340–343.

7. Graf CJ, Rossi NP: Catecholamine response to intracranial hypertension. J Neurosurg 1978;49:862–868.

8. Clifton GL, McCormick WF, Grossman RG: Neuropathology of early and late deaths after head injury. Neurosurgery 1981;8:309–314.

9. Brown RS, Mohr PA, Carey JS, et al.: Cardiovascular changes after cranial cerebral injury and increased intracranial pressure. Surg Gynecol Obstet 1967;125:1205–1211.

10. LaBrosse EH, Cowley RA: Tissue levels of catecholamines in patients with different types of trauma. J Trauma 1973;13:61–64.

11. Langfitt T, Weinstein J, Kassell N: Cerebral vasomotor paralysis produced by intracranial hypertension. Neurology (Minneap) 1965;15:622–641.

12. Cottrell J, Patel K, Ransohoff J, et al.: Intracranial pressure changes induced by sodium nitroprusside in patients with intracranial mass lesions. J Neurosurg 1978;48: 329–331.

13. Overgaard J, Skinhoj E: A paradoxical cerebral hemodynamic effect of hydralazine. Stroke 1975;6:402–404.

14. Clifton G, Ziegler M, Grossman R: Circulating catecholamines and sympathetic activity after head injury. Neurosurgery 1981;8:10–14.

15. Schulte am Esch J, Murday H, Pfeifer G: Haemodynamic changes in patients with severe head injury. Acta Neurochir (Wien) 1980;54:243–250.

16. Popp AJ, Gottlieb ME, Paloski WH, et al.: Cardiopulmonary hemodynamics in patients with serious head injury. J Surg Res 1982;32:416–421.

17. Morgan B, Crawford E, Hornbein T, et al.: Hemodynamic effects of changes in arterial carbon dioxide tension during intermittent positive pressure ventilation. Anesthesiology 1967;28:866–873.

18. Theye R, Michenfelder J: Effect of hypocapnia on cardiac output during anesthesia. Anesthesiology 1966;27:778–782.

19. Hackenberry LE, Miner ME, Rea GL, et al.: Biochemical evidence of myocardial injury after severe head trauma. Crit Care Med 1982;10:641–644.

20. Hunt D, Gore I: Myocardial lesions following experimental intracranial hemorrhage: prevention with propranolol. Am Heart J 1972;83/2:232–236.

21. Miner ME, Kaufman HH, Graham SH, et al.: Disseminated intravascular coagulation and fibrinolysis following head injury in children: Frequency and prognostic implications. J Pediatr 1982;100:687–691.

22. Kaufman HH, Moak JL, Olson JD, et al.: Delayed and recurrent intracranial hematomas related to disseminated intravascular clotting and fibrinolysis in head injury. Neurosurgery 1980;7:445–450.

CHAPTER 17

Management of Spinal Cord Trauma

Dennis R. Kopaniky and Elizabeth A.M. Frost

CLINICAL SPINAL CORD INJURY

Epidemiology

Traumatic spinal cord injury (SCI) is a low-incidence catastrophic illness. Recent data encompassing over 6000 SCI patients (1) estimates its frequency to be 30 to 35 individuals per million population per year. Approximately 8000 spinal cord injuries occur yearly in the United States, and the majority of these occur in the young. In the cited study, SCI occurred most frequently at age 19. Approximately 80% of all SCI patients are under the age of 40, and almost 50% are in the 14- to 24-year age range.

Vehicular or pedestrian-related accidents account for the majority of traumatic spinal cord injuries (48%). Sports (15%), falls (15%), and penetrating wounds (14%) account for most of the rest. The majority of spine and spinal cord pathology occurs in the low cervical region and at the thoracolumbar junction, the most mobile areas of the spine.

In our assessment of SCI as a major medical problem, it is clear that an increasing number of patients with SCI are surviving the immediate injury and transportation to major medical centers. Furthermore, the proportion of incomplete SCI, which carries a better overall prognosis than does complete injury, has increased significantly in recent years. These changes can be attributed almost entirely to the added sophistication of emergency medical services across the nation. Remarkably, within the medical profession itself, it has been only within recent decades that SCI has been looked upon as a disease that we can effectively treat with the expectation that the patient will have a life of reasonable fulfillment.

Clinical Assessment

A significant number of patients with SCI have serious associated injuries involving limb fractures and intrathoracic, intraabdominal, and head injuries (2).

Thus, the management plan for these patients requires knowledge of all injuries and their complications.

The initial assessment must include the respiratory and circulatory status as well as level of consciousness. When respiratory and circulatory systems have been stabilized, the SCI and function of other systems are assessed. During this time the patient is immobilized with the spine in neutral position if the potential for SCI exists.

Pain along the spine and loss of sensation or motor control in an injured individual suggest SCI. Pain along the spine without neurologic deficit is regarded as *potential* SCI until proven otherwise. Immobilization may most effectively and simply be done with a combination of hard board, sandbags, and taping of the head until appropriate traction devices have been applied.

Once injury to the spinal cord has occurred, the degree of potential recovery depends on three major factors: the extent of pathologic changes in the spinal cord induced by trauma; the successful prevention of further trauma to the spinal cord during rescue and hospitalization; and the successful prevention of complications that may further compromise the function of neural tissue, such as hypoxia and hypotension. Medical and surgical intervention cannot reverse the first and most critical factor, so the latter two become most significant to the medical community.

When the neurologic level for all function has been established clinically, x-ray examination of the involved vertebral areas should be done. Radiographic examination of cervical injuries must include views of the craniocervical and cervicothoracic junctions. It is not necessary to turn the patient to obtain these films. To rule out hidden fractures in areas of neurologic deficit, standard x-ray views should be taken of the unaffected areas of the spine and of the extremities and pelvis when indicated.

Other diagnostic tools include standard and computed tomographic studies of the spine at the level of injury (3). These may prove useful when standard radiographs do not suffice to define the injury. Myelography seems to be most useful in investigating disorders of the spinal cord from causes other than trauma. Exceptions may include spine trauma with neurologic deficit but no identifiable ligamentous or bone injury. In these cases, myelography is used to exclude the diagnosis of traumatic disk rupture.

Acute injuries involving the spine may be classified according to the mechanism of injury or the appearance of the spine on radiographs (4); however, there is no general agreement as to the management of acute spine injuries based upon these classifications. For practical purposes, classification has been formulated on the notion that each type of injury is caused by a pure mechanism of injury (rotation, flexion, extension, vertical compression, distraction) or a combination of the pure forces (flexion-rotation, etc.) (5,6).

It is equally important to be aware of the degree of stability of the lesion, as this will be a factor in determining the need for surgery. For example, anterior subluxation in the cervical region has a reported 21% incidence of late instability

(7,8), heavily favoring surgical stabilization for adequate treatment. Certain surgical procedures, such as laminectomy in the cervical region, may render the fracture site even less stable (9). Stability refers to maintenance of the integrity of the ligamentous and skeletal components of the spine following trauma, such that further controlled motion has a low risk of producing cord or nerve root damage (10). The unstable fracture allows actual or potential abnormal excursion of one vertebral segment upon another, implying potential or actual compromise of neural elements (11). Many clinicians (10,12,13) relate stability to the integrity of the posterior ligamentous complex, such that an intact posterior complex suggests a stable fracture. Others (14) contend that additional damage must involve portions of the anterior ligamentous structures as well.

Most fracture-dislocations of the cervical spine require cervical traction using skull tongs. Care must be taken, however, to identify unstable lesions that may overdistract with traction and further damage the spinal cord.

Surgical Indications

Surgical management of acute traumatic SCI remains highly controversial (15). Contradictory modes of treatment for SCI as espoused by various recognized experts in the field range from the nonoperative approach (16–18) to aggressive operative programs involving emergent decompressive surgery (19,20). Despite the controversy, controlled studies comparing surgical and nonsurgical treatments have not been done. Those who advocate surgery suggest that (a) anatomic bone alignment is restored, (b) neural tissue is decompressed, (c) the spine is stabilized by fusion or instrumentation, and (d) earlier mobilization of the patient is achieved. Others counter those arguments with the following: (a) reduction and alignment can be obtained by traction and closed manipulation, (b) removal of bone fragments or disk material from the spinal canal has never been satisfactorily demonstrated to assist recovery of neurologic function, and (c) significant mobilization of patients confined to a bed may be obtained by active physiotherapy. Whether there exist specific advantages to routine early surgery for acute SCI remains controversial (21–27), and the decision to operate should be made after weighing the possible advantages against the inherent risks of surgery in the spinal cord injured and perhaps multiply traumatized patient. Reasonable indications for early or emergent surgery include: (a) failure to achieve reduction of a fracture-dislocation or restore alignment by closed methods; (b) presence of a highly unstable fracture, such that traction or movement of the patient may further jeopardize the neural structures; (c) penetrating wounds or compound spinal fracture; and (d) progressive neurologic deficit. Except for progressive neurologic deficit, surgical treatment is intended to correct an abnormality of the bone structure of the spine and minimize the risk of late deformity, infection, or instability.

Intraoperative Considerations and Intensive Care of SCI

The management of SCI in the operating room or intensive care unit requires primary attention to dysfunction of other organ systems caused by spinal cord pathophysiology. It is apparent that these secondary problems of SCI may have more of an effect on morbidity and mortality than does injury to the spinal cord itself.

Transection of the cervical spinal cord results in cessation of cerebral interaction with voluntary motor, sensory and inhibitory activity in areas innervated by the cord distal to the site of the lesion; the sacral parasympathetic system; and the sympathetic pathways that synapse in the paravertebral ganglionic chain. These events result in loss of electrical activity in the cord distal to the lesion (spinal shock), muscle paralysis, intensification of vagal activity uncompensated by sympathetic tone, and obliteration of descending inhibitory pathways with consequent favoring of facilitation.

Cardiovascular Complications

Cardiovascular complications are inherent in individuals with spinal cord injuries at the T6 level or above, secondary to loss of sympathetic tone. The peripheral sympathetic outflow occurs between T1 and L2, and injury to the descending sympathetic tracts in the spinal cord results in hypotension and bradycardia, so-called neurogenic shock. Thus, it is common in patients with SCI to have the systolic blood pressure stabilize at 90 to 100 mm Hg, which is adequate for tissue perfusion in the supine position for most young patients. The emphasis is on "adequate" because the margin may be small, and careful fluid administration and possibly use of hypertensive agents, such as dopamine, may be required if the blood pressure continues to fall or the patient becomes symptomatic. Fluid therapy must be given cautiously to avoid overload, as pulmonary edema is a common hazard after spinal cord injury.

Sinus bradycardia in previously healthy individuals with SCI will generally not require treatment. The bradycardia is initiated by unopposed vagal tone on the sinoatrial node, so that increased vagal stimulation, as during improper tracheal suctioning, must be avoided. Intermittent use of anticholinergic drugs, such as atropine (0.4 mg), may be necessary, or, in a small number of cases, a transvenous pacemaker may be required until the cardiovascular system accommodates.

There is reported degenerative damage to the myocardium rapidly following experimental SCI (28). This damage plus the loss of sympathetically mediated compensatory cardiovascular reflexes resulting from the sympathectomy effect of acute SCI results in a myocardium that may be marginally competent. Electrocardiographic (ECG) changes consistent with subendocardial ischemia have been observed both clinically and experimentally following cord transection at C5–6 (29). Other changes in the ECG may include sinus pauses, shifting sinus pacemaker, nodal escape beats, runs of atrial fibrillation, multifocal premature ventricular contractions, ventricular tachycardia, and ST- and T-wave changes.

Coupled with the necessity for controlled ventilation during resuscitation and anesthesia, a failing myocardium can compromise venous return, cardiac output, systemic blood pressure, and tissue perfusion. Since the spinal cord injured patient lacks the ability to compensatorily increase venous return when intrathoracic pressure is raised during controlled ventilation, an expiratory pause may be required to allow adequate venous return (30). It has been shown that a high intrathoracic pressure during inspiration is better tolerated when expiration is at least twice as long as inspiration (31).

Following SCI, there ensues a period of spinal cord shock during which no spinal cord function exists below the level of the lesion. This state may remain for days to several weeks following injury, after which the spinal reflexes return. Autonomic hyperreflexia (34,35) may then occur as the result of afferent somatic and visceral sensory impulses entering the isolated spinal cord and initiating sympathetic and somatic (mass) reflexes uninhibited by higher centers. Initiating stimuli include distention of a hollow viscus such as bladder or gut, noxious stimulation of skin below the level of the lesion, and sudden decreases in arterial pressure during induction of anesthesia (36). The massive sympathetic reflex results in vasoconstriction below the lesion level and hypertension (at times to dangerous levels), with parasympathetic countereffects (flushing, sweating, headache, bradycardia and blurred vision) above the lesion level. Treatment requires immediate sedation; usually general endotracheal anesthesia is indicated. If necessary, nitroprusside, 0.01% solution, may be required. Pretreatment with α-adrenergic blocking drugs may be successful in preventing onset of this syndrome prior to changing bladder catheters or performing other maneuvers such as cystoscopy or colonoscopy.

Fluid and Electrolyte Balance

Fluid and electrolyte balance in the acutely spinal cord injured patient may be disturbed by pathophysiologic or iatrogenically induced respiratory and metabolic changes in acid/base balance such as respiratory acidosis owing to alveolar hypoventilation, metabolic alkalosis from vomiting or gastric suction, and hypokalemia caused by loss from or into a dilated gut. In patients with an intact renal system, electrolyte and fluid maintenance in the majority of cases will be achieved by judicious administration of appropriately balanced fluids. Alterations in fluid and electrolyte components in SCI patients, caused by changes in renin and aldosterone, have been reviewed (32). For some months after high cord injury there is disturbance of the rhythmic pattern of sodium and potassium excretion or aldosterone secretion normally associated with diurnal postural changes. While intact central and sympathetic nervous systems are necessary for the rhythmic secretion of aldosterone, levels may continue to respond to sodium shifts. Afferent sensory stimuli arising from above the level of the cord transection exert a decreased influence on ACTH secretion. The isolated adrenal cortex still responds to ACTH stimulation. The "vacancy" state sometimes seen in quadriplegic patients may be due to this low basal output of the adrenal cortex, which causes hyponatremia, eosinophilia, hypotension, and a stuporous state (30). Patients with SCI, and consequently reduced sympathetic tone, have an expanded intravascular space, and pulmonary edema is a common complication. When difficulty is encountered, placement of a Swan-Ganz catheter will provide direct measurement of pulmonary artery diastolic pressure and wedge pressure, changes of which may be early indications of developing pulmonary edema (33). Information obtained from the Swan-Ganz catheter has a distinct advantage over central venous pressure changes, which become apparent only after cardiopulmonary decompensation is well advanced.

Pulmonary Complications

Pulmonary complications may develop at any time following cervical or high thoracic cord injuries, but are particularly likely to occur in the acute stage.

Respiration is impaired secondary to loss of intercostal and diaphragmatic function (37). The phrenic nerve rootlets originate at C3 through C5, and levels of injury at C5 and above will cause paralysis of the diaphragm. Secondary to hemorrhage and edema, however, the level of neurologic dysfunction often ascends as high as two spinal cord segments above the initial injury, and delayed deterioration in respiratory function is not unusual in lower cervical lesions. Unusual but potentially catastrophic injuries to cervical cord segments C2-4 may be associated with sleep apnea (Ondine's curse), which can be enhanced by central nervous system depressive agents (30). With loss of intercostal muscles (which may account for 60% of the tidal volume) (38,39), there is impaired cough effectiveness, with consequent pulmonary fluid accumulation, and decreased vital capacity. In addition, these patients have an increased physiologic arteriovenous shunt or ventilation/perfusion mismatching. These patients require intensive respiratory therapy, including intermittent positive-pressure breathing, chest percussion, postural drainage, and assisted cough. These measures must be used prophylactically, since SCI patients are at continued high risk for catastrophic pulmonary complications.

The forced vital capacity appears to be a good indicator of respiratory reserve, and sequential measurements may aid in a determination of need for intubation or continued ventilatory assistance. Intubation of patients with cervical spine injury requires maintaining the neck in neutral position with the assistance of sandbags or traction with skull tongs for stabilization of the neck. Movement of the cervical spine may be minimized by use of a fiberoptic laryngoscope for insertion of the tube. While sedation frequently is indicated prior to intubation, muscle relaxant drugs such as succinylcholine and even diazepam should be avoided, as bony fragments may be maintained in alignment only by muscle spasm. Tracheostomy may be necessary, but often is avoided, as it interferes with an anterior approach to the cervical spine. Nevertheless, the long-term requirements for intense pulmonary toilet and ventilatory assistance for many cord injury patients should weigh heavily in the decision concerning tracheostomy.

Gastrointestinal Problems

Gastrointestinal dysfunction after SCI occurs as a result of spinal shock. There is cessation of peristalsis, usually lasting from three to five days; however, extensive retroperitoneal hemorrhage, as with thoracolumbar fracture or intraabdominal trauma, may sustain an ileus for several weeks. Until good bowel motility returns, nasogastric suction should be continued. Bowel distention, with consequent increase in intraabdominal pressure, may further decrease pulmonary reserve.

Gastrointestinal bleeding and ulcer disease may develop in patients with SCI (40) and may be enhanced by the use of steroids. Cimetidine has been advocated as prophylaxis against acid peptic disease. Use of steroids for the acute treatment of SCI continues to be debated (41,42). Although work in experimental SCI appears to suggest an advantage to this use (43), usefulness in the clinical situation in human beings is not apparent (44).

Nutritional Difficulties

The nutritional complications of the spinal cord injured patient may be disastrous (45,46). Secondary to muscle denervation, inactivity, and severely increased metabolic demands, these patients immediately enter an obligatory phase of negative nitrogen balance. It is clear, however, that not only the skeletal muscle mass, but also the visceral mass of the body enters a catabolic phase. The muscular diaphragm, upon which many patients with SCI have sole dependence for respiratory effort, is also weakened by protein catabolism. Furthermore, the association of the general nutritional state of the patient with multiple bodily dysfunctions has been clearly documented. Examples may include the association of poor nutritional state and the development of pressure sores, an incompetent immunologic state (47–49), or compromise of cardiac and respiratory function (50).

To deliver adequate caloric requirements, parenteral nutrition (51,52) may be needed when the patient has sustained multiple trauma in addition to SCI. Nasogastric (53) rather than intravenous feeding may be preferable because of the potential complications; however, the input route must ensure that adequate caloric requirements are met.

Genitourinary Dysfunction

Genitourinary dysfunction results from injury to the descending autonomic tracts. Contractile ability of the bladder is lost during the initial phase of spinal shock (areflexic bladder). An indwelling Foley catheter is required in the initial phase; however, in an effort to eliminate bacteriuria, intermittent catheterization may be used at a later time, when the patient's fluid input and output have been stabilized.

Musculoskeletal Dysfunction

Musculoskeletal dysfunction is primarily associated with malalignment of the spine secondary to trauma. The importance of immediate immobilization has been addressed. Continued immobilization while diagnostic tests are being performed for evaluation of the bone injury or during surgical procedures is an absolute necessity. Several problems of intubation have been discussed earlier. Induction and maintenance of anesthesia often includes the use of muscle relaxants. Individuals with unstable fracture-dislocations of the spine may have additional instability imposed by relaxation of paraspinous muscles that, while in spasm, may be splinting the injury site. Relaxant agents must be judiciously selected. In the severely traumatized patient, succinylcholine administration may result in a rise in serum potassium sufficient to cause cardiac arrest, so that use of this agent is contraindicated in SCI (54).

Sensory evoked potentials are the electrophysiologic response of the nervous system to sensory stimuli and may be used to assess neural function in anesthetized patients (55–57). The majority of work in spinal surgery has been done with somatosensory evoked potentials, which have been recorded from scalp (58), bone (59), posterior spinous ligaments (60), or from the epidural space (61), following stimulation of peripheral nerve below the surgical spinal cord level. Although these recordings reflect primarily dorsal column function, sensory and motor functional changes correspond reasonably well (62). Variations on these techniques have been reported (63,64). Based on noted changes in the evoked potentials, surgical decisions concerning degree of decompression, continued stability of spine fracture during turning or positioning of a patient, and surgical manipulation of neural or vascular structures may be made immediately. A steady pharmacologic and physiologic state must be ensured so that the changes in evoked potentials are attributable to the manipulation of interest. The necessary anesthetic management and pitfalls during electrophysiologic monitoring have been reviewed by Grundy (55) (see Chapter 4).

Skin Problems

Complications of the integument are by far the costliest of all complications of spinal cord injury. Pressure ulcers developing over bony prominences are the single most frequent cause of extension of hospitalization and increased medical costs to the spinal cord injured patient. It is clear that prevention of pressure sores must begin at the time the patient is admitted to the hospital, since one half hour of skin ischemia may result in ulceration. The consequent risks of infection, additional nutritional requirements, and difficulty of nursing care imposed by the presence of pressure ulcers are self-evident.

A standard nursing bed, with appropriate traction devices, and an astute nursing care team to turn patients frequently and attend to their special needs cannot be replaced by any of the mechanical beds that have become available. The mechanical beds, however, do have a place in nursing patients with multiple trauma and grossly unstable fractures of the spine or extremities.

Temperature Control

Cord transection above C7 abolishes sweating. Thus, quadriplegic patients become poikilothermic. Oxygen demand is increased, which may prove fatal if alveolar ventilation cannot be increased. Localizing a site for infection may be extremely difficult in a patient with absent or decreased sensory perception. Nursing these patients in an ambient temperature of about 21 °C allows the body to stabilize at approximately 35 °C, which reduces oxygen consumption by 20%.

Anesthetic Management

Emergency Care

The patient with an acute cord injury—especially in the upper cervical levels—who is a surgical candidate is a major anesthetic risk. The effects of all anesthetic techniques and drugs are enhanced in a patient who has completely or partially lost central, inhibitory, and integrative control and modulation of most voluntary and reflex functions.

Preanesthetic evaluation should be divided into a general overview and a systems review. In a multiple trauma victim, an apparently normal blood pressure may be misleading, especially in a young patient with concomitant head injury (see Chapter 15). Measurement from a pulmonary artery catheter may be necessary to recognize the true state of dehydration. All patients presenting for emergency surgery should be considered to have a full stomach. Loss or diminution of protective pharyngeal reflexes makes aspiration an ever-present hazard.

Neck injuries following blunt trauma, lacerations, or bullet wounds cause rapid formation of edema, which may lead to respiratory obstruction.

In assessing respiratory status, the lowest uninvolved cord segment should be recorded preoperatively. If the lowest functioning segment is at or below C6, diaphragmatic ventilation is intact but ventilation is reduced because of total intercostal paralysis. Transection at C5 causes partial diaphragmatic denervation with marked ventilatory reduction. At C4, alveolar ventilation is grossly impaired. In the absence of intercostal action (which accounts for about 60% of tidal volume), paradoxical respiration develops and coughing is ineffective. Other causes of decreased alveolar ventilation are:

1. Intercostal paralysis
2. Interruption of diaphragmatic innervation
3. Paradoxical respiration
4. Aspiration of stomach contents
5. Excessive secretions
6. Pulmonary edema
7. Multiple trauma
8. Sleep induced apnea
9. Paralytic ileus
10. Pulmonary embolism

If the tidal volume is less than 3 ml/kg and the vital capacity below 1 liter, the need for postoperative ventilatory assistance is almost a certainty.

If at all possible, surgery should be delayed for 24 to 48 hours to attempt to increase respiratory reserve with such maneuvers as machine-assisted intermittent mandatory ventilation, continuous positive airway pressure, rocking bed, resisted diaphragmatic breathing, postural drainage, percussion massage, and incentive spirometry. Patient cooperation is imperative and intensive professional psychological support invaluable.

As mentioned already, in the acute phase after cervical cord injury, cardiovascular reflexes are absent. Bradycardia and hypotension develop as a result of sympathetic hypofunction. Tracheal suctioning or intermittent ventilatory assistance, especially in association with varying degrees of hypoxia, may result in reflex bradycardia or even cardiac arrest owing to an unopposed vagovagal reflex. Similarly, mechanical irritation of vagal sensory receptors in the trachea during intubation may also cause bradycardia. These complications may be blocked by prior administration of atropine, 0.6 mg intravenously.

The choice of preanesthetic sedation is limited by the patient's emotional need, the risk of inducing sleep apnea, and the availability of adequate monitoring capabilities after administration of any drugs.

As has been already stressed, tracheal intubation may be extremely difficult. The head and neck may be immobilized with skull traction calipers, traction on adhesive tape, or using a VAC-PAK collar (Howmedica Ltd., Rutherford, New Jersey). This last device is a flexible bag containing polystyrene balls that becomes rigid after evacuation of air. The collar is molded into position with the patient conscious and is then evacuated. Sedation using thiopental or small doses of narcotics in combination with local anesthesia may be used. Muscle relaxants, especially depolarizing agents, should be avoided. In cases of extreme instability, a blind awake nasotracheal intubation may be indicated. If at all possible, the anesthesiologist should obtain all the skilled assistance available before attempting tracheal intubation in these patients. Anesthesia may then be maintained with an inhalation or narcotic technique.

Careful intraoperative positioning is essential. The prone position allows good access to the cervical, thoracic, and lumbar areas—but the patient must be positioned to avoid pressure on the anterior abdominal wall, which would obstruct venous return by diverting blood from the inferior vena cava to the valveless low-pressure vertebral veins, where it causes engorgement of extradural veins.

During cervical laminectomy, the head may be gently flexed to open up the intervertebral spaces. It is then placed in a horseshoe brow rest with attention paid to avoidance of pressure on the eyes. For operations on the thoracic spine, the arms should be extended with the elbows flexed to allow the scapulas to fall away from the surgical field. A posterolateral approach with removal of a rib may be necessary for adequate exposure. This imposes the added risk of pneumothorax.

In the lateral position there is good access to the thoracic and lumbar spine, but increased abdominal compression, especially if the patient is obese, increases bleeding.

Occasionally the preferred approach is via a sitting position. In the acutely or severely traumatized patient, this position, with its attendant complication of hypotension, should be adopted only after very careful consideration.

Anterior approaches to the spine include the Cloward procedure and transthoracic approaches. Rarely, as following a gunshot wound in the mouth causing an unstable atlanto-occipital joint, a transoral approach may be used after preliminary tracheostomy.

Standard monitoring requires continuous ECG and arterial pressure recording. Fluid input and output must be carefully charted. As already indicated, prior placement of a baloon flotation pulmonary artery catheter provides an invaluable guide to appropriate fluid management in the patient with a high cervical cord lesion.

Extubation should be delayed pending complete return to consciousness and assurance of adequate respiratory status. If there is a possibility that postoperative edema may further compromise respiration, the endotracheal tube should be left in place.

Postoperative pain usually is not severe after cervical spine fusion. If narcotic administration becomes necessary and if ventilation is no longer assisted, effects on respiratory rate, tidal volume, and arterial blood gas estimations must be carefully monitored.

Impairment of temperature regulatory mechanisms may result in hypothermia and delayed recovery after general anesthesia. Care must be taken in rewarming, since loss of sensation prevents self-protection from burning.

Loss of sensory and proprioceptive input increases the incidence of hallucinations. If possible, these patients should be kept in contact with auditory and visual stimuli (e.g., a radio by the bedside or clear vision to a clock or through a window).

Chronic Care

In the chronic phase of cord injury, the cardiovascular system becomes more unstable as a result of autonomic hyperreflexia. Sudden decreases in arterial pressure on induction of anesthesia can be followed by sudden severe hypertension (65). An increase in arterial pressure of more than 50 mm Hg was described in 42% of patients with lesions above T5 with associated appearance of dysrhythmias, which included ventricular ectopic beats and heart block (66). Halothane (65) and trimethaphan have both been used successfully to block this response. A spinal technique has also been recommended for control of hyperreflexia (67). It has been argued, however, that spinal and extradural anesthesia is contraindicated in the presence of unpredictable vascular tone and hypovolemia (65). A recent study of 78 procedures performed on 50 spinal cord injured patients at risk of developing autonomic hyperreflexia indicated that either general or spinal anesthesia provided equal protection (35). These investigators found that the suggestion that spinal anesthesia might be difficult to perform or control, ineffective, or cause hypotension was not substantiated. It should be noted, however, that 79% of patients operated under topical anesthesia, sedation, or no anesthesia became hypotensive intraoperatively.

A ganglionic blocking agent that has been widely used to control hypertension in these patients is pentolinium, which is no longer available (68). Sodium nitroprusside is generally effective, although there is a case report of failure with this agent in a quadriplegic parturient who was then successfully controlled with epidural anesthesia (69).

The general status of these patients is poor. Anemia is frequently present and may require preoperative transfusion. Electrolyte balance may be disturbed by vomiting, repeated enemas, ileal conduits, or diuretic therapy. Patients are frequently in severe negative nitrogen balance. Renal failure may be present owing to infection or renal amyloidosis. Drug interaction during anesthesia must be considered as these patients frequently are receiving such agents as antibiotic, psychotropic, and antihypertensive drugs, which may cause a delayed return to consciousness or prolonged neuromuscular blockade (70).

EXPERIMENTAL SPINAL CORD INJURY

Pathophysiologic Mechanisms of SCI

Traumatic SCI implies mechanical neural tissue distortion or disruption, vascular ischemia (71), and neurochemical interruption of neurotransmitters (72,73). All these effects are interrelated in many respects. Mechanical tissue damage is followed by release of lysosomal enzymes (74) and gross focal metabolic changes (75,76). Spinal cord blood flow at the area of injury has been shown to decrease dramatically (77), with the gray matter being involved more than white matter (78).

The continued role of neural tissue distortion after the injury has not been clarified. For this reason, consideration continues to be given to decompressive surgery following SCI. Comments have already been made on the surgical and nonsurgical approaches to this problem. This remains a significant area for further laboratory and clinical research.

Multiple histologic studies of traumatized spinal cord tissue have been done in many species, including humans (79–82). A general pattern of structural changes has been defined. Immediately following traumatic impact to the spinal cord, disruption of vascular structures (83) is followed by development of hemorrhagic necrosis (81) initially in the gray matter, with spread to the peripheral white matter within 10 minutes. Significant edema within hours has been described with focal axonal swelling tending to form microcysts, which later rupture into the extracellular space, creating large cavities in the cord (84).

The precise mechanisms that block electrical conduction in the compressed spinal cord are unclear. Two mechanisms already implicated are compression-related structural changes and mechanical disruption in axons and other neural elements at the cellular or subcellular levels; and spinal cord ischemia, with resultant metabolic deficiencies. Some authors argue that spinal cord blood flow (SCBF) is the determining factor (85), while others suggest that mechanical trauma, but not ischemia, is the cause of the conduction block (86). The controversy surrounding this issue is unresolved. A major problem appears to be inability to separate the mechanical and ischemic conditions. For example, to name but a few of the many possibilities, extracellular potassium released from cells or entry of calcium into cells, which may result in a sudden increase in membrane permeability of compressed cells to the bursting point, may cause a conduction block as well as a change in blood flow.

Although the direct mechanical effects of spinal cord compression may be obvious, there is an increasing body of literature suggesting an important role for ischemia. Anoxia or compression applied along any local segment of the peripheral nerve will halt conduction across that segment, but conduction along the remainder of the axon remains intact, indicating that the ability to conduct is a local phenomenon. Similar studies have shown that conduction of action potentials in the spinal cord is also a local phenomenon (87).

Indirect evidence that maintenance of SCBF might be necessary for conduction to continue in the compressed cord has been shown in a feline acute compression model (88). The authors observed somatosensory evoked potentials (SEP) during submaximal cord compression or hypotension. In either case, the SEP was unchanged. If both submaximal stimuli were applied simultaneously, however, the influence of each was additive and the SEP was blocked. Furthermore, if compression was applied to the spinal cord so that the SEP was blocked, elevating the systemic blood pressure to hypertensive levels reversed the conduction block despite continued compression. These experiments, using compression and blood pressure as elements of cord perfusion pressure, were thought to influence SCBF at the compression site. Indeed, in this laboratory, measurement of SCBF by a microsphere technique indicates that cord compression severe enough to block conduction is associated with a significantly reduced SCBF, and elevation of the blood pressure sufficient to cause return of conduction is associated with return of SCBF to at least control levels, despite continued compression (89).

In the long axons of peripheral nerve, complete anoxia resulted in loss of the ability to conduct action potentials in 10 to 20 minutes (90). By manipulating systemic blood pressure in spinal cord compression, a time delay of 10 to 20 minutes has been observed prior to loss of conduction in the dorsal funiculus (88). A similar time delay was found in nontraumatized ischemic (91), anoxic, and compressed (82) spinal cord, which would suggest a common mechanism for loss of conduction. Conduction in spinal cord axons or peripheral nerve is dependent upon oxidative phosphorylation through the energy-requiring sodium pump, which may be the common pathway.

In ischemic but nontraumatized spinal cords, it has been found that conduction in the dorsal funiculus remained intact at ischemic levels of 20% of normal SCBF (91). If ischemia was increased further, conduction was blocked after at least 10 minutes. Others have found (92) a gradual decline in amplitude of cord-evoked potentials as cord compression was increased, while SCBF was maintained over the range of autoregulation. After the lower limit of autoregulation was passed, there was a closely correlated decline in both SCBF and evoked potential amplitude. On the other hand, another author (93) found evoked potential amplitude to be maintained until a high degree of compression was attained, when the evoked potential was abruptly blocked. Thus, the results obtained by these various authors are inconsistent, perhaps as a consequence of the use of different animal models with different methods of compression.

As in cerebral tissue, autoregulation has been identified in spinal cord (94). Also similar to cerebral tissue, contusion injury to spinal cord destroys autoregulation and carbon dioxide responsiveness (95). It is unclear whether *sustained* compression resulting in loss of conduction also results in loss of autoregulation and carbon dioxide responsiveness. The role of the sympathetic nervous system on the response to contusion injury to the spinal cord has been studied (96). Paravertebral thoracic sympathectomy is associated with loss of autoregulation in spinal cord. Furthermore, sympathectomy appeared to be associated with maintenance of blood flow to the injured segment of spinal cord and a return of the evoked potential. The effects of α - and β -adrenergic blockade upon autoregulation of SCBF have been studied (97,98). At lower systemic blood pressure, the α -adrenergic component of the sympathetic system appears to mediate autoregulation through progressive vascular constriction in response to blood pressure elevation, whereas the β -adrenergic component is involved with breakthrough of autoregulation by initiating vasodilation and consequent increase in SCBF. The precise degree to which the sympathetic system controls autoregulation and SCBF is unclear. Furthermore, it remains unclear whether attempts at maintenance of SCBF following injury will assist in preserving neurologic function. In the subacute or chronic phases of SCI, where regeneration mechanisms might be operational, it is clear from animal experimentation and from work in humans that, following severe injury, vascular perfusion at the focus of injury may not only be suboptimal, but may be absent altogether. These matters have prompted the experimental use of revascularization procedures following SCI, such as a vascularized pedicle of omentum placed in the area of injury (99).

Experimental Pharmacologic Treatment

A multitude of vasoactive drugs have been used experimentally in an attempt to minimize the vascular changes in an area of SCI. One of the most promising pharmaceutical treatments from a clinical standpoint may be the narcotic antagonist naloxone. In experimental animal models of SCI, cats treated with naloxone regained neurologic function substantially faster than those not treated (100). Naloxone may have a direct effect on SCBF through the endorphin system, although this has not been demonstrated (101,102). It may act indirectly through its ability to block the drop in systemic arterial blood pressure usually seen immediately following spinal cord trauma. Other possibilities include nonopiate mechanisms, such as stabilizing lysosomal membranes (103) and inhibition of free radical reactions (104). Considerable research is still required on the use of this drug in SCI, but the preliminary studies have prompted several institutions in the United States to engage in clinical studies of the effect of naloxone on SCI in humans.

Dimethyl sulfoxide (DMSO), when given to animals with SCI, has been associated with accelerated return of motor function when compared with other treatments (105). Furthermore, electron microscopic studies have suggested that DMSO given one hour following injury protected the myelin sheaths and axons of spinal cord nerves while reducing the associated tissue swelling.

The detailed mechanism of action of DMSO in trauma to the central nervous system is not entirely clear. It is thought to act by inhibiting platelet aggregation, thus preventing vascular occlusion to the neural tissue (106). DMSO interacts with cyclic adenosine monophosphate, prostaglandins and thromboxane A_2, a powerful platelet aggregator. Thus, DMSO may have an effect on SCBF through various platelet aggregating mechanisms (107) and through various mechanisms that relate to vasospasm or vasoconstriction (108). In addition, DMSO has a protective effect on cell and subcellular membranes (109).

Regeneration

The factors mediating central nervous system regeneration are particularly unclear. Once transected, the spinal cord does not undergo a process of regeneration as does peripheral nerve. It is of note that similar to peripheral nerve regeneration, cut axons in the central nervous system initiate a sprouting process, but this is aborted after three to ten days. A multiplicity of factors are involved in lack of regeneration in the spinal cord. The two most prominent are lack of specific growth factors and lack of adequate vascular supply.

Growth factors may mean neurotrophic substances, neurotransmitters, hormones, or other neurosecretory materials. They may also refer to morphologic components that may produce a favorable tissue environment for regeneration, as opposed to conditions that might form a barrier to such a process, such as glial scar, tissue necrosis, and cavitation (80,84). The entire process, however, cannot proceed without adequate vascular perfusion, oxygen, and obligatory nutrients required for a regenerative process.

Many other therapeutic approaches to SCI have been studied experimentally and clinically (110). Reported results have often been disappointing or incongruous, so that many of these therapeutic modalities have not developed into routinely used clinical tracks. These include (a) norepinephrine inhibitors (α -methyltyrosine) (111), (b) osmotic diuretics (112), (c) hyperbaric oxygen (113,114), (d) hypothermia (115,116), (e) aminocaproic acid (117), and (f) enzymes (118,119).

The research efforts discussed are but a small fraction of the total number of therapeutic modalities considered for acute SCI. It is critical to note that the quality of life for patients with SCI is significantly improved when great care is taken by medical professionals to optimize management by preventing common complications. This remains the "state of the art" in medical care for SCI and is a compelling reason for continued efforts in SCI research and development of regional SCI centers countrywide in order to provide maximum service to these patients.

REFERENCES

1. Young JS, Burns PE, Bowen AM, et al.: Spinal cord injury statistics. Experience of the Regional Spinal Cord Injury Systems, Good Samaritan Medical Center, Phoenix, Arizona, 1982.
2. Tator CH (ed): Early management of acute spinal cord injury. New York, Raven Press, 1982, pp 53–58.
3. White RR, Newberg A, Seligson D: Computerized tomographic assessment of the traumatized dorsolumbar spine before and after Harrington instrumentation. Clin Orthop 1980;146:150–156.
4. Harris JH Jr: The radiology of acute cervical spine trauma. Baltimore, Williams & Wilkins, 1978.
5. Holdsworth FW: Fractures, dislocations, and fracture-dislocations of the spine. J Bone Joint Surg [Am] 1970;52:1534–1551.
6. Whitesides TE, Ali Shah SG: On the management of unstable fractures of the thoracolumbar spine. Rationale for use of anterior decompression and fusion and posterior stabilization. Spine 1976;1:99–107.
7. Cheshire DJE: The stability of the cervical spine following the conservative treatment of fractures and fracture-dislocations. Paraplegia 1969;7:193–203.
8. Green JD, Harle TS, Harris JH Jr: Anterior subluxation of the cervical spine: Hyperflexion sprain. AJNR 1981;2:243–250.
9. Shields CL Jr, Stauffer ES: Late instability in cervical spine fractures secondary to laminectomy. Clin Orthop 1976;119:144–147.
10. Apley AG: Fracture of the spine. Ann R Coll Surg Engl 1970;46:210–223.
11. Fielding JW, Hawkins RJ: Roentgenographic diagnosis of the injured neck, in AAOS Instructional Course Lectures, St. Louis, CV Mosby, 1976, vol 25, pp 149–170.
12. Holdsworth F: Fractures, dislocations and fracture-dislocations of the spine. J Bone Joint Surg [Am] 1970;52:1534–1551.
13. Beatson TR: Fractures and dislocations of the cervical spine. J Bone Joint Surg [Br] 1963;45:21–35.
14. Bedbrook GM: Stability of spinal fractures and fracture-dislocations. Paraplegia 1971;9:23–32.
15. White RJ: Advances in the treatment of cervical cord injuries. Clin Neurosurg 1979;26:556–569.
16. Guttman L: Spinal cord injuries: Comprehensive management and research, ed 2. Oxford, Blackwell Scientific Publications, 1976.
17. Bedbrook GM: The care and management of spinal cord injuries. New York, Springer-Verlag, 1981.
18. Guttman L: Initial treatment of traumatic paraplegia. Proc R Soc Med 1954; 47:1103–1109.
19. Schneider RC, Crosby EC, Russo RH, et al.: Traumatic spinal cord syndromes and their management. Clin Neurosurg 1973;20:424–492.
20. Verbiest H: Anterolateral operations for fractures or dislocations of the cervical spine due to injuries or previous surgical interventions. Clin Neurosurg 1972;20: 334–366.
21. Heiden JS, Weiss MH, Rosenberg AW, et al.: Management of cervical spinal cord trauma in Southern California. J Neurosurg 1975;43:732–736.

22. Maynard FM, Reynolds GG, Fountain S, et al.: Neurological prognosis after traumatic quadriplegia. Three year experience of California Regional Spinal Cord Injury Care System. J Neurosurg 1979;50:611–616.

23. Harris P, Karimi MJ, McClemont E, et al.: The prognosis of patients sustaining severe cervical spine injury (C_2-C_7 inclusive). Paraplegia 1980;18:324–330.

24. Bedbrook G, Clark WB: Thoracic spine injuries with spinal cord damage. J R Coll Surg Edin 1981;26:264–271.

25. L'Laoire SA, Thomas DGT: Surgery in incomplete spinal cord injury. Surg Neurol 1982;17:12–15.

26. Wagner FC, Chehrazi B: Early decompression and neurological outcome in acute cervical spinal cord injuries. J Neurosurg 1982;56:699–705.

27. Durward QJ, Schweigel JF, Harrison P: Management of fractures of the thoracolumbar and lumbar spine. Neurosurgery 1981;8:555–561.

28. Greenhoot JH, Shiel FO, Mauck HP Jr: Experimental spinal cord injury: electrocardiographic abnormalities and fuchsinophilic myocardial degeneration. Arch Neurol 1972;26:524–529.

29. Greenhoot JH, Reichembach D: Cardiac injury and subarachnoid hemorrhage: A clinical pathological correlation. J Neurosurg 1969;30:521–531.

30. Quimby CW Jr, Williams RN, Griefenstein FE: Anesthetic problems of the acute quadriplegic patient. Anesth Analg (Cleve) 1973;52:333–340.

31. Morgan BC, Martin WE, Hornbein TF, et al.: Hemodynamic effects of intermittent positive pressure respiration. Anesthesiology 1966;27:584–590.

32. Claus-Walker J, Halstead LS: Metabolic and endocrine changes in spinal cord injury: II (section 2). Partial decentralization of the autonomic nervous system. Arch Phys Med Rehabil 1982;63:576–580.

33. Troll GF, Dohrmann GJ: Anesthesia of the spinal cord injured patient: cardiovascular problems and their management. Paraplegia 1975;13:162–171.

34. Erickson RP: Autonomic hyperreflexia: pathophysiology and medical management. Arch Phys Med Rehabil 1980;61:431–440.

35. Lambert DH, Deane RS, Mazuzan JE: Anesthesia and the control of blood pressure in patients with spinal cord injury. Anesth Analg (Cleve) 1982;61:344–348.

36. Walters FJM, Nott MR: The hazards of anaesthesia in the injured patient. Br J Anaesth 1977;49:707–720.

37. Frost EAM: The physiopathology of respiration in neurosurgical patients. J Neurosurg 1979;50:699–714.

38. Bergofsky EH: Mechanism for respiratory insufficiency after cervical cord injury. Ann Intern Med 1964;61:435–447.

39. DeTroyer A, Heilporn A: Respiratory mechanics in quadriplegia. The respiratory function of the intercostal muscles. Am Rev Respir Dis 1980;122:591–600.

40. Leramo OB, Tator CH, Hudson AR: Massive gastroduodenal hemorrhage and perforation in acute spinal cord injury. Surg Neurol 1982;17:186–190.

41. Bowen JC, Fleming WH, Thompson JC: Increased gastrin release following penetrating central nervous system injury. Surgery 1974;75:720–724.

42. Epstein N, Hood DC, Ransohoff J: Gastrointestinal bleeding in patients with spinal cord trauma: Effects of steroids, cimetadine and mini-dose heparin. J Neurosurg 1981;54:16–20.

43. Anderson DK, Means ED, Waters TR, et al.: Microvascular perfusion and metabolism in injured spinal cord after methylprednisolone treatment. J Neurosurg 1982;56:106–113.

44. Albin MS: Resuscitation of the spinal cord. Crit Care Med 1978;6:270-276.
45. Peiffer SC, Blust P, Leyson JFJ: Nutritional assessment of the spinal cord injured patient. J Am Diet Assoc 1981;78:501-505.
46. Silberman H, Eisenberg D, Shofler R, et al.: Nutrition-related factors in acutely injured patients. J Trauma 1982;22:907-909.
47. Mullin TJ, Kirkpatrick JR: The effect of nutritional support on immune competency in patients suffering from trauma, sepsis, or malignant disease. Surgery 1981;90: 610-615.
48. Nair KS, Garrow JS: Depression of cellular immunity as an index of malnutrition in surgical patients. Br Med J 1981;282:698.
49. Miller SE, Miller CL, Trunkey DD: The immune consequences of trauma. Surg Clin North Am 1982;62:167-181.
50. Hodges RE: Nutrition in medical practice. Philadelphia, WB Saunders, 1980, pp 254-264.
51. Dudrick SJ, MacFayden BV, Van Buren CT, et al.: Parenteral hyperalimentation—metabolic problems and solutions. Ann Surg 1972;176:259-264.
52. Deitel M, Kaminsky V: Total nutrition by peripheral vein—the lipid system. Can Med Assoc J 1974;111:152-154.
53. Heymsfield SB, Bethel RA, Ansley JD, et al.: Enteral hyperalimentation: An alternative to central venous hyperalimentation. Ann Intern Med 1979;90:63-71.
54. Brooke MM, Donovan WH, Stolov WC: Paraplegia: succinylcholine-induced hyperkalemia and cardiac arrest. Arch Phys Med Rehabil 1978;59:306-309.
55. Grundy BL: Monitoring of sensory evoked potentials during neurosurgical operations: Methods and applications. Neurosurgery 1982;11:556-575.
56. Yates BJ, Thompson FJ, Mickle JP: Origin and properties of spinal cord field potentials. Neurosurgery 1982;11:439-450.
57. Power SK, Bolger CA, Edwards MSB: Spinal cord pathways mediating somatosensory evoked potentials. J Neurosurg 1982;57:472-482.
58. Grundy BL, Nash CL Jr, Brown RH: Arterial pressure manipulation alters spinal cord function during correction of scoliosis. Anesthesiology 1981;54:249-253.
59. Brown RH, Nash CL Jr: Current status of spinal cord monitoring. Spine 1979;4: 466-470.
60. Lueders H, Gurd A, Hahn J, et al.: A new technique for intraoperative monitoring of spinal cord function: Multichannel recording of spinal cord and subcortical evoked potentials. Spine 1982;7:110-115.
61. Macon JB, Poletti CE, Sweet WH, et al.: Spinal conduction velocity measurement during laminectomy. Surg Forum 1980;31:453-455.
62. Spielholz NI, Benjamin MV, Engler G, et al.: Somatosensory evoked potentials and clinical outcome in spinal cord injury, in Popp AJ, Bourke RS, Nelson LR, et al. (eds): Neural trauma. New York, Raven Press, 1979, pp 217-222.
63. Lueders H, Hahn J, Gurd A, et al.: Surgical monitoring of spinal cord function: Cauda equina stimulation technique. Neurosurgery 1982;11:482-485.
64. Yates GJ, Thompson FJ, Mickle JP: Origin and properties of spinal cord field potentials. Neurosurgery 1982;11:439-450.
65. Desmond J. Paraplegia: Problems confronting the anaesthesiologist. Can Anaesth Soc J 1970;17:435-451.
66. Alderson JD, Thomas DG: The use of halothane anaesthesia to control autonomic hyperreflexia during transurethral surgery in spinal cord injury patients. Paraplegia 1975;13:183-188.

67. Ciliberti BJ, Goldfein J, Rovenstine EA: Hypertension during anesthesia in patients with spinal cord injuries. Anesthesiology 1954;15:273–279.

68. Texter JM, Reece RW, Hranowsky EA: Pentolinium in the management of autonomic hyperreflexia. J Urol 1976;116:350–351.

69. Ravindran RS, Cummins DF, Smith IE: Experience with the use of nitroprusside and subsequent epidural analgesia in a pregnant quadriplegic patient. Anesth Analg (Cleve) 1981;50:51–53.

70. Nagashima H: Drug interaction in the recovery room. Int Anesthesiol Clin 1983; 21(1):93–105.

71. Wagner F, Taslitz N, White RJ, et al.: Vascular phenomena in the normal and traumatized spinal cord patient. Anat Rec 1969;163–281.

72. de la Torre JC: Chemotherapy of spinal cord trauma, in Windle WF (ed): The spinal cord and its reaction to traumatic injury. New York, Marcel Dekker, 1980, pp 291–310.

73. Smith BN, Kornblith PL: Axoplasmic transport and neurological surgery. Neurosurgery 1982; 10:268–276.

74. Kakari S, Decrescito V, Tomasula JJ, et al.: Distribution of biogenic amine in contused feline spinal cord. J Histochem Cytochem 1973;21:403–404.

75. White A, Handler P, Smith EL: Principles of biochemistry. New York, McGraw-Hill, 1968, p 389.

76. Kelly DL Jr, Lassiter KRL, Vongsvivut A, et al.: Effects of hyperbaric oxygenation and tissue oxygen studies in experimental paraplegia. J Neurosurg 1972;36:425–429.

77. Senter JH, Venes JL: Altered blood flow and secondary injury in experimental spinal cord trauma. J Neurosurg 1979;50:198–206.

78. Sandler AN, Tator CH: Effect of acute spinal cord compression injury on regional spinal cord blood flow in primates. J Neurosurg 1976;45:660–676.

79. Kakulas BA, Bedbrook GM: A correlative clinico-pathologic study of spinal cord injury. Proc Aust Assoc Neurol 1969;6:123–132.

80. Kakulas BA, Bedbrook GM: Pathology of injuries of the vertebral column, in Vinken PJ, Bruyn GW (eds): Handbook of clinical neurology, vol 25. New York, John Wiley and Sons, 1976, pp 27–42.

81. Balentine JD: Pathology of experimental spinal cord trauma. I. The necrotic lesion as a function of vascular injury. Lab Invest 1978;39:236–253.

82. Balentine JD: Pathology of experimental spinal cord trauma. II. Ultrastructure of axons and myelin. Lab Invest 1978;39:254–266.

83. Sasaki S: Vascular change in the spinal cord after impact injury in the rat. Neurosurgery 1982;10:360–363.

84. Kao CC, Chang LW, Bloodworth JMB Jr: The mechanism of spinal cord cavitation following spinal cord transection: Electron microscopic observations. J Neurosurg 1977;46:745–756.

85. Goodging MR, Wilson CB, Hoff JT: Experimental cervical myelopathy: Effects of ischemia and compression of the canine cervical spinal cord. J Neurosurg 1975;43:9–17.

86. Gelfan S, Tarlov IM: Physiology of spinal cord, nerve root and peripheral nerve compression. Am J Physiol 1956;185:217–229.

87. Deecke L, Tator CH: Neurophysiological assessment of afferent and efferent conduction in the injured spinal cord of monkeys. J Neurosurg 1973;39:65–74.

88. Brodkey JS, Richards DE, Blasingame JP, et al.: Reversible spinal cord trauma in cats: Additive effects of direct pressure and ischemia. J Neurosurg 1972;37:591–593.

89. Kopaniky DR, Brodkey JS: Unpublished data, 1983.

90. Leone J, Ochs S: Axonic block and recovery of axoplasmic transport and electrical excitability of nerve. J Neurobiol 1978;9:229–245.

91. Kobrine AI, Evans DE, Rizzoli HV: The effects of ischemia on long tract neural conduction in the spinal cord. J Neurosurg 1979;50:639–644.

92. Griffiths IR, Trench JG, Crawford RA: Spinal cord blood flow and conduction during experimental cord compression in normotensive and hypotensive dogs. J Neurosurg 1979;50:353–360.

93. Schramm J, Hashizume K, Fukushima T, et al.: Experimental spinal cord injury produced by slow graded compression: Alterations of cortical and spinal evoked potentials. J Neurosurg 1979;50:48–57.

94. Kobrine AI, Doyle TF, Rizzoli HV: Spinal cord blood flow as affected by changes in systemic arterial blood pressure. J Neurosurg 1976;44:12–15.

95. Smith AJK, McCreery BD, Bloedel JR, et al.: Hyperemia, CO_2 responsiveness, and autoregulation in the white matter following experimental spinal cord injury. J Neurosurg 1978;48:239–251.

96. Young W, DeCrescito V, Tomasula JJ, et al.: The role of the sympathetic nervous system in pressor responses induced by spinal injury. J Neurosurg 1980;52:473–481.

97. Kobrine AI, Evans DE, Rizzoli HV: The effect of alpha adrenergic blockade on spinal cord autoregulation in the monkey. J Neurosurg 1977;46:336–341.

98. Kobrine AI, Evans DE, Rizzoli HV: The effects of beta adrenergic blockade on spinal cord autoregulation in the monkey. J Neurosurg 1977;47:57–63.

99. Goldsmith HS, Steward E, Chen WF, et al.: Application of intact omentum to the normal and traumatized spinal cord, in Kao CC, Bunge RP, Reier PJ (eds): Spinal cord reconstruction. Proceedings of the First International Symposium on Spinal Cord Reconstruction. New York, Raven Press, pp 235–244.

100. Faden AI, Jacobs TP, Holaday JW: Opiate antagonist improves neurologic recovery after spinal injury. Science 1981;211:493–494.

101. Flamm ES, Young W, Demopoulos HB, et al.: Experimental spinal cord injury: Treatment with naloxone. Neurosurgery 1982;10:227–231.

102. Faden AI, Jacobs TP, Mougey E, et al.: Endorphins in experimental spinal injury: Therapeutic effect of naloxone. Ann Neurol 1981;10:326–332.

103. Curtis MT, Lefer AM: Protective actions of naloxone in hemorrhagic shock. Am J Physiol 1980;239:H416–H421.

104. Demopoulos HB, Flamm ES, Pietronigro DD, et al.: The free radical pathology and the microcirculation in the major central nervous system disorders. Acta Physiol Scand [Suppl] 1980;492:91–119.

105. Kajihara K, Kawanaga M, de la Torre JC, et al.: Dimethyl sulfoxide in the treatment of experimental acute spinal cord injury. Surg Neurol 1973;1:16.

106. Tateson JE, Moncada S, Vane JR: Effects of prostacyclin (PGX) on cyclic AMP concentrations in human platelets. Prostaglandins 1977;13:389–397.

107. de la Torre JC, Johnson CM, Goode DJ, et al.: Pharmacologic treatment and evaluation of permanent experimental spinal cord trauma. Neurology (Minneap) 1975;24:508–514.

108. Rao CV: Differential effects of detergents and dimethyl sulfoxide on membrane prostaglandin E_1 and F_2 receptors. Life Sci 1977;20:2013–2022.

109. Lim R, Mullan S: Enhancement of resistance of glial cells by dimethyl sulfoxide against sonic disruption. Ann NY Acad Sci 1975;243:358–361.

110. de la Torre JC: Spinal cord injury. Review of basic and applied research. Spine 1981;6:315–335.

111. de la Torre JC, Johnson CM, Harris LH, et al.: Monoamine changes in experimental head and spinal cord trauma: Failure to confirm previous observations. Surg Neurol 1974;2:5-11.
112. Reed JE, Allen WE, Dohrmann GJ: Effect of mannitol on the traumatized spinal cord: Microangiography, blood flow patterns and electrophysiology. Spine 1979; 4:392-397.
113. Bedbrook G: Spinal injuries and hyperbaric oxygen. Med J Aust 1979;2:618-619.
114. Sukoff MH, Ragatz RE: Hyperbaric oxygenation for the treatment of acute cerebral edema. Neurosurgery 1982;10:29-38.
115. Albin MS, White RJ, Acosta-Rua G, et al.: Study of functional recovery produced by delayed localized cooling after spinal cord injury in primates. J Neurosurg 1968; 29:113-120.
116. Andrioli GC, Iob I, Doldo G: Significance of local extradural cooling on cervical spinal cord (experimental study). J Neurol Sci 1980;24:13-16.
117. Naftchi NE, Demeny M, DeCrescito V, et al.: Biogenic amine concentrations in traumatized spinal cords of cats. Effect of drug therapy. J Neurosurg 1974;40:52-57.
118. Magness AP, Barnes KL, Ferrario CM, et al.: Effect of hyaluronidase on acute spinal cord injury. Surg Neurol 1980;13:157-159.
119. Guth I, Albuquerque EX, Deshpande SS, et al.: Ineffectiveness of enzyme therapy on regeneration in the transected spinal cord of the rat. J Neurosurg 1980;52:73-86.

PART IV

Postoperative and Intensive Care

CHAPTER 18

Recovery Room Care
Elizabeth A.M. Frost

Increased use of the operating microscope and understanding of cerebrovascular pathology has resulted in many more and sicker patients becoming operative candidates.

The combination of preexisting central nervous system disease, operative intervention, and the depressant effect of anesthetic drugs has the potential to cause serious complications in the recovery room. Many of these complications can be avoided or successfully treated with early detection. Vigilant care is required in a recovery area staffed with personnel conversant with the special complications inherent to neurosurgery. Moreover, the quality of neurologic recovery is dependent also on excellence in immediate postoperative management.

Close interaction of the respiratory and cardiovascular systems with the central nervous system means that dysfunction of one adversely affects the others. In addition, preexistent neurologic disease frequently is associated with abnormal cardiac (e.g., after subarachnoid hemorrhage) or respiratory (e.g., brain-stem injury) functions (1). Immediate postoperative care must therefore focus on close monitoring of the three systems. In interpreting any changes in vital signs, the interaction and feedback mechanisms must be appreciated.

TRANSFER TO THE POSTANESTHETIC AREA

Following elective procedures, a patient who was conscious preoperatively should be responsive and breathing adequately with intact upper airway reflexes. The trachea should be extubated prior to discharge from the operating room. Anesthesiologists and surgeons find this technique appealing, as an immediate success of surgery is realized and it is easier to detect subsequent deterioration in the neurologic status should vasospasm, edema, or a hematoma develop. In addition, increases in intracranial pressure (ICP) caused by stimulation or bucking related to the endotracheal tube are eliminated; however, any inadequacy in respiratory function could lead to hypoxia, hypercapnia, and aspiration, which may prove catastrophic in this group of patients. Thus, although early extubation of the trachea is ideal, it could be hazardous in patients in whom airway or pulmonary decompensation existed preoperatively and in those in whom operative intervention involved encroachment on the vital centers in the brain stem. In these situations, if early extubation is planned, team consultation and assessment of the patient's self-supportive respiratory capabilities are essential.

During transportation, patients should be maintained in a 30-degree head-up position unless contraindicated (as in shunt procedures), supplemental oxygen should be given, and basic vital signs such as heart sounds and respiration should be monitored. Oscilloscopic display of the blood pressure tracing if an arterial cannula is in place is desirable. A capnograph, although bulky, is useful equipment since it serves as a constant visual reminder of adequacy of ventilation.

INITIAL EVALUATION

In the recovery room, vital signs are immediately measured. Serum electrolyte estimations, hemoglobin, arterial blood gas values, and skull films are obtained. A basic neurologic assessment consists of determination of the level of consciousness, the degree of motor activity, and the size, quality, and reaction to light of the pupils. A more complete neurologic assessment in the immediate postoperative period may be compromised by residual anesthetic effect. In addition, early evaluation of mental status and response is often remarkably subjective, especially between anesthesiologists, neurosurgeons, and recovery room nurses. The Glasgow Coma Scale was devised initially as a prognostic indicator after head injuries but has also been used to assess the postoperative neurologic status (2). A more elaborate record is composed of a coma scale with the addition of an assessment of pupil reaction, respiratory rate, and lateralization of muscle movement and strength.

Pupillary size and light response are useful signs of intracranial integrity, especially in the unconscious patient (3). Regional increases in ICP and herniation of the uncus around the tentorium cause the pupil on the same side to dilate. In cases of midbrain lesions, the pupils constrict. Atropine, trimethaphan, and epinephrine cause pupillary dilation. Narcotics cause pupillary constriction, which is reversed by naloxone. Anisocoria and stabismus, which may be seen as residual effects of all potent inhalational anesthetics, generally resolve promptly with return of consciousness.

Localizing neurologic signs indicative of supratentorial or brain-stem dysfunction may be present preoperatively or occur immediately after neurosurgical intervention, although the development of such signs after recovery from anesthesia suggests hematoma formation, vasospasm, or regional edema formation. Immediate evaluation is essential. The early detection of focal muscle weakness is the most useful clinical indication of supratentorial lesions.

Postoperatively, neurosurgical patients should be nursed in a 30-degree head-up position unless surgically contraindicated, as after lumbar laminectomy, ventriculoperitoneal shunting, and carotid endarterectomy. This position facilitates venous drainage from the brain and improves oxygenation by increasing the functional residual capacity (4). Other contraindications to the use of this position include hypotension and brain-stem injury with absence of protective pharyngeal reflexes.

SYSTEMS REVIEW

"Mens sana in corpore sano"—sed corpus sano necessitit mensam sanam.
Efficient functioning of the body requires the integrity of numerous systems interactions.

Intracranial Dynamics

Maintenance of adequate blood perfusion to brain tissues is essential. The cerebral perfusion pressure (CPP) is defined according to the equation:

$$CPP = SABP - ICP$$

where SABP is mean systemic arterial blood pressure and ICP is intracranial pressure. The normal range is 70 to 100 mm Hg. Any factors that decrease the SABP or increase the ICP will decrease cerebral perfusion.

Hypotension is an uncommon complication in the postneurosurgical patient and usually is due to inadequate volume replacement or intraoperative catastrophe. Intracranial hypertension is encountered more frequently. Normally ICP is less than 15 mm Hg. The rigid cranium contains brain tissue (84%), cerebrospinal fluid (CSF) (12%), and venous and arterial blood (4%). Once the spatial buffer in the intracranial compartment is exhausted, any further increase in volume of any of these intracranial components will increase ICP. Brain bulk is increased by cerebral edema, which is maximal within the first 12 hours after surgery and again after 24 to 48 hours. The magnitude of edema depends on the amount of resection, dissection, and retraction of the brain tissues.

Hematoma formation either from the operative site or associated with administration of aspirin (5), dilantin (6), or dextran also increases ICP.

The intracranial blood volume approximates 200 ml in an adult. A decrease in return of the venous blood from the cranium to the thorax may be caused by twisting the neck, lowering the head below the heart level, or increasing the intrathoracic pressure as in coughing, bucking, and during tracheal suctioning. The total blood volume is also increased by the use of drugs such as nitroglycerin and nitroprusside, which decrease cerebrovascular resistance, and by systemic hypertension if autoregulation is impaired. Hypercapnia, hypoxia, and acidosis all increase cerebral blood flow and hence ICP.

Tension pneumocephalus associated with gravitational effects of the sitting position, iatrogenic intraoperative decrease in brain size, or use of nitrous oxide may also cause sudden, persistent, and even catastrophic intracranial hypertension (7).

Arterial vasospasm, a serious complication after obliteration of aneurysms or arteriovenous malformations, may cause ischemia, edema, and infarction. Spasm, which may be limited to the main artery on which the defect is located or may spread to the entire arterial tree, may develop immediately or be delayed for hours or days. Initial spasm may be due to mechanical irritation of the nerve plexus of the adventitia, dissection or to blood elements. Serotonin or other vasoactive substances released from decaying platelets may cause delayed spasm (8). Arterial spasm has also been described following other intracranial procedures such as removal of pituitary adenomas (9). The diagnosis is suspected by observation of lateralizing muscle signs or by decrease in consciousness. Angiography offers confirmatory evidence.

Although alterations in cerebral hemodynamics may be reflected by changes in clinical signs, the relationship is neither precise nor immediately recognized in many instances. The classic triad of raised ICP, systemic hypertension, and bradycardia was described by Harvey Cushing in 1901. The reflex involved is that of compression of the blood supply to the medulla, which results in an increased catecholamine release from the brain stem in an attempt to restore cerebral blood flow. As systemic pressure increases, the arterial baroreceptors cause a reflex bradycardia. Unfortunately, this sequence of events is rarely recognized quite so simply in the recovery room. In an experimental model, the sequence of alterations in the vital signs during an acute increase in ICP was described as changes in the ipsilateral electroencephalogram followed by a decrease in respiratory rate, ipsilateral pupillary dilation, and only late increases in systemic pressure as ICP approximated the diastolic pressure. Significant bradycardia was noted terminally as systemic pressure and ICP declined (10). It is apparent that accurate assessment and thus therapy of altered intracranial dynamics can be made only if ICP is measured directly. Frequently a ventriculostomy opening has been required during surgery, and this port may be conveniently used to record ICP trends postoperatively. Should sudden deterioration warrant emergency pressure recording, we have found that insertion of a three-way stopcock to the subarachnoid space affords a fast and reasonably accurate measure of ICP.

Although continuous recording of ICP provides considerable information, neurologic deterioration may not always correlate with increasing pressure. Lesions in the medial temporal lobe are life threatening because of their proximity to the brain stem. ICP may remain normal until death (11).

Therapy of raised ICP in the recovery room begins with prompt and accurate diagnosis by skull film, arterial blood gas estimation, and computed tomographic (CT) scan. Hematoma formation requires surgical reexploration and evaluation of coagulation profiles. Pneumocephalus, depending on its size, can be released by burr hole craniotomy and fluid displacement (7). Cerebral edema is treated with hyperventilation, diuretics, steroids, anticonvulsants, and barbiturates.

Cardiovascular System

Cardiovascular instability is a common complication immediately postoperatively in neurosurgical patients. Either hypotension or hypertension may develop. The most frequently encountered causes of hypotension are:

1. Hypovolemia
2. Hypothermia
3. Persistent anesthetic effect
4. Hypoventilation
5. Myocardial damage
6. Electrolyte imbalance
7. Adrenal failure
8. Intraoperative catastrophe

Hypovolemia usually is caused by underreplacement of vascular volume in patients who may have received several doses of both osmotic and loop diuretics. Preoperative administration of steroids to reduce cerebral edema surrounding a brain tumor may cause increased diuresis. Diabetes insipidus is a rare complication of head injury and pituitary surgery. Chronic hypovolemia is also commonly found in patients controlled on long-term antihypertensive medications.

Hypothermia frequently develops during prolonged surgery. Although normal systemic arterial pressure may be recorded initially, as the body becomes warmer, peripheral vasodilation causes hypotension. An accurate assessment of fluid intake-output, urine volume and osmolarity, central venous pressure and, in appropriate situations, cardiac output and pulmonary capillary wedge pressure measurements, will help in the diagnosis and therapy (12).

Hypertension probably is the most common nonneurologic abnormality of the postoperative period and usually is precipitated by

1. Fluid overload
2. Hypothermia, vasoconstriction
3. Emergence from anesthesia with pain and shivering
4. Hypoventilation, hypercapnia
5. Cushing reflex, raised ICP
6. Rebound hypertension, acute or chronic
7. Medications

Rebound hypertension owing to interference with the renin-angiotensin system may occur following the intraoperative use of hypotensive agents such as nitroprusside (13). The phenomenon may also be seen in hypertensive patients who have been receiving long-term antihypertensive medications. Frequently, blood pressure decreases following admission to hospital and enforced bed rest, and therefore drugs that may have been required as a daily routine are either forgotten or deemed unnecessary. During stress, rebound hypertension occurs. The complication is less likely to prove dangerous if chronic medications are continued until the day of surgery and are reestablished as soon as possible postoperatively. Patients receiving short-acting agents such as clonidine, which is not readily available in parenteral form, should have their blood pressure controlled by some other means preoperatively.

Several medications such as naloxone (14), ketamine, and dextran have been implicated in a hypertensive response. Following carotid endarterectomy, hypertension occurs in approximately 20% of patients (80% of these patients were hypertensive preoperatively). Denervation of the carotid baroreceptors has been implicated (15); however, alterations of cerebral flow must also be a factor, as similar hypertensive responses are observed following other cerebral revascularization techniques.

Apart from adding stress to the myocardium, hypertension can raise ICP by increasing the tendency to bleed at the operative site through disruption of hemostatic plugs and by impairing autoregulation, either globally or regionally. Moreover, damage to the blood-brain barrier by surgical intervention, compounded by arterial hypertension, increases the leak of intravascular contents and causes vasogenic edema.

Blood pressure increases to above 20% to 25% of preoperative levels require therapy. One cause of hypertension is the Cushing response, which is a protective mechanism to improve cerebral perfusion; therefore, accurate diagnosis is essential. Appropriate treatment includes adequate ventilation, diuretics, or intravenous administration of hydralazine (5 to 10 mg), propranolol (1 to 2 mg), or diazoxide (50 mg) (16). In patients with normal ICP, such as occurs following carotid endarterectomy, nitroprusside infusion may be required and the pressure maintained around 160 mm Hg systolic, although the ideal blood pressure for this group of patients is not known. In the treatment of vasospasm following aneurysm surgery, induced hypertension has been recommended in addition to correction of any blood volume deficits (9).

Electrocardiographic (ECG) abnormalities, usually bradycardia or supraventricular arrhythmias, may be related to intracranial pathology, to hypokalemia caused by diuretic therapy aggravated by respiratory alkalosis, or to concurrent cardiac disease (17). Acute ECG changes (e.g., T-wave inversion, ST-segment elevation) similar to those associated with myocardial ischemia have been observed in neurosurgical patients, especially following head trauma and ruptured cerebral aneurysm (18). Suggestions for causes of these changes have included high blood epinephrine levels causing myocardial necrosis, central autonomic stimulation, or ischemia owing to vascular spasm at cortical, hypothalamic, or brain-stem levels (18). Occasionally, tachycardia rather than bradycardia may be associated with hypertension and rising ICP. A useful sign that has been shown to correlate with decreasing brain compliance is an increasing sinus arrhythmia index (SAI). This number is calculated by:

$$SAI = \frac{\text{Maximum heart rate} - \text{minimum heart rate}}{\text{Mean heart rate}}.$$

Changes in the index have been observed with little or no alteration in the mean heart rate (19).

Respiratory System

Arterial hypoxemia commonly occurs postoperatively. Close correlation is seen between increasing age and the degree of hypoxemia and probably is a reflection of the inverse relationship that exists between age and arterial oxygen tension (20). Although these changes may have negligible deleterious effects on general surgical candidates, such results in the neurosurgical patient could be catastrophic.

The most common causes of postoperative respiratory difficulties are listed below.

1. Residual anesthetic effect (from drugs, diffusion hypoxia, prolonged hyperventilation, or shivering)
2. Surgical intervention (brain stem or carotid body)
3. Airway obstruction
4. Pulmonary pathology (acute or chronic)
5. Neurogenic pulmonary edema

The residual effects of inhalation and narcotic agents and neuromuscular blocking drugs may extend well into the postoperative period. Immediately on discontinuing nitrous oxide, diffusion hypoxia occurs and lasts some 15 to 20 minutes. Prolonged intraoperative hyperventilation reduces carbon dioxide stores, which are replenished slowly by spontaneous hyperventilation when hypoxia may develop (21). Hypocapnia, hypothermia, and transfusion of stored blood all shift the oxygen dissociation curve to the left, making oxygen less available to tissues. Shivering, which may increase oxygen requirements by up to 400%, occurs in about 20% of patients anesthetized with halothane or isoflurane and is related to the lowest body temperature recorded in the operating room. The condition usually lasts only a few minutes, but if it persists, small intravenous doses of methylphenidate (Ritalin) may prove beneficial (1).

Change or irregularity in respiration usually is a comparatively late sign of brain-stem dysfunction, although hyperventilation may be the first indication of bleeding in the posterior fossa or of edema formation. Surgical intervention may also damage the carotid body, which is the chemoreceptor responsible for reflex increase in ventilation in response to arterial hypoxemia or acidosis. Recovery of this function is very slow, and thus patients should breathe a high inspired oxygen concentration (FIO_2 0.3 to 0.4) in the early postoperative period, especially if bilateral surgery has been performed during the past several months or if there is preexisting cardiac or pulmonary disease.

Airway obstruction due to edema of the neck or tongue following positional changes, especially in the sitting position, has been described (22,23).

Hypoxia may also be caused by pulmonary pathology. Acutely, aspiration pneumonia, a frequent problem in patients with absent gag reflexes, may be due to cranial nerve palsy. Intraoperative air embolism is seen postoperatively as lung scan defects. The size of the defects is directly proportional to the amount of air infused. Large volumes of air can cause pulmonary edema and require respiratory support. Decortication patterns and segmental defects also occur and may be mistaken for pulmonary thromboembolism. These lesions resolve without heparin treatment, however.

Chronic lung pathology may also contribute to respiratory dysfunction. A close association between cerebrovascular disease and heavy smoking has been well documented and may cause considerable problems postoperatively (16).

A rare cause of postoperative hypoxia resulting from lung damage is neurogenic pulmonary edema, which has been reported in a variety of neurologic conditions. A sudden syndrome of respiratory distress due to massive pulmonary edema occurs. This may be a centrally mediated massive sympathetic discharge, causing a generalized vasoconstriction that results in a shift of blood from the systemic circulation to the low-resistance pulmonary circulation, leading to pulmonary edema (24).

Basic measurements in the management of respiratory dysfunction require trend recording of respiratory rate, tidal volume, inspiratory force, and arterial blood gas estimations. Chest film should be obtained routinely on admission to the recovery area. Postoperative hypoxia from most causes will effectively respond to oxygen therapy of 0.3% to 0.4% inspired oxygen fraction with either nasal cannulas or face masks. Tracheobronchial toilet and chest physiotherapy will help to prevent or reverse any atelectasis and airway collapse.

If one or more of the criteria listed in Table 18.1 persist, they should be regarded as an indication of ventilatory problems, and tracheal intubation with respiratory support probably is necessary.

Patients with preoperative pulmonary problems, gross obesity, or following high cervical laminectomy require closer respiratory observation and may require ventilatory support for a variable period in the postoperative period. Extubation may usually be safely performed when the conditions listed in Table 18.2 prevail.

Table 18.1 Important Measurements in the Diagnosis of Respiratory Insufficiency

If one or more of these criteria are met, ventilatory problems exist:

Rate of respiration	$>40/\text{min}$, $<8/\text{min}$
Tidal volume	<3.5 ml/kg
Vital capacity	<15 ml/kg
V_D/V_T	>0.5
Maximal inspiratory force	<-25 cm H_2O
% pulmonary shunt	$>15\%$
$PaCO_2$	>45 mm Hg
Respiratory pattern	Irregular

V_D/V_T = ratio of physiological dead space to tidal volume.

Table 18.2 Criteria for Extubation

If the following conditions are realized, extubation may be safely accomplished:

History	Awake preoperatively; smooth intraoperative course
Respiratory rate	12–35/min
Respiratory pattern	Regular
Vital capacity	$> -30 \text{ cm H}_2\text{O}$
Maximal inspiratory force	$> -20 \text{ cm H}_2\text{O}$
$V_D V_T$	< 0.5
Pulmonary shunt	$< 12\%$
$PaCO_2$	30–45 mm Hg
PaO_2	> 75 mm Hg ($FiO_2 = 0.3$)

Thermoregulatory System

Accidental hypothermia caused by heat loss convection, conduction, and radiation during long procedures may be compounded by infusion of cold intravenous fluids. A technique of profound, deliberate hypothermia to allow a period of cardiac slowing or arrest to afford brain protection during clipping of basilar tip aneurysms is rarely used now.

Compensatory mechanisms, which are initiated from the hypothalamus, are suppressed during general anesthesia. In the immediate postoperative period, as the hypothalamus regains function, shivering rebuilds the lost heat by increasing oxygen consumption. Vasoconstriction and arterial hypertension occur. Other undesirable effects of hypothermia include a shift to the left of the oxygen dissociation curve and potentiation of general anesthetic and muscle relaxant effect.

Neurogenic hyperthermia is associated with brain-stem or hypothalamic damage and usually is a consequence of severe head injury, although it may occur after removal of a large pituitary tumor or craniopharyngioma. It is usually associated with blood in the ventricular or subarachnoid spaces.

Gastrointestinal System

Decreased gastric motility is associated with increased ICP. It is therefore wise in such situations to empty the stomach by passage of a nasogastric tube prior to extubation of the trachea.

Gastrointestinal bleeding occurs in about 2% of neurosurgical patients (25). The etiology of this complication is associated with damage to the orbital surface of the frontal lobe, hypothalamus, or the tegmental area of the pons rather than to routine steroid administration.

Seizure States

Seizures occur in approximately 13% of patients who have not experienced attacks prior to surgery. In half of these patients, the seizure may be expected to occur within the first 24 hours. If a seizure state preexisted, attacks may be expected in 35% of patients immediately postoperatively (26). An even higher incidence of postoperative seizures is seen in epileptic patients, even with continuation of anticonvulsant therapy. Seizures are more likely to occur if the surgery involved the sensory or motor area of the cortical hemisphere. Prophylactic anticonvulsive therapy will reduce the incidence of postoperative seizures and possibly also the subsequent development of epilepsy and its associated complications of hypoxia and aspiration pneumonia. Diagnostic testing to evaluate postictal neurologic deficit, particularly if the seizure was not observed, can be avoided.

In the control or prevention of seizures, phenytoin is the drug of choice as it has minimal sedative effects. To obtain therapeutic levels, 18 mg/kg, diluted in normal saline (about 50 ml), is infused slowly at 50 mg/min. This dose will maintain a plasma level of about 10 μg/ml for 24 hours. During infusion of the drug, hypotension and arrhythmias can occur, and therefore arterial pressure and ECG should be monitored. Emergency therapy for status epilepticus includes sodium thiopental, succinylcholine, endotracheal intubation, and ventilatory support.

Fluid and Electrolyte Balance

The blood-brain barrier protects the central nervous system against excesses or deficits of sodium and water in isotonic proportions. This mechanism may fail if there is a major shift in osmolality of body fluids or after surgical intervention. Derangements of water, electrolytes, and acid-base homeostasis are manifest frequently as altered sensorium, disorientation, or focal or generalized manifestations. Thus postoperative neurologic assessment may be further complicated. Malfunction of the neurohypophyseal system may occur following subarachnoid hemorrhage, aneurysm surgery, skull fracture, craniofacial trauma, or surgery involving the pituitary and hypothalamic areas. Frank diabetes insipidus, temporary or permanent, may result. Although symptoms do not usually develop for 12 to 24 hours, onset of polyuria may be almost immediate. Diagnosis is confirmed by urine volume (1 to 2 L/hr), urine specific gravity (around 1.001), hemoconcentration, and improvement of symptoms by fluid restriction. Treatment involves accurate fluid intake-output charting, frequent serum electrolyte and osmolality determinations, and replacement of the urine loss with 2.5% to 5% dextrose in water (27). Although the syndrome is self-limiting, it is prudent to treat early with specific therapy (i.e., vasopressin) to prevent development of nonketotic, hyperglycemic coma (28). Suitable preparations include 1-desamino-8-D arginine vasopressin (DDAVP), which is given by intranasal insufflation in the conscious patient, or vasopressin tannate in oil, 5 units intramuscularly.

Other causes of polyuria include solute diuresis owing to diuretics, hyperglycemia, and mineralocorticoid deficiency.

Nerve Dysfunction

Intraoperative malpositioning may result in nerve palsies. Brachial plexus (29) and peroneal nerve (30) palsies have been described in patients after craniotomy in the sitting position. Hypoglossal nerve palsy following carotid endarterectomy may also occur (31). Treatment is supportive as these complications usually resolve spontaneously. Accurate recording of any deficits is essential.

Removal of cerebellopontine angle tumors may be associated with lower cranial nerve paresis (IX, X, XI, XII). Nerve dysfunction may also follow surgery in the fourth ventricle or for syringomyelia. Section of the glossopharyngeal nerve may cause temporary difficulty in swallowing. A nasogastric tube should be inserted to protect the airway. Tracheal intubation may also be indicated. Again, improvement frequently is seen after two to three days.

SPECIAL SITUATIONS

Elective Intracranial Surgery

Postoperative respiratory assessment of the elective neurosurgical patient is simpler than that of the general surgical patient because of fewer complicating factors. There is no diaphragmatic splinting from the pain of an upper abdominal incision. Need for postoperative narcotics is minimal, and the anesthetic technique should have avoided the use of large doses of muscle relaxants or deeper planes of anesthesia.

If the patient was awake and breathing adequately preoperatively, the same state should be realized before or shortly after admission to the recovery room.

Raised ICP is commonly associated with intracranial tumors. Chronic hyperventilatory patterns may occur, and, providing no hypoxia exists, require no therapy. Patients with tumors may present initially with seizures, during which they may aspirate gastric contents. The diagnosis of aspiration pneumonitis is established preoperatively by chest x-ray examination and arterial blood gas analysis.

Following tumor excision, the risk of hemorrhage or cerebral edema remains greatest over the next two days. Should deterioration in consciousness or lateralizing signs occur, an endotracheal tube must be reinserted and hyperventilation established until a definite diagnosis can be made. Close postoperative observation is especially important following needle biopsy without surgical decompression of tumors when development of edema in a patient who already has intracranial hypertension is hazardous. In these cases, the arterial monitor should be preserved into the recovery period to allow continuous blood pressure monitoring and frequent estimation of arterial blood gas values. Vigorous nursing, and respiratory care maneuvers should be kept to a minimum. Patients should be nursed in a 30-degree head-up position and encouraged to breathe deeply. These limitations do not apply as stringently to a patient who has just undergone intracranial aneurysm clipping. Pulmonary care may be given as necessary. Antiembolism stockings, usually removed during controlled hypotensive periods, should be reapplied postoperatively. Occasionally following the use of trimethaphan, return of neuromuscular function is delayed, and apnea or hypoventilation may continue for hours postoperatively (32). Early ambulation is encouraged to prevent pulmonary embolism and atelectasis.

Patients requiring extracranial-intracranial arterial bypass procedures or carotid endarterectomy have often suffered strokes or transient ischemic attacks. Pneumonic processes, aggravated by immobilization and frequently by heavy smoking, are common. Chronic lung disease with decreased arterial oxygen saturation and increased carbon dioxide retention, therefore, commonly occurs in these patients, although little problem may be encountered intraoperatively when ventilation is controlled and a high inspired oxygen concentration is administered. Serious difficulties may be encountered immediately postoperatively when respiratory support has been withdrawn and the depressant effects of anesthetic agents or narcotics combine with inspissated secretions to cause upper respiratory obstruction. Because of the importance of maintaining normal blood gases to preserve cerebral blood flow at optimal levels, careful intraoperative and postoperative monitoring and adjustment of inspired oxygen concentration and ventilatory parameters are imperative.

In patients who have vertebrobasilar ischemia, elevation of the hemidiaphragm on the side ipsilateral to the lesion has been described (33). Documentation of this finding preoperatively could avoid a diagnostic error in the postoperative period. More extensive pulmonary function tests are necessary to define the extent of the lung problems and to establish baseline values.

Hypophysectomy is often performed to alleviate pain in women who have metastatic breast cancer. These patients have often received repeated courses of radiotherapy to the primary lesion, and radiation pneumonitis may be present. Metastatic lung disease may also exist. Careful evaluation of all pulmonary function tests is essential to ascertain whether the patient has sufficient (or at least some) reserve to withstand an anesthetic procedure and a postoperative period of immobility. If a pleural effusion exists, this can be withdrawn immediately preoperatively, possibly after induction of anesthesia but before surgery.

A characteristic finding in acromegaly is macroglossia. While this abnormality may pose some problems during intubation, a more common complication is varying degrees of respiratory obstruction postoperatively. Insertion of an oral or nasal airway usually solves the difficulty.

Pediatric Neurosurgery

Hydrocephalic children in whom the shunt mechanism has become obstructed frequently have "runny" noses, and chest râles may be heard. Rarely can pathogenic organisms be cultured from chest secretions, and the children usually are not febrile. This particular respiratory problem does not appear to be aggravated by anesthesia or improved by the postoperative use of a croup tent.

Cardiac rate should be continuously monitored in babies in whom a ventriculojugular shunt has been placed. Development of tachycardia may herald the onset of congestive cardiac failure from fluid overload. Therapy involves disconnection of the shunt mechanism and possibly external drainage.

Respiratory obstruction causing stridor also occurs in babies who have hydrocephalus and myelomeningocele, and may be due to distortion and traction of the lower brain stem and cranial nerves (34).

Children with cerebral palsy have often had repeated surgical procedures and are bedridden, in negative nitrogen balance, and prone to chest infections and aspiration pneumonitis. Particular attention must be given postoperatively to assessment of pulmonary status and fluid and electrolyte balance.

A hypoplastic jaw and a large tongue are two characteristics of the Pierre-Robin syndrome that combine to cause both chronic and acute respiratory obstruction. Neurosurgeon and anesthesiologist should be aware of the extent of the pathology—particularly of the likelihood that the child's tongue will fall backward and cause complete airway obstruction if the trachea is extubated before the patient is fully recovered from anesthetic effects.

Spinal Column Surgery

The level of the spinal column at which the surgical intervention occurred determines the care necessary and the complications that may be seen in the recovery period.

Lumbar laminectomy usually is performed in otherwise healthy young individuals and seldom presents any particular problems in the recovery room. Because there is minimal danger of respiratory depression, pain may be treated as necessary with appropriate dosages of narcotics. Rarely, a hematoma, recognized by sudden alteration of lower limb function, may develop and compress the cord. Immediate reexploration is indicated. Patients who undergo thoracic laminectomy also are generally young and otherwise healthy. The usual indications for this procedure are tumor, arteriovenous malformations, or scoliosis. Tumors usually are meningiomas. The major postoperative considerations involve observation of neurologic signs for possible hematoma development in the tumor bed.

Arteriovenous malformations of the cord may be extensive and require prolonged microsurgical dissection. Blood loss and replacement are frequently one or more blood volumes. Postoperative requirements include careful attention to cardiovascular stability and clotting parameters, correction of hypothermia, and frequent neurologic examinations. If the surgical intervention was below the level of the sixth thoracic vertebra, there is little danger of respiratory depression by narcotic administration for pain relief.

Adolescent patients with idiopathic scoliosis who undergo Harrington rod instrumentation occasionally have respiratory impairment preoperatively. Severe postoperative pain and the need for large amounts of narcotics in the early recovery phase may further increase respiratory difficulties. Administration of a high inspired oxygen concentration must be routine. The major neurologic complication, although rare, is damage to the spinal cord causing paresis or paralysis. A method of testing to ensure intact lower motor neuron function is to elicit ankle clonus bilaterally.

Pathology of the upper thoracic and lower cervical spine levels (T5-C3) may be accompanied by any or all of the complications listed in Table 18.3. After elective fusions performed for spondylosis, observation must be made for new or increasing neurologic deficit. Respiratory embarrassment is usually not problematic. Extubation should be delayed until consciousness has returned, however, as the presence of a cervical collar makes emergency reintubation difficult.

Traumatic cervical spinal cord injuries are associated with many more complications. Intercostal muscle activity is lost if there is complete transection around the fifth cervical vertebra. The patient is then dependent on other means of increasing the chest wall excursion, such as contraction of the sternocleidomastoid muscle and other axillary muscles and diaphragmatic respiration. If the vital capacity was less than 1 liter preoperatively, assisted ventilation is necessary postoperatively to prevent respiratory failure. Occasionally, patients present with marginal respiratory function preoperatively. Following anterior cervical spine fusion, sufficient spasm and edema develop in surrounding tissues to precipitate ventilatory failure. The use of continuous positive pressure must be carefully evaluated as, by increasing the functional residual capacity, diaphragmatic action is hampered and vital capacity decreased.

Hypoxemia secondary to neuromuscular deficit is found in about 50% of patients with high cord injury (35). Tracheal suctioning or intermittent ventilatory assistance may result in reflex bradycardia or even cardiac arrest owing to a

Table 18.3 Conditions Complicating Injury at the Cervical and Upper Thoracic Levels of the Spinal Column

Complication	Sequelae
Respiratory distress	Pneumonia
	Atelectasis
	Decreased sensorium
Cardiovascular instability	Positional hypotension
	Bradycardia
Gastric distention	Regurgitation
	Aspiration
Sensory deficits	Pressure sores
	Sepsis
Bladder distention	Infection
Temperature impairment	Hypothermia
Psychiatric disturbances	Hallucinations
	Denial of injury

vagovagal reflex in sympathectomized patients (36). Mechanical irritation of vagal sensory receptors in the trachea during intubation may also cause bradycardia. The reflex is blocked by prior administration of atropine, 0.6 mg intravenously.

Postoperative pain is not usually severe, but if narcotics are required, careful monitoring of respiratory response, especially in the extubated patient, is essential.

A rare but very serious postoperative respiratory complication is development of sleep-induced apnea (Ondine's syndrome). Descending axons from cortical sites travel in the dorsolateral columns and autonomic pathways and are carried in tracts of the ventral quadrant. After severe high spinal cord injury or following bilateral percutaneous cervical cordotomy performed to relieve pain, there is interruption of ascending spinothalamic pathways transmitting pain sensation and also a block of involuntary respiratory tracts in the ventral quadrant of the cord. Although adequate respiratory exchange occurs in the waking state, patients cease to breathe during sleep (37). An apnea alarm must be attached and prophylactic intubation or tracheostomy performed. The disease is self-limiting over 1 to 2 weeks.

Cardiovascular instability caused by diminished sympathetic tone leads to hypotension and bradycardia. Intravascular volume replacement is often used intraoperatively to treat hypotension. Because of reduced sympathetic action, however, the vascular space already is expanded and pulmonary edema is a common complication (38). Direct measurement of pulmonary artery pressure through a Swan-Ganz catheter detects early rises in pulmonary diastolic pressure before edema develops (39). Central venous pressure changes become apparent only when cardiopulmonary decompensation is well advanced because of sympathetic hypofunction and increased venous capacitance (40). Bradycardia is treated with atropine, 0.6 mg intravenously, as necessary.

Gastric distention and loss or diminution of protective pharyngeal reflexes make aspiration an ever-present hazard. Temperature regulatory mechanisms are impaired and hypothermia delays recovery after general anesthesia. Care must be taken in rewarming as loss of sensation prevents self protection from burning.

Loss of sensory and proprioceptive input increases the incidence of hallucinations. Wherever possible, the patients should be kept in contact with auditory and visual stimuli such as are provided by a radio or window.

The late complication of autonomic hyperreflexia is seen in patients who have sustained transverse lesions in the area of the fifth thoracic vertebra. This syndrome consists of hypertension, bradycardia, headache, sweating, and flushing of the upper part of the body. The hypertension, which may be prolonged, may cause cardiac or intracerebral damage. The origin of this mass reflex probably is stimulation of autonomic afferent fibers no longer under higher control, which causes massive vasoconstriction below the level of the lesion with a simultaneous rise in plasma norepinephrine and dopamine β -hydroxylase. Hypersensitivity to catecholamines in adrenergic structures distal to the site of transection has been demonstrated. Because the afferent part of the baroreflex is still intact, hypertension causes bradycardia. The syndrome is precipitated by stimulation below the level of the injury—as, for example, following urologic intervention without anesthesia. General anesthesia or spinal or epidural blockade have been advocated to control autonomic hyperreflexia. Hypotensive agents and pentolinium (5-mg dose) also offer good control of blood pressure.

REFERENCES

1. Frost EAM: The physiopathology of respiration in neurosurgical patients. J Neurosurg 1979;50:699–714.
2. Teasdale G, Jennett B: Assessment of coma and impaired consciousness. A practical scale. Lancet 1974;2:81–83.
3. Marsh ML, Marshall LF, Shapiro HM: Neurosurgical intensive care. Anesthesiology 1977;47:149–163.
4. Hsu HO, Hickey RF: Effect of posture on functional residual capacity postoperatively. Anesthesiology 1976;44:520–521.
5. Merriman E, Bell W, Long DM: Surgical postoperative bleeding associated with aspirin ingestion. J Neurosurg 1979;50:682–684.
6. O'Reilly RA, Hamilton RD: Acquired hemophilia, meningioma, and diphenylhydantoin therapy. J Neurosurg 1980;53:600–605.
7. Thiagarajah S, Frost EAM, Singh T, et al.: Cardiac arrest associated with tension pneumocephalus. Anesthesiology 1982;56:73–75.
8. Arutinunov AI, Baron MA, Majorova NAJ: Experimental and clinical study of the development of spasm of the cerebral arteries related to subarachnoid hemorrhage. J Neurosurg 1970;32:617–625.
9. Mawk JR, Ausman JI, Erickson DL, et al.: Vasospasm following transcranial removal of large pituitary adenomas. J Neurosurg 1979;50:229–232.
10. Hekmatpanah J: The sequence of alterations in the vital signs during acute experimental increased intracranial pressure. J Neurosurg 1970;32:16–20.
11. Cooper PR, Ransohoff J: Limitations of intracranial pressure monitoring, in Morley TP (ed): Current controversies in neurosurgery. Philadelphia, WB Saunders, 1975, pp 658–666.
12. Lappas DG, Powell WM, Jr, Dagett WM: Cardiac dysfunction in the perioperative period: pathophysiology, diagnosis and treatment. Anesthesiology 1977;47:117–137.
13. Khambatta HJ, Stone JG, Khan E: Hypertension during anesthesia on discontinuation of sodium nitroprusside-induced hypotension. Anesthesiology 1979;51:127–130.
14. Azar I, Turndorf H: Severe hypertension and multiple atrial premature contractions following naloxone administration. Anesth Analg (Cleve) 1979;58:524–525.
15. Town JB, Bernhard VM: The relationship of postoperative hypertension to complications following carotid endarterectomy. Surgery 1980;88(4):575–580.
16. Frost EAM: Anesthetic management of cerebrovascular disease. Br J Anaesth 1981;53:745–756.
17. Lawson NW, Butler GH, Ray CT: Alkalosis and cardiac arrhythmias. Anesth Analg (Cleve) 1973;52(6):951–954.
18. Hersch C: Electrocardiographic changes in subarachnoid hemorrhage, meningitis, and intracranial space-occupying lesions. Br Heart J 1964;26:785–789.
19. Campkin VT, Turner JM: Postoperative and intensive care, in Campkin VT, Turner JM: Neurosurgical and intensive care. London and Boston, Butterworths, 1980, p 240.

20. Raine JM, Bishop JM: a-a difference in O_2 tension and physiologic dead space in normal man. J Appl Physiol 1963;18:284-288.

21. Sullivan SF, Patterson RW: Posthyperventilation hypoxia. Anesthesiology 1968;29:981-986.

22. Ellis SC, Bryan-Brown GW, Hyderally H: Massive swelling of the head and neck. Anesthesiology 1975;42:102-103.

23. McAllister R: Macroglossia a positional complication. Anesthesiology 1974;40:199-200.

24. Theodore J, Robin ED: Pathogenesis of neurogenic pulmonary edema. Lancet 1975;2:749-751.

25. Takaku A, Tanaka SM, Mori T, et al.: Postoperative complications in 1000 cases of intracranial aneurysms. Surg Neurol 1979;12(2):137-144.

26. Matthew E, Sherwin AL, Weiner K, et al.: Seizures following intracranial surgery: Incidence in the first postoperative week. Can J Neurol Sci 1980;7:285-290.

27. Shucart WA, Jackson I: Management of diabetes insipidus in neurosurgical patients. J Neurosurg 1976;44:65-71.

28. Freidenberg GR, Kosnik EJ, Sotos JF: Hyperglycemic coma after suprasellar surgery. N Engl J Med 1980;303:863-865.

29. Saady A: Brachial plexus palsy after anesthesia in the sitting position. Anaesthesia 1981;36:194-195.

30. Keyrhah MM, Rosenberg H: Bilateral footdrop after craniotomy in the sitting position. Anesthesiology 1979;51:163-164.

31. Bageant TE, Tondini D, Lysons D: Bilateral hypoglossal nerve palsy following a second carotid endarterectomy. Anesthesiology 1975;43:595-596.

32. Miller R, Tausk HCC: Prolonged anesthesia associated with hypotension induced by trimethaphan. Anesthesiol Rev 1974;5:36-37.

33. Korczyn AD: Respiratory and cardiac abnormalities in brain stem ischaemia. J Neurol Neurosurg Psychiatry 1975;38:187-190.

34. Bell WE, McCormack WF: Increased intracranial pressure in children. Major problems in clinical pediatrics, Philadelphia, WB Saunders, 1972, vol 8, p 70.

35. Sinha RP, Ducker TB, Perot PL Jr: Arterial oxygenation. Findings and its significance in central nervous system trauma patients. JAMA 1973;224:1258-1260.

36. Welply NC, Mathias CJ, Frankel HL: Circulatory reflexes in tetraplegics during artificial ventilation and general anaesthesia. Paraplegia 1975;13:172-182.

37. Severinghaus JW, Mitchell RA: Ondine's curse—failure of respiratory center automaticity while awake. Clin Res 1962;10:122.

38. Wolman L: The disturbance of circulation in traumatic paraplegia in acute and late states: A pathologic study. Paraplegia 1965;2:213-226.

39. Troll GF, Dohrmann GJ: Anaesthesia of the spinal cord-injured patient. Cardiovascular problems and their management. Paraplegia 1975;13:162-171.

40. Civetta JM, Gabel JC: Flow directed pulmonary artery catheterization in surgical patients. Indications and modifications of technic. Ann Surg 1972;176:753-756.

CHAPTER 19

Chronic Supportive Care
Elizabeth A.M. Frost

Failure of extracranial organ systems adversely affects the injured brain. Such complications as hypoxemia, hypercapnia, hypotension, severe hypertension, coagulation abnormalities, hyperthemia, sepsis, pain, renal failure, and malnutrition can all add to the initial insult, increase cerebral edema and ischemia, and result in further neurologic deficit (1). Thus, chronic supportive care must be aimed at systematic monitoring and support of each body system.

MONITORING

Physiologic monitoring of the neurosurgical patient with multisystem disease requires a team approach that combines the efforts of physicians of different specialties, specially trained nursing personnel, and ancillary medical staff (including social worker, dietician, respiratory therapist, and physical therapist) in an intensive care setting. Mandatory intensive care monitoring of neurosurgical patients should include continuous electrocardiographic (ECG) monitoring, intracranial pressure (ICP), and cerebral perfusion pressure (CPP) as indicated, frequent recording of arterial blood pressure (preferably with an indwelling cannula), respiratory rate, temperature, heart rate, and fluid input-output charts. Use of an alarmed apnea monitor is valuable in comatose patients and in those with high spinal cord injuries who are not artificially ventilated. Hypotensive patients require central venous pressure monitoring. If there is coexistent cardiopulmonary disease, pulmonary artery catheterization is highly desirable. Hourly recording of coma scale level affords an indication of improvement or deterioration in the disease process.

Complete monitoring necessitates immediate access to a laboratory that can rapidly perform blood gas measurements, osmolalities, directly measured spectrophotometric oxygen saturation levels, colloid osmotic pressure, hemoglobin and hematocrit, serum electrolyte concentrations, arterial lactate, and toxicologic levels.

RESPIRATORY SYSTEM

Although the need to reestablish and maintain respiration in the resuscitation of comatose patients has been realized for many centuries, it is only relatively recently that the importance of continued ventilatory support to improve neurologic outcome has been stressed. In 1901, Walter B. Cannon noted, "Severe concussion frequently causes paralysis of the respiratory center; respiration entirely ceases although the heart continues beating for some time. If artificial respiration is persisted in, the respiratory center may wholly recover its function" (2).

Some 70 years later, studies of large groups of patients showed that ventilation controlled to maintain arterial carbon dioxide ($PaCO_2$) levels between 25 and 30 mm Hg not only increased actual numbers of survivors but also improved the quality of life (3,4).

Respiratory Patterns

Plum and Posner (5) theorized that specific abnormalities of respiratory rate and pattern may be correlated with the level of the central nervous system lesion. These associations are not precise, however, and more severe aberrations of respiratory pattern probably are associated with larger or bilateral lesions (6,7). There does appear to be a clear link between ataxic breathing and medullary damage (8). Trend recording of respiratory patterns is important as they may indicate the extension or improvement of a cerebral lesion.

In general, five respiratory patterns have been described in association with intracranial injury (Table 19.1). Eupneic breathing indicates a small, unilateral lesion and the patient is usually awake. Cheyne-Stokes respiration or periodic breathing is associated with destructive bilateral lesions in the cerebral hemispheres or basal ganglia and may indicate an expanding supratentorial mass such as a hematoma. This pattern has been related to an increased ventilatory response to carbon dioxide, which causes hyperventilation and hypocapnia. Apnea supervenes, which permits carbon dioxide to reaccumulate until the threshold is exceeded and the cycle repeats itself. Prognosis is grave (mortality over 50%) (9). Cheyne-Stokes variant has been used to describe phasic variations in depth of respiration without apneic periods. Under these circumstances, the lesions are usually unilateral, the patients can be aroused, and the prognosis is good. Central neurogenic hyperventilation may be due to a pontine lesion, systemic hypoxia, or metabolic acidosis. Sustained hyperventilation results in a high pH and a shift of the oxygen dissociation curve to the left, which makes oxygen less available to the tissues. Moreover, the intense work of breathing increases the metabolic rate and aggravates the hypoxic state. Transtentorial herniation frequently occurs and the patients usually die. Management requires tracheal intubation and ventilation adjustment.

Adding extra "dead space" is often not effective as the respiratory centers are not responsive to decreased $PaCO_2$ levels. Neuromuscular blocking agents will control ventilation but obscure neurologic assessment, which is unacceptable to many neurosurgeons. Small doses of narcotics (fentanyl, 25 to 50 μg, demerol, 25 mg) decrease ventilatory drive sufficiently to allow ventilator control. This action can be rapidly reversed by narcotic antagonists should neurologic deterioration be suspected. Prognosis again is poor.

Table 19.1 Abnormal Respiratory Patterns following Head Injury

Respiratory Pattern		Level of Consciousness	Lesion	Prognosis
Normal	⌇	Awake	Small Unilateral	Good
Cheyne-Stokes	⌇	Comatose	Large Bilateral Supratentorial	Poor
Cheyne-Stokes variant	⌇	Arousable	Large Unilateral	Good
Central neurogenic hyperventilation	⌇	Comatose	Large Bilateral Partial	Poor
Apneustic	⌇	Comatose	Large Bilateral Midpontine	Poor
Ataxic	⌇	Comatose	Large Bilateral Posterior fossa	Fatal
Hiccough	⌇	Arousable	Variable High medulla Low pontine	Fair

SOURCE: From Frost EAM: Head trauma and the anesthesiologist. Weekly Anesthesiology Update, vol 2, lesson 10, 1979. (Reprinted by permission.)

Apneustic breathing is a rare abnormality usually associated with pontine infarction owing to basilar artery occlusion. It may also be related to drug intoxication, hypoglycemia, or anemia. Ataxic respiration is seen with rapidly expanding lesions in the posterior fossa that have caused medullary compression. The outcome usually is fatal.

Causes of Respiratory Insufficiency

If one or more of the criteria listed in Table 19.2 are met, a diagnosis of respiratory insufficiency may be made. Causes, which may be central or peripheral, are listed in Table 19.3. Intracranial pathology may cause hypoxia because of raised ICP or interruption of nervous pathways around the brain stem. Head-injured patients must be considered to be hypoxic until proven otherwise. In our series of 86 patients (10), 60% had an increased ventilatory shunt with no apparent cause other than the head injury. If the ventilation/perfusion abnormality was less than 9%, most patients did well; but if it exceeded 15%, most patients, especially those over the age of 55, died.

Drug overdose frequently is associated with head injury. Should coma be protracted in a narcotic addict, symptoms of withdrawal, including mucosal hyperemia and further upper airway obstruction, may develop. Diagnosis depends on history, serum alcohol or barbiturate levels, and response to small intravenous injections of naloxone hydrochloride.

Aspiration is associated with sudden deceleration or diving injuries, loss of protective reflexes from medullary or pontine lesions, decreased gastric motility owing to increased ICP, inept attempts at artificial ventilation or endotracheal intubation, seizure states, or stroke.

Pulmonary edema may result from increased ICP. Theodore and Robin (11) have theorized that neurogenic pulmonary edema (NPE) is caused by a centrally mediated massive sympathetic discharge caused by hypothalamic damage, which shunts blood from the higher-resistance systemic circulation into the lower-

Table 19.2   Criteria for Diagnosing Respiratory Insufficiency

Respiratory rate	>40/minute; <10/minute
Respiratory pattern	Irregular
Vital capacity	<15 ml/kg
Maximal inspiratory force	<−20 cm H_2O
V_D/V_T	>0.5
Percentage pulmonary shunt	>15%
$PaCO_2$	>45 mm Hg; <25 mm Hg

SOURCE: From Frost EAM: Head trauma and the anesthesiologist. Weekly Anesthesiology Update, vol 2, lesson 10, 1979. (Reprinted by permission.)

NOTE: If one or more of these criteria exists, respiratory insufficiency is present and plans should be made immediately for intubation and assisted ventilation.

Table 19.3 Causes of Respiratory Insufficiency Associated with Head Injury

Central Causes	Peripheral Causes
Head trauma	Aspiration
Drug overdose	Pulmonary edema
	Disseminated intravascular coagulopathies
	Fat embolism
	Chest trauma
	Iatrogenic causes

resistance pulmonary circulation. Pulmonary edema may also be caused by fluid overload, especially in elderly patients with cardiac disease who may also have received rapid, large-volume infusions of mannitol. Newborns similarly tolerate injection of osmotic agents very poorly, and pulmonary edema may be readily caused by a 10 to 15 ml infusion. In cases of NPE, the edema is related to altered capillary permeability and the protein content approaches that of plasma. Pulmonary edema related to simple increases in pulmonary capillary pressure is associated with fluid of relatively low protein content.

Fat embolism is a complication of long-bone fractures in 10% to 25% of multiple trauma victims. In large autopsy studies, 80% to 100% of patients who die of various causes after fractures of long bones have fat emboli in their lungs (12). Szabo, Lerenyi, and Kocsar (13) studied the mean number of fat emboli in patients dying less than one week after fracture and found 1017 ± 257/cu mm, compared with 89 ± 24/cu mm in patients expiring after more than one week. It therefore appears that not only does fat embolism occur more commonly than was previously thought, but it mainly occurs early after trauma (14). No matter where the fat globules arise, their embolization to the lungs causes major insult. Clinical diagnosis is made by the presence of tachycardia, ECG changes, fever, and progressive signs of respiratory distress (tachypnea, râles, bronchospasm, increasing hypoxemia). Therapy is both supportive and specific. Ventilation and cardiac output must be maintained. Evidence suggests that hypotension aggravates the situation greatly. Steroids, narcotics, aminophylline, alcohol, and (by some workers) heparin have all been advocated, as has the use of the membrane heart-lung machine. Low-molecular-weight dextran is also used to prevent aggregation of blood components and sludging.

Impact against the steering column and windshield frequently causes both chest and head trauma. Pneumothorax or flail chest is treated by endotracheal intubation, respiratory support, and chest tube placement as indicated.

Among the iatrogenic causes of respiratory problems in neurosurgical patients are pneumothorax after rib fracture in overly vigorous resuscitation attempts or injudicious subclavian vein cannulation (15). Angiography by way of carotid puncture may cause hematoma formation and tracheal displacement. Malposition, obstruction, and kinking of endotracheal tubes are not infrequent occurrences.

Respiratory Therapy

Early recognition and prompt, aggressive treatment of respiratory dysfunction are of major importance in supportive neurologic care. Respiration should be assisted or controlled in all patients exhibiting abnormal respiratory patterns or if one or more criteria listed in Table 19.2 are met. It is far preferable to intubate the trachea of a patient who has marginal difficulty and remove the endotracheal tube shortly than to risk a delay that may have catastrophic consequences.

As already noted, controlled hyperventilation to maintain $PaCO_2$ between 25 and 30 mm Hg appears to have beneficial effects in most patients (3). Small increases of $PaCO_2$, even within a range considered at the lower limits of normal, may cause large increases in ICP, especially in patients with reduced intracranial compliance (Fig. 19.1). There has been controversy as to the value of continued hyperventilation as a means of reducing ICP. As cerebrospinal fluid pH readjusts to a higher level, vascular responses to carbon dioxide may be lost, but this is far from simply realized clinically. Lack of response to hyperventilation generally correlates with poor condition. If clinical condition improves, response to carbon dioxide may return at any time (16). Thus no general rules can be made. Each patient must be tested by observing changes in ICP with hyperventilation throughout the intensive care period.

Intermittent positive-pressure breathing (IPPB), once widely used preoperatively and postoperatively for prophylaxis and for maintenance of adequate ventilation in comatose and semicomatose patients, will result in significantly decreased oxygen levels on discontinuing therapy (17,18). In patients with reduced

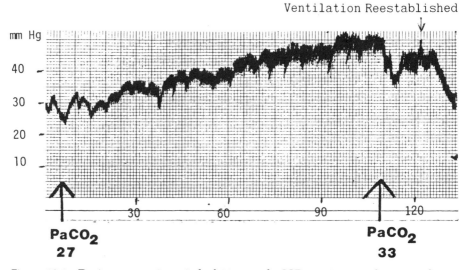

Figure 19.1 During an apneic period of 90 seconds, ICP may increase by 100% despite maintenance of hypocapnia. (From Frost EAM: Head trauma and the anesthesiologist. Weekly Anesthesiologist Update, vol 2, lesson 10, 1979. Reprinted by permission.)

intracranial compliance, IPPB may cause a sudden rise in ICP and even initiate prolonged plateau waves (Fig. 19.2).

Positive end-expiratory pressure (PEEP) added to the expiratory limb during controlled ventilation increases $PaCO_2$ and decreases the alveolar-arterial oxygen tension gradient (A-aDO_2) by increasing mean airway pressure, which in turn augments functional residual capacity (19). In most instances, it is then possible to reduce a high, potentially toxic inspired oxygen concentration while maintaining an adequate arterial oxygen tension (PaO_2). Normally, 5 cm H_2O PEEP is added initially and, depending on stability of vital signs and neurologic status, may be increased by increments of 2 cm H_2O. Levels of PEEP above 20 cm H_2O (super PEEP) are usually not employed, as not only is little improvement seen in oxygenation but the danger of pulmonary bullous rupture is significantly increased.

The advantages and disadvantages of the use of PEEP in patients with intracranial hypertension have been debated (20,21). If this respiratory modality is indicated because of lung disease and reduced pulmonary compliance, ICP does not increase if the patient is nursed in a 30-degree head-up position and cardiovascular stability is maintained. Marked improvement in intracranial compliance may be seen if hypoxemia can be corrected (Fig. 19.3).

Continuous positive airway pressure (CPAP) in a spontaneously breathing patient will provide higher mean airway pressures and therefore increase lung volumes (especially functional residual capacity). This is now the mode of choice for assisted ventilation to improve oxygenation in neurosurgical patients who are breathing spontaneously but either have some lung dysfunction already or

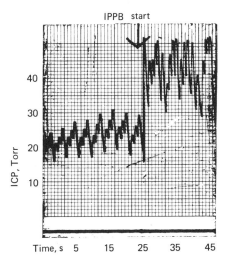

Figure 19.2 Sudden addition of IPPB to a spontaneously breathing patient may increase ICP.

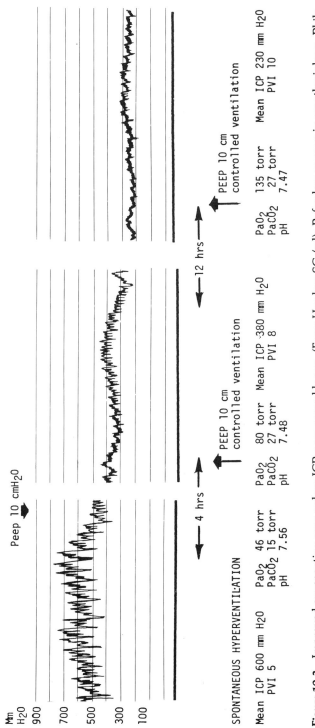

Figure 19.3 Improved oxygenation may reduce ICP over several hours. (From Hershey SG (ed): Refresher courses in anesthesiology. Philadelphia, Lippincott, 1979. Reprinted by permission.)

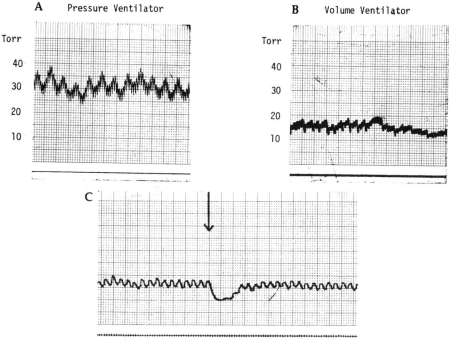

A   Pressure Ventilator

B   Volume Ventilator

Little increase in ICP is seen with the addition of CPAP

Figure. 19.4 (A,B) Decrease in ICP may be seen by controlling respiration with a volume rather than a pressure cycled ventilator. (C) Little increase in ICP is seen with the addition of CPAP.

have the potential for developing atelectasis. Little if any change is observed in ICP (Fig. 19.4). As with PEEP, however, CPAP should also be increased gradually with attention to vital signs, ICP, and neurologic status. CPAP usually causes a prompt rise in PaO_2 and a reduction in pulmonary shunting (22).

Intermittent mandatory ventilation (IMV) was introduced as a valuable technique to wean patients from ventilatory support (23). It is a useful means of augmenting spontaneous ventilation rather than providing total support, and is often used in conjunction with CPAP (24). Graded withdrawal of mechanical support and slow decrease in IMV rate permit normalization of pulmonary function and improvement of oxygenation.

Prolonged controlled ventilation (i.e., for weeks to months) may be essential in the supportive care of the patient with Guillain-Barré syndrome or the patient who is apneic from brain-stem compression or ischemia. A technique of reduction of intracranial hypertension by total muscle paralysis and controlled ventilation is not often employed now. Not only may ICP be reduced usually more readily by other pharmacologic or surgical means, but complete body paralysis renders neurologic testing impossible.

Negative-pressure modes of ventilation are also seldom employed because they are generally less effective in improving hypoxic states, the chance of brain-stem herniation is increased if ICP is increased, and there is an added danger of air embolism if the vasculature is opened.

Pulmonary toilet is an important maneuver for any patient who requires mechanical ventilation. Suctioning is not only a noxious stimulus, however, but $PaCO_2$ also rises when ventilation is discontinued. A dramatic rise in ICP may occur. This effect is even more apparent if PEEP is required. The abrupt termination of PEEP augments venous return, which increases heart rate and systemic blood pressure. Moreover, fluid layered within alveoli accumulates, thus causing apparently more secretions, and suctioning may have to be prolonged. Intravenous and topical lidocaine, sodium thiopental, succinylcholine, Althesin, and prior hyperventilation have all been used in patients with raised ICP to avoid further elevations during catheterization and clearing of airways. Above all, suctioning should be accomplished quickly and as aseptically as possible.

If prolonged ventilation is indicated, decision may be made to perform tracheostomy although endotracheal intubation can usually be safely tolerated for 2 to 3 weeks or longer. Tracheostomy increases the comfort for the patient, decreases the chances of trauma to the mouth, lips, and larynx, and facilitates suctioning, oral nutrition, and mobilization (25). Complications usually are due to ischemia of the tracheal mucosa and can be reduced by using a high-compliance, low-pressure cuff (maintaining a cuff-to-tracheal wall pressure less than 30 cm H_2O). Hypotension can cause tracheal ischemia without increments in cuff pressure since cuff to tracheal pressures are then increased. The incidence of tracheal stenosis following tracheostomy has been variously reported as 2% to 20% (26,27). Symptomatic tracheal stenosis (reduction in tracheal diameter of 75%) usually occurs in four to nine weeks and presents as wheezing, exertional dyspnea, and stridor (28). Other complications of tracheostomy include tracheoesophageal fistula, hemorrhage from erosion of the innominate artery, or local tracheal erosion and perforation (28).

CARDIOVASCULAR SYSTEM

Maintenance of adequate CPP, between 70 and 110 mm Hg, is essential to avoid brain ischemia. Head injuries are often associated with considerable blood loss. Control of intracranial hypertension usually includes administration of diuretic agents. Thus patients are often hypovolemic, hypokalemic, and hypochloremic. A satisfactory hematocrit must be assured in the later stages of head injury. The oxygen-carrying capacity of the blood is directly proportional to the amount of hemoglobin contained. If the hemoglobin is reduced to 10 gm/dl, 95% oxygen saturation would be equivalent only to 63% oxygen saturation if the hemoglobin were a normal 15 mg/dl.

Hypovolemia frequently is unrecognzied initially, especially if right atrial and pulmonary capillary wedge pressures and cardiac output are not measured, because patients are usually young with healthy vasculature that compensates well (29). Moreover, intracranial damage often causes arterial hypertension. A multi-institutional study reported a 20% incidence of systolic blood pressure higher than 160 mm Hg after severe head injury (30). As ICP may also be elevated, this factor should be taken into consideration before antihypertensive medication is started. Although autoregulation is often preserved despite severe intracranial injury, this protective effect may be lost at any time during recovery (31). Therefore, an increase in arterial blood pressure can cause brain edema in injured cerebral tissue, a further increase in ICP, and reduction of CPP (32). Individual therapy therefore requires precarious balancing between the risk of ischemia caused by too low CPP and the danger of edema from systemic arterial hypertension. Moderate hypertension (150/90 to 180/100) does not require therapy and probably is beneficial to the injured brain; however, levels above 180/100 to 200/115 are hazardous to the brain and heart. Although sodium nitroprusside and nitroglycerin are excellent and immediate-acting hypotensive agents, they should be avoided when the skull and dura are closed because as cerebral vascular resistance decreases, ICP may increase by 200% to 300%. Verapamil appears to cause less alteration of intracranial dynamics and be an effective antihypertensive drug.

Although cardiac arrhythmias should never automatically be attributed to primary neurosurgical disease, many abnormal patterns may be associated with intracranial pathology. Almost any cardiac arrhythmias may be seen with ischemia of the brain stem and compromise of the vasomotor centers. Raised ICP characteristically causes hypertension and bradycardia, but multifocal ventricular premature contractions and even ventricular tachycardia can occur. Therapy requires prompt reduction of ICP (hyperventilation, diuretics, barbiturates, or narcotics). Sudden reduction of raised ICP such as occurs when cerebrospinal fluid is withdrawn may also cause traction on the brain stem and bizarre ventricular arrhythmias or extreme bradycardia. Therapy may require replacement of some of the removed fluid.

Blood in the subarachnoid space (as after rupture of an aneurysm) occasionally causes ECG changes resembling myocardial infarction (ST-segment elevation and T-wave inversion) (33). The reasons for the occurrence of these ECG abnormalities are not clear, but high serum catecholamine levels causing myocardial necrosis, central autonomic stimulation or ischemia from vascular spasm at cortical, hypothalamic, or brain-stem levels have been cited (34). Because curative therapy of cardiac abnormalities associated with intracranial pathology is limited, it behooves the physician to seek other causes for the arrhythmias that may be more easily treated. Such problems as cardiopulmonary disease, certain iatrogenic metabolic abnormalities, hypoxia, hypoglycemia, acidosis, alkalosis, hypokalemia, fluid overload, digitalis toxicity, and abnormalities of magnesium, phosphorus, or calcium metabolism, are all common complications in the intensive care unit.

INTRAVASCULAR COAGULOPATHIES

As discussed more fully in Chapter 16, disseminated intravascular coagulopathy (DIC) may occur in the head-injured patient or postoperatively because of the release of brain tissue thromboplastin (35). Disseminated intravascular coagulation (DIC) probably is a much more common complication of intracranial damage than was originally believed, since the brain is a very rich source of thromboplastin (12). Eeles and Sevitt (36) postulated that it is caused by a breakdown in the homeostatic mechanism between hypercoagulability and thrombolysis, which occurs during the first 48 to 72 hours after trauma when large amounts of tissue thromboplastin are released. Microthrombosis and accelerated clotting may be due to vascular entry or activation of thromboplastic substances released in large amounts from the injured brain (36). It is also a complication in the patient with multiple trauma and acute respiratory distress syndrome, sepsis, shock, fat embolism, burns, or following transfusion of O-negative or type-specific blood in emergency situations. Some minor variations in clotting parameters (such as abnormalities of partial thromboplastin time) may be detected in approximately 60% to 70% of patients seen in the emergency room after major head injury (37). Hypofibrinogenemia, thrombocytopenia, elevation of fibrin degradation products, and a prolonged thrombin time that does not "correct" with the addition of normal plasma to the test specimen may also be found. The peripheral blood smear contains schistocytes. Progress of the disease in the early stages may be halted by administration of fresh-frozen plasma. Rarely, severe hemorrhage occurs and requires platelet transfusion (10 to 12 units), fresh-frozen plasma (in increments of 4 units). Cryoprecipitate (three to six bags) is indicated if the serum fibrinogen level is less than 60 mg/dl. Only fresh blood should be transfused, as older blood is deficient in coagulation factor activity.

Serial coagulation studies should always be performed to assess the effects of the blood component therapy. The role of heparin is controversial (38). One unit of heparin may be added to each milliliter of blood component transfused (plasma, platelet concentrates, cryoprecipitate, blood) to activate plasma antithrombin III present in these components. Antithrombin III is deficient in patients with DIC and is necessary for inhibition of coagulation factor consumption. Transfusion of concentrates containing factors III, VII, IX, and X (Proplex, Conyne) should be avoided since their use has been associated with exacerbation of DIC, probably owing to the presence of procoagulants in the preparations. The incidence of hepatitis approximates 50% in patients who receive Proflex or Conyme. In the more severe form of this syndrome, the patient characteristically is brought to the hospital comatose. Initial respiratory assessment and arterial blood gas determinations are normal, as is the hematocrit level. At operation, severe tissue destruction and generalized brain edema usually are observed. Postoperatively the hematocrit falls dramatically, often to 10% to 15%, without overt signs of bleeding. Transfusion at this time rarely raises the hematocrit significantly, although a small but significant increase may be seen after an infusion of low-molecular-weight dextran. Copious blood-stained secretions are obtained from the pulmonary tree. Prothrombin times, fibrinogen and split product levels, and partial thromboplastin times are all abnormal. Arterial blood gases and respiratory changes noted subsequently are typical of the respiratory distress syndrome. If the patient survives longer than 24 to 48 hours, acute renal failure may develop. If the patient can be supported, the disease is apparently self-limiting and reverses after about three to four days.

Coagulopathies caused by hemorrhagic loss of coagulation factors may develop in patients who receive multiple transfusions, especially if the blood is not warmed. Hemorrhage continues after correction of the surgical lesion because banked blood is deficient in coagulation factor activity and platelets. Correction can usually be made by transfusing fresh-frozen plasma in 4-unit increments. If the platelet count is less than $60,000/mm^3$, the patient should be given 10 to 12 units of platelet concentrate.

RENAL SYSTEM

Acute renal failure remains one of the most dreaded complications in any intensive care setting (39). Common causes of this complication in neurosurgical patients include infection, sepsis and hypotension. Many drugs used in the intensive care unit are nephrotoxic (e.g., some broad-spectrum antibiotics), and appropriate dose reduction in the presence of established renal insufficiency may prevent complete renal failure.

Overzealous use of diuretics in the treatment of intracranial hypertension causes dehydration and hyperosmolality and may precipitate renal shutdown. Induction of barbiturate coma may further reduce renal perfusion and compromise function. Most renal complications may be avoided by aseptic technique, fluid input-output balancing, hemodynamic stabilization, maintenance of serum osmolality at less than 320 mOsm/L, and monitoring of serum electrolytes and creatinine.

FLUID MAINTENANCE

Disturbances in fluid and electrolyte balance are not uncommon following intracranial procedures. Approximately 3 liters per day of a balanced electrolyte solution such as 5% dextrose in lactated Ringer's solution to which 40 mEq/L of K^+ is added is required for the average 70 kg man. Adjustments must be made daily according to output, vital signs and electrolyte determinations. Two abnormalities that occur in neurosurgical patients require special mention: the syndrome of inappropriate antidiurectic hormone secretion (SIADH) and diabetes insipidus (DI).

Syndrome of Inappropriate ADH Secretion

ADH secretion is associated with central nervous system trauma, brain tumors, encephalitis, pneumonia, pulmonary tuberculosis, or bronchogenic carcinoma. Diagnosis depends on: (a) hyponatremia and renal salt wasting, (b) elevated urine osmolality in excess of plasma, (c) presence of normal renal and adrenal function, and (d) normal blood pressure with absence of dehydration (40). As the serum sodium concentration falls below 120 mEq/L, confusion and delirium develop and the clinical picture progresses to seizures, tremors, aphasia, hyporeflexia or hyperreflexia, hemiparesis, generalized rigidity, and even coma. An acute decrease of the serum sodium below 125 mEq/L can cause irreversible brain damage within 12 hours, and therefore restoration of sodium levels must be rapid. The amount of sodium necessary to correct the deficit can be estimated according to the equation:

$$(\text{Desired Na}^+ \text{ conc.} - \text{initial Na}^+ \text{ conc.}) \times 0.5 \text{ (body weight in kg)} = \text{mEq Na}^+ \text{ required}$$

The sodium may be given as 3% to 5% saline, which should be preceded by an intravenous injection of furosemide, 20 mg, to promote negative water balance. Fluid restriction is required (41). The use of hypertonic saline to restore the serum sodium concentration to the normal range (136 to 145 mEq/L) has been associated with acute pulmonary edema and intracerebral hemorrhage. Careful monitoring is essential.

Diabetes Insipidus

DI caused by the decreased pituitary secretion of antidiuretic hormone results in polyuria and progressive dehydration and hypernatremia. It is associated with severe, diffuse head injury or intracranial surgery involving the pituitary-hypothalamic axis (42). Diagnosis is made when polyuria (excretion of more than 200 to 300 ml of urine per hour not associated with diuretic administration or fluid challenge), hypernatremia, and low urine osmolality and specific gravity develop. Muscle irritability, seizures, and loss of consciousness occur at serum sodium levels over 160 mEq/L. Urinary output should be replaced hourly with hypotonic solutions such as 5% dextrose/0.25% sodium chloride with additional potassium chloride. If the polyuria exceeds 150 ml/hr the patient should be given pitressin tannate in oil, 5 units subcutaneously (43). Control can usually be obtained within five to ten minutes in cooperative patients by nasal insufflation of 1-desamino-8-D-arginine vasopressin (DDAVP).

The syndrome usually resolves spontaneously in 72 hours. If the condition has been diagnosed only after severe hypernatremia has developed, however, too rapid correction of the hyperosmolar state should be avoided as fatal cases of cerebral edema or irreversible brain damage may develop if total correction is made within 24 hours. As symptoms of water intoxication can occur with large volume replacement at high serum sodium concentrations, half of the calculated free water deficit should be replaced within the first 24 hours, and the remainder over the next one to days (in addition to each day's normal maintenance fluid requirements). The decreased total body water as a result of dehydration can be estimated as follows:

$$\text{Actual body water} = \frac{\text{(desired serum Na}^+)}{\text{(actual serum Na}^+)} \times \frac{\text{normal total body water}}{\text{(60\% of body wt. in kg)}}$$

If very large volumes of dextrose solution are given, nonketotic hyperglycemic coma may develop. This syndrome is characterized by sudden loss of consciousness, focal tonic-clonic seizures, and even respiratory arrest. Laboratory values show serum sodium levels in the range of 145 to 155 mEq/L, serum osmolality of 350 to 380 mOsm/kg, and serum glucose around 1000 mg/dl (44). Therapy includes pitressin, withdrawal of dextrose-containing solutions, and small doses of regular insulin. As the neurologic sequelae of this complication of the therapy of diabetes insipidus are so severe, prevention by using 2.5% dextrose solutions and early administration of pitressin are warranted.

TEMPERATURE CONTROL

Hyperthermia is likely to develop in patients with head injuries, especially if lesions involve the brain stem or hypothalamic region or if there is blood in the ventricular system. Children are particularly susceptible to this complication. Pyrexia, not related to infection, may occur in 15% of patients (30). As any increase in temperature increases oxygen consumption and cerebral metabolic rate, therapy including alcohol sponging, acetaminophen suppositories, ice packs, and antishivering infusions (thorazine, phenergan, demerol) should be rigorously instituted. Aspirin, which may alter coagulability, is probably best avoided if possible (45).

The patient's temperature may be a critical factor in interpreting blood gas result, although this has been disputed. More sophisticated blood gas analyzers allow for temperature adjustment, but older machines give results based on a normal temperature of 37°C. In an otherwise healthy patient with fever related to the head injury, the measured $PaCO_2$ should be corrected upward or downward by 4.4% for each degree Celsius increase or decrease in the patient's temperature. The PaO_2 is corrected by a factor of 7.2% per degree Celsius, and the pH is reduced or increased by 0.015 unit for each degree Celsius rise or fall from 37°C. Oxygen saturation is based on measured pH and PaO_2 at 37°C and is also affected by temperature, which gives a series of oxygen/hemoglobin dissociation curves. (Other factors that shift the oxygen/hemoglobin dissociation curves in critically ill patients include 2,3-diphosphoglycerate, anemia, serum phosphorus, and acid-base imbalance.)

Hypothermia has long been advocated as a means of preserving the injured brain. The cerebral metabolic rate decreases approximately 7% per degree Celsius drop (46). The ideal level of hypothermia or the time at which the therapy should be started or terminated has not been determined, however (see Chapter 20).

SEIZURES

Without anticonvulsant therapy, approximately 12% of patients develop seizures within the first week following intracranial surgery. A preoperative history of seizures increases this incidence to 35% (47). In both of these groups there is a greatly increased risk of experiencing recurrent seizures, especially if surgery involved the sensory or motor area of the cortical hemispheres.

Poorly controlled epilepsy was cited as the second most commonly occurring intracranial factor contributing to death after head injury (48). In fact, status epilepticus was regarded as the sole cause of death in two children, mildly injured but who were shown to have extensive hypoxic and ischemic damage at autopsy.

Reluctance to give sedative drugs after neurosurgical procedures may delay appropriate therapy and expose the patient not only to hypoxic risk but also to the complications of aspiration. In the control or prevention of seizures, especially in the conscious patient who does not require ventilatory support, phenytoin is probably the drug of choice since it has minimal sedative effect as compared to phenobarbital. To obtain therapeutic levels rapidly, 18 mg/kg diluted in approximately 50 ml of normal saline is infused at 50 mg/min. This dose will maintain a plasma level of approximately 10μg/ml for 24 hours (49). During infusion of the drug, especially in elderly patients, hypotension and arrhythmias can occur and therefore careful monitoring is essential. Emergency therapy for status epilepticus includes sodium thiopental, succinylcholine, endotracheal intubation, and ventilatory support. Phenobarbital is still frequently the drug of choice of many neurosurgeons and it certainly is not contraindicated in patients who require prolonged respiratory assistance; however, the drug (like diazepam) is long acting and has accumulative properties. It is important to consider drug effect in assessing the level of consciousness. Successful weaning of a patient from ventilatory support may be hampered by even small doses of phenobarbital (30 mg four times per day).

SEPSIS

Infection in neurosurgical patients in an intensive care setting is due to the initial injury, invasive monitoring, and antibiotic and steroid therapy. The most frequent infecting organisms are *Staphylococcus epidermis*, *Staphylococcus aureus*, *Escherichia coli*, β -hemolytic streptococci, and *Klebsiella*. Viruses, fungi, protozoa, and rickettsia may also be involved. A large series of intravascular catheterizations showed an 8% infection rate. Arterial cannulation carried a 4% infection rate with no significant difference between the arterial sites used. Central venous catheterization had a 20% infection rate if insertion was in the antecubital vein, 12% in the internal jugular vein, and 7% in the subclavian vein. The researchers reported a 29% infection rate for pulmonary artery catheters passed through the internal jugular site compared to 7% via subclavian routes (50). Catheter infection and related septicemia may be minimized by good dressing technique of the insertion site and frequent changing of the tubing, stopcocks, transducers, and domes (51).

Although the pathophysiology of septicemia is poorly understood, the clinical, metabolic, and hemodynamic consequences of sepsis have been identified. An increased metabolic rate occurs with reduction of oxygen consumption owing to perfusion failure and cellular block to oxygen uptake. The hemodynamic consequences occur in two phases. The first is an early hyperdynamic phase with normal or decreased total peripheral vascular resistance, low arteriovenous oxygen content differences, and low oxygen consumption rate. Arterial blood gases reflect a mixed respiratory alkalosis and mild metabolic acidosis with some hypoxemia. Successful outcome can be expected with aggressive therapy including oxygenation, hydration, appropriate antibiotic therapy, correction of nutritional deficiencies, and placement, as indicated, of a transvenous inferior vena cava umbrella to prevent the development of thromboembolic phenomena. Thrombolytic therapy with steptokinase or urokinase or transvenous catheter extraction of pulmonary emboli may also be necessary (52). Heparinization, although advantageous in many surgical patients, probably is not indicated in most neurosurgical patients. The second phase of sepsis is a late hypodynamic situation with hypotension, low cardiac output, increased peripheral vascular resistance, tachycardia, arteriovenous differences of less than 3.5%, and increased oxygen consumption rate. This phase is characterized by shock, decreased consciousness, oliguria, and severe metabolic acidosis. Treatment requires aggressive volume replacement, maximal dose of broad-spectrum antibiotics, and intravenous steroids (methylprednisolone, 30 mg/kg every four hours for 48 hours). Optimum oxygen-carrying capacity is maintained by blood transfusion. Inotropic vasoactive drugs such as dopamine or dobutamine may also be used for hypotension in the hypodynamic phase after volume expansion is achieved, although mortality, which occurs in about 80% of cases, is rarely prevented.

NUTRITIONAL SUPPORT

Trauma, prolonged surgery, starvation, and anesthesia are all detrimental to good nutritional status. The stress of trauma and infection is characterized by accelerated tissue catabolism, hypermetabolism, and erosion of essential protein. A further complicating factor that increases the effects of starvation and aggravates a negative nitrogen balance is diarrhea, which has been reported to have a 41% incidence after severe intracranial injury. A significant increase in the incidence of diarrhea is associated with nasogastric feeding and cimetidine but not with antibiotic therapy (53). Therapy includes gastric instillation of lomotil, replacement of cimetidine with magnesium/aluminum antacid, and a slow rate of nasogastric feeding. Nutritional support aims to diminish losses of vital protein by reducing the components of injury and sepsis and the appropriate provision of adequate calories and nutrients to replenish body composition. Although the nutritional requirements of critically ill patients differ quantitatively, they are qualitatively the same as in normal subjects. Minerals, vitamins, trace elements, and all required nutrients must be provided daily (54). Approximately 3600 calories must be delivered to an average 70-kg patient.

Hyperalimentation should start immediately through a central venous or through the "dietary lumen" of the triple-lumen pulmonary artery presure catheter.

A recommended parenteral formula combines a mixture of 500 ml of 50% dextrose in water with 500 ml of amino acids such as Aminosyn 7% or Freeamine II. To each liter of this solution should be added sodium chloride, 40 to 60 mEq, potassium chloride, 10 to 20 mEq, potassium phosphate, 1 to 20 mEq, magnesium sulfate, 8 mEq, folic acid, 1.0 mg, and multivitamins. Calcium chloride or gluconate may also be added to the solution, or may be infused through a peripheral vein in an initial dose of 1 gm/24 hr. Vitamin supplementation must include vitamin B_{12}, 100 g intramuscularly weekly, and vitamin K (Aquamephyton), 15 mg intramuscularly weekly. Trace elements should be added to the hyperalimentation solution. When indicated, 2.5 to 4.0 mg of zinc should be given to the stable adult patient daily. An additional 2.0 mg daily is recommended in acute catabolic state. Copper supplementation is suggested at the rate of 0.5 to 1.5 mg/day, chromium at 10 to 15 g/day and manganese at 0.15 to 0.8 mg/day.

Parenteral hyperalimentation should be started at a rate of 50 ml/hr for eight hours, increased to 100 ml/hr for eight hours if no hyperglycemia has occurred, and subsequently increased to a plateau of 125 ml/hr, at which time a nitrogen balance study is performed. Should a negative balance persist, a higher concentration of amino acids such as Aminosyn, 8.5% or 10%, may be substituted.

Complications of total parenteral nutrition include hyperglycemia, hypokalemia, hypophosphatemia, hypomagnesemia, and catheter-related sepsis. Fatty acid deficiency may occur with long-term parenteral hyperalimentation and can be prevented by infusing Intralipid, 500 ml three times weekly via a peripheral vein. Positive nitrogen balance is impaired in neurosurgical patients receiving steroids as these drugs exhibit catabolic effects and inhibit protein synthesis, facilitate amino acid release from skeletal muscle, and reduce the renal tubular reabsorption of amino acids. Total avoidance of steroids or early tapering is recommended.

PAIN MEDICATION

Pain is rarely a major complaint following craniotomy. In patients who have suffered severe craniofacial trauma, however, sedation may be essential to prevent ICP elevation or occurrence of plateau waves. If narcotics are used, careful monitoring of respiratory and neurologic status is essential. If doubt as to the integrity of either of these systems exists, an endotracheal tube should be placed and ventilation assisted.

REFERENCES

1. Bleyaert A, Safar P, Nemoto E, et al.: Effect of postcirculatory arrest life support on neurological recovery in monkeys. Crit Care Med 1980;8:153.
2. Cannon WB: Cerebral pressure following trauma. Am J Physiol 1901;VI,II;91–121.

3. Crockard HA, Coppel DL, Morrow WFK: Evaluation of hyperventilation in treatment of head injuries. Br Med J 1973;4:634–640.

4. Gordon E: The management of acute head injuries, in Gordon E (ed): A basis and practice of neuroanesthesia. New York, Excerpta Medica, 1975, pp 249–265.

5. Plum F, Posner JB: The diagnosis of stupor and coma, ed 3. Philadelphia, FA Davis, 1980.

6. Jennett S, Ashbridge K, North JB: Post hyperventilation apnoea in patient with brain damage. J Neurol Neurosurg Psychiatry 1974;37:288–296.

7. Lee MC, Klassen AC, Heaney LM, et al.: Respiratory rate and pattern disturbances in acute brain stem infarction. Stroke 1976;7:382–385.

8. North JB, Jennett S: Abnormal breathing patterns associated with acute brain damage. Arch Neurol 1974;31:338–344.

9. Rout MW, Lane DJ, Wollner L: Prognosis in acute cerebral vascular accidents in relation to respiratory patterns and blood gas tension. Br Med J 1971;3:7–9.

10. Frost EAM, Arancibia CU, Shulman K: Pulmonary shunt as a prognostic indicator in head injury. J Neurosurg 1979;50:768–772.

11. Theodore J, Robin ED: Pathogenesis of neurogenic pulmonary oedema. Lancet 1975; 2:749–751.

12. Herndon JM: The syndrome of fat embolism. South Med J 1975;68:1577–1584.

13. Szabo G, Lerenyi P, Kocsar L: Fat embolism: Fat absorption from the site of injury. Surgery 1963;54:756–760.

14. Swank RL, Sugger GS: Fat embolism: A clinical and experimental study of mechanisms involved. Surg Gynecol Obstet 1954;98:641–652.

15. Shapira M, Stern WZ, Frost EAM: Complications and pitfalls of subclavian vein cannulation. An update. Conn Med 1977;41(3):140–143.

16. Marshall WJ, Jackson JLF, Langfitt TW: Brain swelling caused by trauma and arterial hypertension hemodynamic aspects. Arch Neurol 1969;21:545–553.

17. Fouts JB, Brashear RE: Intermittent positive-pressure breathing. A critical appraisal. Postgrad Med 1976;59:103–107.

18. Wright FG Jr, Foley MF, Downs JB, et al.: Hypoxemia and hypocarbia following intermittent positive pressure breathing. Anesth Analg (Cleve) 1976;55:555–559.

19. Kumar A, Falke KJ, Geffin B, et al.: Continuous positive pressure ventilation in acute respiratory failure. Effects on hemodynamics and lung function. N Engl J Med 1970;283:1430–1436.

20. Aidinis SJ, Shapiro HM, Van Horn K: Effects of positive end-expiratory pressure (PEEP) on intracranial pressure, sagittal sinus and cerebral perfusion pressures during experimental intracranial hypertension in cats, abstract 58. Proceedings of the American Association of Neurologic Surgeons. 43rd Annual Meeting, April 1975, p 94.

21. Frost EAM. Effects of positive end-expiratory pressure on intracranial pressure and compliance in brain injured patients. J Neurosurg 1977;47:195–200.

22. Garg GP, Hill GE: The use of spontaneous continuous positive airway pressure (CPAP) for reduction of intrapulmonary shunting in adults with acute respiratory failure. Can Anaesth Soc J 1975;22:284–290.

23. Downs JB, Klein EF Jr, Desaultels D, et al.: Intermittent mandatory ventilation: A new approach to weaning patients from mechanical ventilators. Chest 1973;64:331–335.

24. Downs JB, Perkins HM, Modell JH: Intermittent mandatory ventilation: An evaluation. Arch Surg 1974;109:519–523.

25. Aass A: Complications of tracheostomy and long term intubation. Acta Anaesthesiol Scand 1975;19:127–133.

26. Harley H: Laryngotracheal obstruction complicating tracheostomy or endotracheal intubation with assisted respiration. Thorax 1971;26:493–533.

27. Andrews M, Pearson F: Incidence and pathogenesis of tracheal injury following cuffed tube tracheostomy with assisted ventilation. Ann Surg 1971;173:249–263.

28. Dane T, King E: A prospective study of complications after tracheostomy for assisted ventilation. Chest 1975;67:398–404.

29. Lassen NA: Control of cerebral circulation in health and disease. Circ Res 1974;34: 749–759.

30. Jennett B, Teasdale G, Galbraith S, et al.: Severe head injuries in three countries. J Neurol Neurosurg Psychiatry 1977;40:3291–3298.

31. Enevoldsen EM, Jensen FT: Autoregulation and CO_2 responses of cerebral blood flow in patients with acute severe head injury. J Neurosurg 1978;48:689–703.

32. Marshall WJ, Jackson JLF, Langfitt TW: Brain swelling caused by trauma and arterial hypertension: Hemodynamic aspects. Arch Neurol 1969;21:545–553.

33. Hersch C: Electrocardiographic changes in subarachnoid hemorrhage, meningitis and intracranial space occupying lesions. Br Heart J 1964;26:785–793.

34. Hackenberry LE, Miner ME, Rea GL, et al.: Biochemical evidence of myocardial injury after severe head trauma. Crit Care Med 1982;10:641–644.

35. Astrup T: Assay and content of tissue thromboplastin in different organs. Thrombosis et Diathesis Haemorrhagica 1965;14:401–416.

36. Eeles G, Sevitt S: Coagulation and fibrinolysis in injured patients. J Clin Pathol 1964;17:1–13.

37. Kaufman HH, Olson JD, Makela ME, et al.: Disseminated intravascular coagulation and fibrinolysis in head injury, abstracted. American Association Neurologic Surgeons, Boston, 1981, pp 131–132.

38. Gosch HH, Kindt GW: Head injury. Some current concepts in management. Univ Mich Med Center 1971;37:274–279.

39. Sladen RN: Renal function and critical care. Sem Anesth 1982;1(4):323–332.

40. Deutsch S, Goldberg M, Dripps RD: Postoperative hyponatremia with the inappropriate release of antidiuretic hormone. Anesthesiology 1966;27:250–256.

41 Bartter RC, Schwartz WB: The syndrome of ADH. Am J Med 1967;42:790.

42. Griffin JM, Hartley JH, Crow RW, et al.: Diabetes insipidus caused by craniofacial trauma. J Trauma 1976;16(12):979–984.

43. Shucart WA, Jackson I: Management of diabetes insipidus in neurosurgical patients. J Neurosurg 1976;44:65–71.

44. Freidenberg GF, Kosnik EJ, Sotos JF: Hyperglycemic coma after suprasellar surgery. N Engl J Med 1980;303:863–865.

45. Merriman E, Bell W, Long DM: Surgical postoperative bleeding associated with aspirin injection. J Neurosurg 1979;50:682–684.

46. Rose J, Valtonen S, Jennett B: Avoidable factors contributing to death after head injury. Br Med J 1977;2:615–617.

47. Matthew E, Sherwin AL, Welner SA, et al.: Seizures following intracranial surgery: Incidence in the first postoperative week. Can J Neurol Sci 1980;7(4):285–290.

48. Reivich M: Regulation of cerebral circulation. Clin Neurosurg 1968;16:378–418.

49. Cranford RE, Leppik IE, Patrick B, et al.: Intravenous phenytoin: Clinical and pharmacokinetic aspects. Neurology (NY) 1978;28:874–880.

50. Pinilla JC, Ross DF, Martin T, et al.: Study of the incidence of intravascular catheter infection and associated septicemia in critically ill patients. Crit Care Med 1983;11 (1):21–25.

51. Cleri DG, Corrado ML, Seligman SJ: Quantitative culture of intravenous catheters and other intravascular inserts. J Infect Dis 1980;141:781.

52. Frost EAM. The intensive care of the neurosurgical patient. Sem Anesth 1982;1(4):L 340–353.

53. Kelly TWJ, Patrick MR, Hellman KM: Study of diarrhea in critically ill patients. Crit Care Med 1983;11(1):7–9.

54. Hyman AI, Rodriguez J, Weissman C: Nutritional support of the critically ill patient. Sem Anesth 1982;1(4):354–361.

CHAPTER 20

Therapy following Major Brain Insult
Elizabeth A.M. Frost

The earliest attempts at resuscitation were directed at rescue breathing and reestablishment of respiration. It was not until the 1960s that resuscitation manuals began to emphasize the importance of both cardiac and pulmonary supportive efforts. In recent years, increased understanding of the pathophysiology of brain hypoxia and ischemia has combined with laboratory findings to indicate that improved neurologic outcome after major cerebral insult is feasible. A successful outcome to cardiopulmonary cerebral resuscitation (CPCR) depends not only on the speed and quality of emergency help but also on long-term intensive care and support of the brain.

Differentiation should be made between brain protection, which implies treatment initiated before or during the insult, and resuscitation, which signifies implementation of therapy following injury. From all practical points of view, brain resuscitation is usually the only realistic clinical approach.

IS THERE A RATIONALE FOR INITIATING RESUSCITATION?

Global ischemia causes depletion of oxygen stores within a few seconds and depletion of glucose and glycogen stores with cessation of low-energy-producing anaerobic metabolism within four minutes. High-energy phosphate charges (adenosine triphosphate, ATP) are exhausted, which stops all energy-dependent reactions within five minutes (1). As it is rarely possible to start resuscitation within this time frame, the feasibility of starting therapy at all might be questioned. If the circulation is not halted completely, however, it is known that cells may be neurophysiologically silent for relatively long periods of decreased perfusion. Duration of viability and critical flow level (probably between 12 and 20 ml/100 gm/min) are unknown, but return of normal function may occur with restoration of flow. The concept of "idling neurons" indicates the need for early and aggressive therapy (2).

Were the primary target of ischemia the cerebral vasculature, then attempted restoration of cerebral flow would be ineffective. In animal models, initial damage has been shown to be neuronal, and situations of no reflow rarely develop even after 30 minutes of hypoxia-ischemia (3). Much experimental work has indicated that increased cerebral damage can occur during periods of reflow. No histologic changes within the brain substance have been seen when studies were performed immediately after clinical death (4). Vacuolization of neurons may be demonstrated after five minutes of ischemia, but these changes are reversible (5). Irreversible histologic changes may be delayed for several minutes to hours after circulation has been reestablished, indicating that permanent tissue damage is a late phenomenon (4).

The cerebral circulation undergoes several changes during resuscitation. Restoration of flow is accompanied by a relatively short hyperperfusion period (6). Cerebral blood flow then decreases and is followed by a prolonged course of hypoperfusion (7). Reperfusion occurs nonhomogeneously in the brain because of variable resistance caused by degrees of vasospasm or intravascular clotting or tissue edema. The situation of no or poor reflow can be improved by sufficiently high cerebral perfusion pressure (8).

It has been shown experimentally that drugs that decrease vasospasm and influence pial vessels improve low-flow states (4). Amelioration of neurologic deficit has also been demonstrated in the laboratory following administration of several drugs, hypertension induced by intraarterial dextan 40, hemodilution, and heparinization if these therapies are initiated during resuscitation. These beneficial actions would further support the hypothesis that a significant portion of the neurologic deficit ultimately sustained can occur after restoration of circulation and would endorse a program of aggressive or perhaps even prophylactic therapeutic intervention.

Finally, the interaction of the body systems means that the failure of extracranial organ function must influence the brain. Hypotension, hypoxemia, hyperthermia, pain, "stress," sepsis, and renal failure all add to the initial insult and intensify the neurologic deficit. Thus the need for total-body supportive care during cerebral resuscitation is underscored.

CLINICAL INTERPRETATION OF LABORATORY DATA

There are many problems in transferring information from brain resuscitation laboratory experiments to the clinical setting. Although global brain anoxia of more than five minutes generally causes permanent brain damage or death in human beings, in animal models this threshold may be considerably higher, averaging 15 minutes and perhaps even as high as 60 minutes (9). Great difficulty exists in creating comparable tests of neurologic function, particularly those pertaining to higher cerebral function such as speech and memory. There are many species differences in collateral circulation and metabolism. Lesion production in the animal model can be standardized and controlled, which is not possible clinically. The quality and timing of postinjury intensive care are very variable between patients and animals.

Perhaps the biggest difference between the two situations is that of age, as laboratory models are usually young with healthy, intact organ systems. It has been shown that the human infant brain has reduced sensitivity to ischemic-anoxic insults, probably owing to incomplete maturation of central nervous system neurotransmitters (10). Ischemic catastrophies in humans afflict mainly the older segment of the population, and cerebral metabolic studies in older subjects have shown significant decrease in glucose consumption relative to oxygen utilization (11). In normally aged rats, however, a moderate reduction in cerebral glucose utilization was found only up to the twelfth month of life with a less progressive decline thereafter (12). In addition, older people often have not only generalized vascular disease but multiple organ system dysfunction.

PATHOPHYSIOLOGY

Integrity of neuronal function depends on tight coupling between cerebral blood flow and metabolism, which is achieved by neurotransmitters. Failure of any one of these three factors—blood flow, metabolism, or neurotransmitter function—either during the initial brain insult or at some later time, will cause cerebral damage.

Pathologic processes that cause neuronal cell dysfunction are severe hypoxia or ischemia (reduction in cerebral blood flow to less than 50% of control), repeated or sustained epileptic seizures, which pathologically enhance neuronal activity, and hypoglycemia with loss of spontaneous or evoked electrical activity (13). Clinical conditions that may cause brain injury are shown in Figure 20.1. The entire brain may become ischemic as during cardiac arrest. Focal ischemia anoxia results in stroke. Cerebral blood flow may be decreased by vasospasm globally (e.g., head injury) or regionally (e.g., after rupture of an intracranial aneurysm). Respiratory failure caused by overwhelming lung disease or muscle paralysis causes cerebral hypoxemia but flow is usually maintained, at least initially. Carbon monoxide poisoning results in hypoxemia-anemia. Encephalopathies may be caused by many factors including hypertension, fluid and electrolyte imbalance, diabetes, drug or plant intoxication, and several infectious organisms. The pathology is one of cerebral edema with intracranial hypertension and decreased cerebral blood flow and cerebral perfusion pressure. Head injury may result in diffuse edema and decreased blood flow or involve a space-occupying lesion such as epidural, subarachnoid, or intracerebral clot formation. Several types of ischemic insults occur, such as the complete ischemia that may occur after cardiac arrest or incomplete ischemia of the type found in hypotensive situations (shock). Temporary ischemia results if cardiac arrest has been followed by successful resuscitation. Permanent ischemia causes regional or global cerebral infarction.

Although the mechanisms of cell damage in the brain are largely unknown, three factors appear to be of particular importance in modulating the extent and degree of neuronal damage. First, the severity of lactic acidosis during ischemia

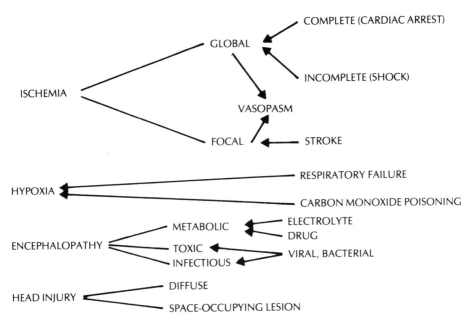

Figure 20.1 The pathology of brain injury may be due to several distinct disease processes.

and hypoxia profoundly affects the cellular disruption incurred (14). Second, cell damage matures and perhaps even develops during a recirculation, preoxygenation period (15). Third, one of the major factors causing cell damage is altered calcium ion homeostasis with release of Ca^{2+} from intracellular sequestration sites and influx from extracellular fluids. Although an increase in the activity of free intracellular Ca^{2+} can activate many catabolic reactions, including those leading to protein degradation, research has mainly involved reactions triggered by lipolysis, which causes breakdown of membrane-bound phospholipids and accumulation of arachidonic acid and other free fatty acids (13).

Possible mechanisms leading to cellular damage following brain insult are outlined in Figure 20.2. Following a major cerebral insult from ischemia, hypoxia, or hypoglycemia, energy failure leads to an influx of Ca^{2+} and Na^+ into cells. As Ca^{2+} sequestering mechanisms are also disrupted, intracellular Ca^{2+} activity increases. An increase in extracellular K^+ causes vasospasm, which enhances the ischemic process. Accumulation of Ca^{2+} activates phospholipases with a rapid accumulation of free fatty acids, especially arachidonic acid. As K^+ and Cl^- are taken up by glial cells, with further oxygen consumption there is edematous expansion of astrocytic processes and compromise of substrate availability. Oxidative metabolism of arachidonic acid during the recirculation, preoxygenation period along cyclo-oxygenase and lipoxygenase pathways forms prostaglandin-like substances and leukotrienes, respectively (13). The former may cause

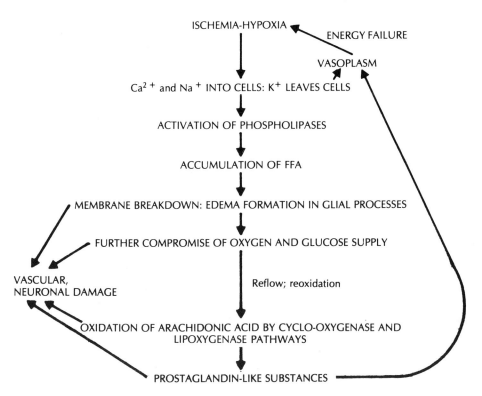

Figure 20.2   Possible mechanisms of cellular damage following brain insult in animals.

vascular and neuronal damage by formation of vasoconstrictory thromboxanes and by inactivation of prostacyclin synthetase and deprivation of an endogenous vasodilator. Other free radicals generated by the oxidative conversion of arachidonic acid may be even more important in causing neuronal damage.

AIMS IN BRAIN RESUSCITATION

Although the chain of events shown in Figure 20.2 has been demonstrated experimentally, it is only speculative that the same holds true in the clinical setting. It would seem reasonable, however, to direct therapy at points that might impede the rate of deterioration. The principal areas where treatment may be undertaken with currently available therapeutic modalities are shown in Table 20.1

Intracranial Homeostasis

Reestablishment of intracranial homeostasis may be achieved by pursuing several routes.

Table 20.1 Principal Therapeutic Maneuvers to Ensure Optimal Brain Resuscitation

Intracranial Homeostasis	Extracranial Homeostasis
Intracranial pressure	Intravascular flow
Cerebral blood flow	Stasis
Edema	Vascular volume
CSF production	Systemic pressure
CSF absorption	Optimal ventilation
Metabolic rate	$PaCO_2$ 25–35 mm Hg
Oxygen	PaO_2 100 mm Hg
Glucose	Normothermia
Free radicals	Fluid and electrolyte balance
Free fatty acids (arachidonic, stearic)	Renal function
Peroxidation	Hyperalimentation
Brain amine	
Drug scavenging (phospholipase :	
lipoxygenase blockade)	
Cellular Ca^{2+} entry	
Ca^{2+} channel blockade	
Seizure activity	
Sympathetic activity	
Central sympathectomy	
Anticholinesterase activity	

Reduction of Intracranial Hypertension

The association of severe intracranial hypertension and poor outcome after cerebral injury has been shown by several investigators (16). The pathophysiology and therapy of intracranial pressure (ICP) have been fully covered in Chapters 3 and 11. Suffice it to say that reduction of ICP may be effected by decreasing the volume of any one of the three intracranial compartments: cerebral blood volume, brain substance, or cerebrospinal fluid. The therapeutic maneuvers available to accomplish these effects include hyperventilation; administration of diuretics and several other specific drugs such as barbiturates, etomidate, and Althesin; cerebrospinal fluid drainage; and operative intervention as indicated.

Decrease in Metabolic Rate

During reflow periods, inappropriate neurotransmitter function may cause abnormal metabolic patterns. If metabolic utilization of oxygen and glucose can be decreased during the time of low perfusion and until recoupling between flow and metabolism is established, neuronal survival may be improved.

Hypothermia has been induced to increase the ischemic threshold by decreasing the cerebral metabolic rate of oxygen utilization ($CMRO_2$) (17). Significant decrease in infarct size was obtained in a dog model of stroke (18) and in a monkey model of global ischemia (19), but subsequent animal studies did not confirm these findings (20,21). Although clinical trials of hypothermia have been disappointing, there is a theoretical advantage, and perhaps a redefining of optimal degree and duration of cooling and method of rewarming is warranted (22).

Several drugs can depress $CMRO_2$. In clinical doses, barbiturates can produce up to a 55% reduction (23). Barbiturates may also offer protection by decreasing the increase in extracellular K^+ (24), reducing cerebral edema (25), scavenging free radicals (26), and diverting blood to ischemic areas by a vasoconstrictive mechanism (27). Controversy continues to exist over the therapeutic effectiveness of iatrogenic barbiturate coma. A clinical review of high-dose barbiturate therapy showed improved survival in patients with head injury and encephalitis, although the ultimate outcome was not altered in patients with stroke or near drowning (28). Continuous pentobarbital therapy was found to be highly successful in the treatment of Reye-Johnson syndrome (29). A more recent report found that barbiturates may not always be necessary to control the intracranial hypertension that characterizes this disease and, even when used, may not always be successful (30). We have failed to demonstrate improvement in outcome in adult patients with intracranial hypertension refractory to other forms of therapy (31). Thus, although barbiturates may protect the brain in models of incomplete ischemia by a metabolic depressant effect, clinical usefulness after global anoxia is less certain. Standardization of dosages and agents, duration of therapy, and indications for use are all required for critical appraisal of the technique; however, as the complications of inducing barbiturate coma are considerable and all the vigilant monitoring necessitated by the anesthetic state are required, present results do not justify uncritical adoption of this therapy.

Depression of $CMRO_2$ is also seen with inhalation anesthetic agents, especially isoflurane (32). γ-Hydroxybutyrate, first described as a useful neuroanesthetic agent, can reduce the cerebral metabolic rate of glucose by 68% in gray matter compared to the 40% reduction seen during surgical anesthesia with barbiturates (33). The drug appears to exert a specific action in high-flow areas with little variation in cerebral lactate levels. Rat studies have shown complete recovery after enormous decreases in metabolic rates.

Free Radical Scavenging

Free radicals are compounds with a single electron in an outer ring, which reacts autocatalytically with neighboring molecules. All aerobic cells form free radicals. Although molecular damage may be caused to DNA, protein, and lipids, the polyunsaturated fatty acids of phospholipids seem to be especially vulnerable to peroxidative attack. Following an ischemic episode there is a sudden, enormous increase in tissue concentrations of free fatty acids, especially arachidonic acid (34).

Much debate has continued over the importance of the concept of free radical damage in ischemia (13). Many drugs, however, including thiopental, promethazine, phenytoin, α-tocopherol, ascorbic acid, mannitol, and glutathione, have all been shown to scavenge free radicals (13). Only some of these agents have been associated with improved neuronal survival, and thus it appears that the protective effects of drugs are not related only to their efficacy in scavenging radicals. In addition, maximal attenuation of the release of free fatty acids with barbiturates occurs at a dose no higher, and perhaps less, than that required for surgical anesthesia. Thus an isoelectric electroencephalogram may not be a valid basis for guiding therapy in cerebral insults, or pharmacologic amelioration of ischemic brain injury may not occur primarily through inhibition of oxidative metabolism (35).

Brain biogenic amines have also been hypothesized as extending the injury process during or after ischemia. Laboratory depletion of these amines can be achieved by a combination of α-methyl p-tyrosine and p-chlorophenylalanine, which causes a decrease in the accumulation of oleic and palmitic acids during an ischemic insult (35). Palmitic, oleic, and stearic acid accumulation may also be reduced by calcium channel blockade (35). Clinically, high-dose narcotics have been used as a means of depressing central amine effect.

Glucocorticoids have been used to induce the synthesis of an intracellular phospholipase inhibitor (15). Other useful drugs might be agents that could inhibit cyclo-oxygenase and lipoxygenase pathways and thus prevent the formation of prostaglandins and other polyunsaturated hydroxy fatty acids. Nevertheless, reproducible neurologic improvement remains to be demonstrated after decrease of free fatty acid concentrations.

Cellular Ca²⁺ Entry Blockade

As abnormal Ca^{2+} entry on reperfusion has been shown to be instrumental in many of the adverse reactions leading to neuronal damage, therapeutic intervention with drugs that block the Ca^{2+} channel would seem to be warranted. Flunarizine, lidoflavine, and etomidate have all demonstrated improved neuronal survival after a hypoxic insult in laboratory animals (36), although reproducible neurologic improvement remains to be confirmed clinically. It would, however, appear that much research should be conducted along these lines.

Decreased Seizure Activity

Hypoxic states may trigger seizure patterns causing intracranial hypertension and enormous increases in brain metabolism (37). A poorly controlled seizure state was listed as the second most common intracranial factor contributing to death in a review of 116 patients with head injury who were admitted conscious but subsequently died (38). Thus, control of this complication is indicated to improve cerebral viability.

The primary action of phenytoin sodium, a commonly employed antiseizure drug, appears to be in the motor cortex where, by promoting sodium efflux from neurons and preventing the rise in intracellular sodium that occurs during hypoxia, it appears to increase the seizure threshold (39). Phenytoin was shown to decrease significantly the neurologic deficit in an animal model of global ischemia (40). It has also been shown to decrease $CMRO_2$ by 40% to 60%, decrease cerebral lactate production, and increase cerebral glucose, probably by depressing insulin secretion (41). Cerebral blood flow is also increased, which is a basic pharmacologic difference between this agent and barbiturates (42). Phenytoin inhibits the $Na^+ + K^+$-ATPase system. Reduction in K^+CSF accumulation occurs in a dose-related manner and is greater than that seen with hypothermia or pentobarbital (43).

Althesin, a steroid combination, is a fast-acting, rapidly excreted intravenous anesthetic agent that decreases ICP without rebound effect. The drug also has marked anticonvulsant properties and has been used successfully in the treatment of refractory status epilepticus (44).

Alteration of Neurotransmitter Function

During reperfusion after a hypoxic insult, neurotransmitter dysfunction may cause further damage. Laboratory evidence has suggested that appropriate pharmacologic manipulation may reverse some of these adverse actions.

Phenoxybenzamine, a long-acting adrenergic blocking agent, can produce and maintain "chemical sympathectomy" and prevent or reverse cerebral vasopasm and improve cerebral blood flow (45). Cerebral edema may also be reduced (46). A preliminary clinical study showed decrease in vasopasm in patients with subarachnoid hemorrhage when phenoxybenzamine was given by intracarotid injection immediately following the injury (47)—an improvement that could not be duplicated in the dog model (48).

Physostigmine, a reversible anticholinesterase drug, effectively increases the concentration of acetylcholine at cholinergic transmission sites and acts as a parasympathomimetic agent. Increased survival time, irrespective of the age of the animal, was demonstrated in the hypoxic rat model following administration of the drug (49).

As the role of anticholinesterase agonist and antagonists is evaluated further, increased therapeutic use of these drugs during cerebral resuscitation is quite possible.

Extracranial Homeostasis

A more detailed review of general supportive care of the brain-injured patient is included in Chapter 16. A few factors, however, are of particular relevance to cardiopulmonary cerebral resuscitation and to brain preservation.

Intravascular Flow

Mean arterial pressure should be maintained at normal or possibly slightly increased levels. In a nonautoregulating situation, such as occurs following hypoxic damage, systemic blood pressure and cerebral blood flow are directly related, and flow becomes a passive function of blood pressure. Sympathomimetically induced hypertension has been shown to improve cerebral blood flow and evoked potentials in baboons after a global ischemic insult (50). Following aneurysm clipping, neurosurgical practice has advocated increasing systemic blood pressure and using blood transfusion to decrease vasopasm (51); however, review of the literature establishes neither an optimal level of induced hypertension nor appropriate duration of therapy. It would appear that with the return of autoregulation, systemic blood pressure variation should no longer exert a critical effect. Indeed, rising blood pressure might increase the incidence and amount of cerebral edema or have other adverse effects such as pulmonary edema (52).

Increase in cerebral blood flow would seem advisable because cellular aggregates form in areas of low flow or hypoperfusion and increase blood viscosity and erythrocyte deformability. Measures to increase flow include hemodilution with low-molecular-weight dextran. Heparin has anticoagulant, antiinflammatory, and antihistaminic properties and may be used to prevent both intracerebral thrombosis and systemic lesions (53,54). In a cat model of global ischemia, heparin given either before or after injury modified the response to anoxia and resulted in a more rapid return of evoked response activity. Neurologic deficit was significantly less than in the control group (55). The heparin was, however, given either immediately before or within a few minutes of the ischemic injury, and thus clinical application of this technique would appear to be extremely limited at this time.

Aspirin has also been used to decrease aggregation of platelets and to block their adhesion to connective tissue or collagen fibers, possibly because of inhibition of collagen glucosyl transferase in platelet membranes (56). It is useful therapy in patients with transient ischemic attacks awaiting surgery for extracranial-intracranial vascular bypass.

Optimal Ventilation

Ventilation should be controlled to maintain the partial pressure of arterial carbon dioxide at 25 to 35 mm Hg and that of oxygen over 100 mm Hg. Improved neurologic outcome in a primate model apparently was due to immobilization and controlled ventilation with neuromuscular blockade, which enhanced venous pooling and decreased control venous pressure and ICP (57). If possible, however, we prefer to avoid the use of muscle relaxants, which obscure neurologic assessment.

Normothermia

Hypothermia, which causes shivering, increases oxygen utilization and should be avoided. Until such time as the therapeutic place of hypothermia is determined, attempts should be aimed at maintaining normal temperature.

Fluid and Electrolyte Balance

During resuscitation, a balanced electrolyte solution such as 5% dextrose in 0.25 to 0.5% saline with potassium added as necessary should be infused at 30 to 50 ml/kg/24 hr. Input/ouput charting is essential. Furosemide may be used to ensure adequate urinary output, although these patients already have frequently received large doses of osmotic diuretics.

EVALUATION OF OUTCOME

A means to evaluate the outcome after resuscitation in terms of quality of life as evident from patient performance capability should be available. The Glasgow outcome categories (1 best to 5 worst) offers a simple mechanism for categorizing performance after head injury. The Glasgow-Pittsburgh cerebral performance categories and overall performance categories separate cerebral from extracerebral disabilities, which is essential for the evaluation of the effect of new treatments of cerebral recovery as opposed to mortality and morbidity from underlying disease (58).

TERMINATION OF RESUSCITATIVE MEASURES

Resuscitation should not be undertaken when the patient is in the terminal stages of an incurable disease or if there is no reasonable chance to restore mentation.

Uncertainty regarding brain death should not deter resuscitative efforts since brain death cannot be determined immediately and, as outlined, treatment can mitigate the damaging effects of ischemia.

CONCLUSION

In reviewing current therapy for brain protection, it is apparent that global and regional cerebral injury require different therapeutic approaches.

Treatment of global hypoxia should include adequate oxygenation, maintenance of or increased blood flow, decrease of cerebral edema and cerebral metabolic rates, free radical scavenging, control of cellular electrolyte balance, and maintenance of systemic arterial blood pressure. This may be equated to controlled ventilation with increased inspired oxygen concentration and administration of dimethyl sulfoxide or other diuretic agents, phenytoin, low-molecular-weight dextran, butyrolactone, and verapamil.

Following a regional hypoxic insult, therapy should aim to decrease local cerebral vasoconstriction and shunt blood to ischemic areas (barbiturates), maintain blood pressure (hemodilution or blood transfusion), prevent platelet aggregation and intravascular sludging (aspirin or heparin), and improve flow (revascularization techniques).

REFERENCES

1. Michenfelder JD, Theye RA: The effects of anesthesia and hypothermia on canine cerebral ATP and lactate during anoxia produced by decapitation. Anesthesiology 1970;33:430–439.
2. Roski R, Spetzler RF, Owen M, et al.: Reversal of seven year old visual field defect with extracranial-intracranial anastomosis. Surg Neurol 1978;10:267–268.

3. Levy DE, Brierley JB, Silvermann DG, et al.: Brief hypoxia-ischemia initially damages cerebral neurons. Arch Neurol 1975;32:450–456.

4. Negovsky VA: General problems of the post-resuscitation pathology of the brain. Resuscitation 1979;7:73–81.

5. Brierley JB, Meldrum BS, Brown AW: The threshold and neuropathology of cerebral anoxic-ischaemic cell change. Arch Neurol 1973;29:367–374.

6. Lassen NA: Cerebral ischemia. Intensive Care Med 1977;3:251–252.

7. Snyder JV, Nemoto EM, Carol RY, et al.: Global ischemia in dogs; intracranial pressure, brain blood flow and metabolism. Stroke 1975;6:21–27.

8. Nemoto EM, Erdmann, W, Strong E: Regional brain PO_2 after 26 minutes global ischemia in monkeys: Evidence for regional variation in critical perfusion pressures. Crit Care Med 1976;4:129–130.

9. Nemoto EM: Pathogenesis of cerebral ischemia-anoxia. Crit Care Med 1978;6: 203–214.

10. Keller HN, Bartholini G, Pletscher A: Spontaneous and drug induced changes of cerebral dopamine turnover during postnatal development of rats. Brain Res 1973;64:371–378.

11. Hoyer S: Normal and abnormal circulation and oxidative metabolism in the aging human brain. J Cer Blood Flow Metab 1982;2(suppl 1):10–13.

12. London ED, Nespor SM, Ohata M: Local cerebral glucose utilization during development and aging of the Fischer-344 rat. J Neurochem 1981;37:217–221.

13. Siesjö BK: Cell damage in the brain: A speculative synthesis. J Cer Blood Flow Metab 1981;1:155–185.

14. Kalimo H, Rehncrona S, Soderfeldt B, et al.: Brain lactic acidosis and ischemic cell damage. 2. Histopathology. J Cer Blood Flow Metab 1981;1: 313–327.

15. Wieloch T, Harris RJ, Siesjö BK: Brain metabolism and ischemia: Mechanism of cell damage and principles of protection. J Cer Blood Flow Metab 1982;2(suppl 1):5–9.

16. Vapalahti M, Troupp H: Prognosis for patients with severe brain injuries. Br Med J 1971;3:404–407.

17. Smith AL, Wollman H: Cerebral blood flow and metabolism: Effects of anesthetic drugs and techniques. Anesthesiology 1972;36:378–400.

18. Rosomoff HL: Hypothermia and cerebral vascular lesions. 1. Experimental interruption of the middle cerebral artery during hypothermia. J Neurosurg 1956;13: 332–343.

19. White RJ, Massopust LA Jr, Wolin LR, et al.: Profound selective cooling and ischemia of primate brain without pump or oxygenator. Surgery 1969;66:224–232.

20. Michenfelder JD: Failure of prolonged hypocapnia, hypothermia or hypertension to favorably alter acute stroke in primates. Stroke 1977;8:87–91.

21. Steen PA, Soule EM, Michenfelder JD: Detrimental effect of prolonged hypothermia in cats and monkeys with and without regional cerebral ischemia. Stroke 1979; 10:522–529.

22. Selman WR, Spetzler RF: Therapeutics for focal cerebral ischemia. Neurosurgery 1980;6:446–452.

23. Pierce EC, Lambertsen JG, Deutsch S: Cerebral circulation and metabolism during thiopental anesthesia and hyperventilation in man. J Clin Invest 1962; 41:1664–1671.

24. Astrup J, Nordstrom CH, Rehncrona S: Rate of rise in extracellular potassium in the ischemic rat brain and the effect of pre-ischemic metabolic rate: Evidence for a specific effect of phenobarbitone. Acta Neurol Scand (Suppl) 1977;56:148–149.

25. Simeone FA, Frazer G, Lawner P: Ischemic brain edema: Comparative effects of barbiturates and hypothermia. Stroke 1979;19:8–12.

26. Flamm ES, Demopoulos HG, Seligman ML, et al.: Possible molecular mechanisms of barbiturate mediated protection in regional cerebral ischemia. Acta Neurol Scand (Suppl) 1977;56:150–151.

27. Brauston NM, Hope T, Symon L: Barbiturates in focal ischemia of primate cortex; effects on blood flow distribution, evoked potential and extracellular potassium. Stroke 1979;10:647–653.

28. Rockoff MA, Marshall LF, Shapiro HM: High dose barbiturate therapy in humans: A clinical review of 60 patients. Ann Neurol 1979;6:194–199.

29. Marshall LF, Shapiro HM, Rauscher, et al.: Pentobarbital therapy for intracranial hypertension in metabolic coma: Reye's syndrome. Crit Care Med 1978;6:1–15.

30. Miller JD: Barbiturates and raised intracranial pressure. Ann Neurol 1979;6(3): 180–193.

31. Frost EAM, Tabaddor K, Chung SK: Induced barbiturate coma—preliminary results. Crit Care Med 1981;9(3):152.

32. Stullken EH, Milde JH, Michenfelder JD, et al.: The nonlinear responses of cerebral metabolism to low concentrations of halothane, enflurane, isoflurane and thiopental. Anesthesiology 1977;46:28–34.

33. Wolfson LI, Sakurada O, Sokoloff L: Effects of gamma-butyrolactone on local cerebral glucose utilization in the rat. J Neurochem 1977;29:777–783.

34. Bazan NG Jr: Free arachidonic acid and other lipids in the nervous system during early ischemia and after electroshock, in Porcellati G, Amaducci L, Galli C (eds): Function and metabolism of phospholipids in the central and peripheral nervous systems. New York, Plenum Press, 1976, pp 317–356.

35. Nemoto EM, Shiu GK, Nemmer JP: Free fatty acids (FFA) in the pathogenesis and therapy of ischemic brain injury. J Cer Blood Flow Metab 1982;2(suppl 1):59–61.

36. Van Neuten JM, Vanhoutte PM: Improvement of tissue perfusion with inhibitors of calcium ion influx. Biochem Pharmacol 1980;29:479–481.

37. Meyer JS, Waltz AG: Arterial oxygen saturation and alveolar carbon dioxide during electroencephalography, in Gastaut H, Meyer JS (eds): Cerebral anoxia and the encephalogram. Springfield, Il, Charles C Thomas, 1961, pp 329–342.

38. Rose J, Valtonen S, Jennett B: Avoidable factors contributing to death after head injury. Br Med J 1877;2:615–618.

39. Pincus JH, Grove I, Marino BB: Studies on the mechanism of action of diphenylhydantoin. Arch Neurol 1970;22:566–571.

40. Cullen JP, Aldrete JA, Jankovsky L, et al.: Protective action of phenytoin in cerebral ischemia. Anesth Analg (Cleve) 1979;58:165–169.

41. Walson P, Trinca C, Bressler R: New uses of phenytoin. JAMA 1975;233:1385–1389.

42. Sokoloff L: The action of drugs on the cerebral circulation. Pharmacol Rev 1959;2:1–8.

43. Artru AA, Michenfelder JD: Anoxic cerebral potassium accumulation reduced by phenytoin: Mechanism of cerebral protection? Anesth Analg (Cleve) 1981;60:41–45.

44. Munari C, Casaroli D, Matteuzzi G, et al.: The use of althesin in drug resistant status epilepticus. Epilepsia 1979;20:4475–4484.

45. Flamm ES, Yasargil MG, Ransohoff J: Control of cerebral vasospasm by parenteral phenoxybenzamine. Stroke 1972; 3:421–426.

46. Nelson SR: Effects of drugs on experimental brain edema in mice. J Neurosurg 1974;41:193–199.

47. Cummins BH, Giffith HB: Intracarotid phenoxybenzamine for cerebral arterial spasm. Br Med J 1971;1:382–383.
48. White RP, Huang SP, Hagen AA, et al.: Experimental assessment of phenoxybenzamine in cerebral vasospasm. J Neurosurg 1979;50:158–163.
49. Katz RL, Scremin AME, Scremin OU: Physostigmine provides protection from cerebral hypoxia, abstracted ed. Proceedings, Anglo-American Meeting, London, September 1980, p 18.
50. Hope DT, Branston NM, Symon L: Restoration of neurological function with induced hypertension in acute experimental cerebral ischemia. Acta Neurol Scand (Suppl) 1977;56:506–507.
51. Kosnik EJ, Hunt WE: Postoperative hypertension in the management of patients with intracranial arterial aneurysms. J Neurosurg 1976;45:148–154.
52. Michenfelder JD: Failure of prolonged hypocapnia, hypothermia, or hypertension to favorably alter acute stroke in primates. Stroke 1977;8:87–91.
53. Dolowitz DA, Dougherty TF: The use of heparin as an antiinflammatory agent. Laryngoscope 1960;70:873–874.
54. Dougherty TF, Dolowitz DA: Physiologic aspects of heparin not related to blood clots. Am J Cardiol 1964;14:18–24.
55. Stullken EH Jr, Sokol MD: The effects of heparin on recovery from ischemic brain injuries in cats. Anesth Analg (Cleve) 1976;55:683–687.
56. Mielke EH, Ramos JC, Britten AFH: Aspirin as an antiplatelet agent: Template bleeding time as a monitor for therapy. Am J Clin Pathol 1973;59:236–242.
57. Bleyaert AL, Safar P, Stezoski SW: Amelioration of postischemic brain damage in the monkey by immobilization and controlled ventilation. Crit Care Med 1978;6:112–113.
58. Safar P: Cardiopulmonary cerebral resuscitation. Philadelphia, WB Saunders, 1981, p 151.

PART V

Cerebral Death

CHAPTER 21

Brain Death
Robert C. Rubin and
Richard Brennan

The medical and legal demise of an individual can now be defined in terms of cerebral, or more specifically, brain-stem death. Inherent in the diagnosis must be its accuracy and, by definition, its irreversibility. The popular fear has always been overdiagnosis, and perhaps willful misuse of diagnosis, for ulterior motives. Inasmuch as cardiorespiratory failure always followed cerebral death and was easier to assess, it assumed primacy in the diagnosis of death. The advent in the 1950s of adequate ventilatory support led to the survival of patients with severe brain dysfunction and the definition of several syndromes of partial brain failure (1). The "locked-in syndrome" was well recognized, as well as various vegetative states, resulting from cortical disconnection injuries. It is the distinction between a host of vegetative brain syndromes—some of them reversible—and brain-stem death that becomes paramount.

Why the fuss over early diagnosis of brain-stem death? After all, if the diagnosis is correct, its confirmation is inevitable and cardiovascular criteria will eventually be fulfilled. Prompt and accurate diagnostic criteria, however, allow the family and relatives increased dignity; physicians, a defined course of liability; hospitals, better utilization of vital resources; and, perhaps most important, the harvest of useful donor organs while they are still viable.

Since 1970 several jurisdictions, beginning with Kansas, have adopted brain death laws. Still other jurisdictions have left preexisting laws unchanged or purposefully vague, leaving the criteria of death ambiguous and up to the discretion of the physician. The President's Commission on Biomedical Ethics in 1981 recommended that all 50 states adopt a Uniform Brain Death Act.

In 1968, "A Definition of Irreversible Coma" was published by the Ad Hoc Committee of the Harvard Medical School to examine the definition of brain death (2). The criteria of the Ad Hoc Committee consisted of documentation of:

1. Unreceptivity and unresponsiveness.
2. No movement or breathing.
3. No reflexes.
4. Flat electroencephalogram (EEG)—isoelectric at maximum gain.

5. All of the above tests should be repeated at least 24 hours later with no change.
6. Temperature should be above 32.2°C.

The requirements subsequently were reduced to 12 hours (3) of isoelectric electroencephalography, and some hospitals reduced this requirement to one hour.

The efficacy of the EEG has subsequently been challenged and its use dropped from many criteria since primarily it is a reflection of cortical neuronal activity. Failure of the brain stem, rather than of cerebral cortex function is better assessed for cerebral death (4–6).

More recently, the Conference of Medical Royal Colleges and their faculties in the United Kingdom issued a statement setting forth more clearly defined criteria for the diagnosis of brain death (7). This conference established "conditions for considering the diagnosis of brain death" (7):

1. The patient is deeply comatose.
    a. There should be no suspicion that this state is due to depressant drugs. Narcotics, hypnotics, and tranquilizers may have prolonged duration of action, particularly when some hypothermia exists. It was therefore recommended that the drug history be carefully reviewed and adequate intervals allowed for the persistence of drug effects to be excluded. This was felt to be of particular importance in patients whose primary cause of coma lay in the toxic effects of drugs followed by anoxic cerebral damage.
    b. Primary hypothermia as a cause of coma should have been excluded.
    c. Metabolic and endocrine disturbances that can cause or contribute to coma should have been excluded. Metabolic and endocrine factors contributing to the persistence of coma must be carefully assessed. There should be no profound abnormality of serum electrolytes, acid base balance, or blood glucose concentrations.
2. The patient is maintained by mechanical ventilation because spontaneous respiration has previously become inadequate or has ceased altogether. Neuromuscular blocking agents and other drugs should have been excluded as a cause of respiratory inadequacy or failure. Equally, persistent effects of hypnotics and narcotics should be excluded as a cause of respiratory failure.
3. There should be no doubt that the patient's condition is due to irremediable structural brain damage. The diagnosis of a disorder which can lead to brain death should have been fully established.

Previous history of severe head injury, spontaneous intracranial hemorrhage, or preceding neurosurgical procedure, such as excision of tumors, and so forth, provides a precondition. Toxic and metabolic insults, such as cardiac arrest, hypoxia, or severe circulatory insufficiency, with an indefinite period of cerebral anoxia, may not be as clearly irreversible and may require a longer time to establish the prognosis.

Present availability of computed tomographic (CT) scanning facilitates the establishment of an anatomic diagnosis with a readily ascertainable prognosis. Spontaneous intracerebral hemorrhages and trauma can thus be easily assessed.

Some tests have been established to confirm brain death (7):

All brain-stem reflexes should be absent.

a. The pupils are fixed in diameter and do not respond to sharp changes in the intensity of incident light.
b. There are no corneal reflexes.
c. The vestibular ocular reflexes are absent. These are absent when no eye movements occur during or after the slow injection of 20 ml of ice cold water into each external auditory meatus, clear access to the tympanic membranes having been established by direct inspection. This test may be contraindicated on one or the other side by local trauma.

No motor response.

d. Responses within the cranial nerve distribution cannot be elicited by adequate stimulation of any somatic area.
e. There is no gag reflex or reflex response to bronchial stimulation by a suction catheter passed down the trachea.
f. No respiratory movements occur when mechanical ventilation is discontinued long enough to ensure that the arterial carbon dioxide tension rises above the stimulating threshold, that is, the P_aCO_2 must normally reach 50 mm mercury. This is best achieved by measuring the blood gases; if this facility is available, the patient should be disconnected when the P_aCO_2 reaches 40 to 55 mm of mercury after administration of 5% CO_2 in oxygen through the ventilator. This starting level has been chosen because patients may be modestly hypothermic (35 degrees centigrade to 37 degrees centigrade), flaccid, and with a depressed metabolic rate, so that the P_aCO_2 rises only slowly in apnea (2 mm of mercury/minute). (Hypoxia during disconnection should be prevented by delivering oxygen at 6 liters/minute through a catheter into the trachea.) If blood gas analysis is not available to measure the P_aCO_2 and P_aO_2, the alternative procedure is to supply the ventilator with pure oxygen for 10 minutes (preoxygenation), then with 5% CO_2 in oxygen for 5 minutes and to disconnect the ventilator for 10 minutes, while delivering oxygen at 6 liters/minute by catheter into the trachea. This establishes diffusion oxygenation and insures that, during apnea, hypoxia will not occur, even in 10 or more minutes of respiratory arrest. Patients with preexisting chronic respiratory insufficiency, who may be unresponsive to raised levels of carbon dioxide and who normally exist on hypoxic drive, are special cases and should be expertly investigated with careful blood gas monitoring.

The Conference of Medical Royal Colleges further recommended that these tests be repeated to ensure that no observer error has occurred. The interval between tests depends on the preexisting cause for brain death and the certainty of the prognosis. The interval may be as long as 24 hours in doubtful cases.

It is recognized that spinal cord function can persist even after irreversible brain-stem death. Spinal reflexes may even return after initial absence in brain-dead patients (8).

In addition to the initial criteria proposed by the Harvard Ad Hoc Committee, other laboratory tests have subsequently been proposed. It was hoped that perhaps one test, but probably more than one, without repetition, would provide definitive diagnostic criteria for brain death. These laboratory studies include (9):

1. Isoelectric EEG (10)
2. Arrest of blood flow at the base of the skull, demonstrated by cerebral contrast angiography or by intracarotid injection of xenon or sodium O-iodohyperate (Hyperan) (11), or other carotid imaging techniques such as digital venous subtraction or contrast bolus CT (12)
3. Lack of response to atropine
4. Lack of vestibular response to caloric tests
5. Lack of brain pulsation in echoencephalography
6. Brain temperature lower than body temperature
7. Intracranial pressure higher than systemic and exceeding 100 mm Hg
8. Negligible cerebral oxygen consumption
9. No visualization of brain in scanning and gamma camera (performed with technetium) (11,12) (CT changes with contrast enhancement also signify the presence of cerebral blood flow.)
10. Lack of cerebrospinal fluid circulation demonstrated by intrathecal injection of radioactive iodinated serum albumin (RISA).

Such studies measure different parameters of cerebral function. The EEG measures the electrical activity of the brain and is primarily a reflection of cortical neuronal activity. In a series of 25 cases meeting the clinical criteria for brain death, all demonstrated isoelectric EEG (13). The EEG is helpful in identifying patients with brain-stem disease, usually infarction or hemorrhage, who might fulfill the clinical criteria of unreceptivity, unresponsiveness, apnea, and absent brain-stem reflexes but with a functioning, nonexpressive cerebral cortex. There are, however, situations such as hypothermia or deep barbiturate coma that also give a flat EEG and must be distinguished from cerebral death. It is in those instances that studies demonstrating cerebral blood flow are most valuable. Evoked potentials may prove valuable in this differential diagnosis (14).

The caloric vestibular test is performed by introducing ice water into the external auditory canal. The absence of tonic deviation of the eyes or nystagmus indicates destruction of vestibular-ocular pathways and also is absent in cerebral death.

The atropine test is based on a different assumption. In the presence of cerebral death there is destruction of the intracranial parasympathetic system; vagal activity has ceased, and therefore intravenous injection of 2 mg of atropine will cause no acceleration of heart rate. The sympathetic nervous system with intact cell bodies in the spinal cord continues to have some function and becomes a primary determinant of cardiac rate. Therefore, the response to isoproterenol should remain. The clinical experience has been somewhat variable (15); however, it has been reported that intravenous administration of 2 mg of atropine produced no effects in 30 cases meeting other criteria for brain death. The atropine test is usually positive in deep coma and becomes negative with the advent of a flat EEG.

Many tests are based on the absence of intracranial blood flow and in some way measure this phenomenon. They vary in accuracy and in the complexity of the instrumentation required. Cerebral blood flow should persist in spite of a flat EEG in such conditions as hypothermia and barbiturate intoxication and some brain-stem lesions. Therefore, such relatively simple studies as radionuclide angiography performed by the intravenous bolus administration of technetium pertechnetate and its detection intracranially by means of a scintillation camera should rule out the diagnosis of cerebral death secondary to barbiturates. The failure to demonstrate cerebral blood flow at a given moment has not been proved to be synonymous with cerebral death. This phenomenon may exist for a short period and still be reversible. Although a "no-reflow" phenomenon may exist, a single determination of no intracranial filling, either angiographically or by radionuclide or oxygen consumption, although suggestive, is not definitive. This of course presumes a technically adequate test, such as proper intraluminal placement of the contrast or isotope bolus, adequate blood pressure, and so forth (11,12).

Some of these tests are cumbersome. Measurement of cerebral brain temperature requires a craniotomy, while measurement of cerebral blood flow requires elaborate equipment and intracarotid injection of xenon or Hippuran. Noncirculation of cerebrospinal fluid, as demonstrated by intrathecal injection of RISA, requires scanning over a prolonged period and is too nonspecific to be valuable in the diagnosis of brain death. The obliteration of cerebrospinal fluid pathways from any cause, such as hydrocephalus or hemorrhage, can yield similar results. Despite the sophistication of the studies, it is presently suggested that they be repeated over an interval encompassing at least one hour in demonstrating no flow of blood.

LEGAL ASPECTS OF BRAIN DEATH

An issue of great social significance arises when, in the course of normal medical events, respiratory measures are instituted that are unsuccessful in maintaining a viable brain. How and when can these measures, that is, the respirator and pressor drugs, be discontinued?

The vaunted *Quinlan* case, (*In Re Karen Quinlan*, 70 N.J. 10, 355 A.2d 647, 1976) did not resolve the issue of what constitutes death. The decision was grounded on the right of privacy, a right that would permit the termination of treatment to a hopelessly comatose and persistently vegetative patient. The opinion did not decide that Karen Quinlan was dead; on the contrary, it merely permitted the cessation of her unendurable life. Accordingly, the *Quinlan* case, while of nationwide interest, is of but limited utility in defining "death."

Because the heart death test, or absence of circulation of the blood, is inappropriate in cases of mechanically sustained respiration, many proposals have been made to adopt a modern definition of death. Many states, perceiving the need for a workable and realistic definition of death, have enacted statutes to achieve this result. These states include Alaska, California, Georgia, Illinois, Kansas, Michigan, New Mexico, Oklahoma, Oregon, Tenneseee, Virginia, and West Virginia. Consistency and uniformity among the several states are desirable goals. A giant step toward that end was taken with the drafting of the 1980 Uniform Determination of Death Act, which provides as follows:

> An individual who has sustained either (1) irreversible cessation of circulatory and respiratory functions, or (2) irreversible cessation of all functions of the entire brain, including the brain stem, is dead. A determination of death must be made in accordance with accepted medical standards.

Brain death, as opposed to cessation of respiration and heart beat, as the criterion for the end of human life is also inexorably finding its way into the civil and criminal law of the several states. In addition to statutory enactments, the courts are issuing decisions in which brain death is preferred over heart death. In the case of Bowman (*In Re Welfare of Bowman*, 617 P.2d 731, Washington, 1980), for example, the Supreme Court of the State of Washington approved the Uniform Determination of Death Act and said that great confusion would exist if a determination of death were not based upon the cessation of brain activity. The following language of the Washington Supreme Court is thought-provoking:

> The numerous legal issues which look to the time and presence of death as determining factors requires a legal response to these new developments. Inheritance, liability for death claims under insurance contracts, proximate cause and time of death in homicide cases, and termination of life support efforts are but a few of the areas in which legal consequences follow from a determination of whether death has occurred.

While certain states have opted for brain death over heart death as the criterion for the end of life, it continues to remain a medical decision irrespective of the criteria used. In other words, the criteria for the diagnosis of death are left to the medical profession. The Uniform Anatomical Gift Act, adopted by most jurisdictions, provides:

> The true time of death shall be determined by a physician who tends the donor at his death, or, if none, the physician who certifies the death. The physician shall not participate in the procedure for removing or transplanting a part.

The question of the meaning of death assumes critical significance in the decision of whether to continue life support systems. Courts are beginning to recognize the Harvard Medical School Ad Hoc Committee's criteria in making this determination. Paramount to the issue is the question of who is to make the decision. The doctor, family, or collegiate groups, such as an "ethics committee," all may be involved.

Of obvious concern to every physician faced with a persistently vegetative patient who is being kept alive mechanically is the potential criminal and civil liability for terminating the life support systems. Civil liability, if it existed, would be manifested in a judgment that a physician caused the "wrongful death" of the patient, and the measure of damages would be the pecuniary or monetary loss to the survivors. Criminal liability, if it existed, would take the form of a judgment that the physician was guilty of homicide, that is, murder or the varying degrees of manslaughter.

A civil action for wrongful death would be premised on the proposition that a physician committed malpractice—a negligent deviation from standard and accepted practice—or upon the proposition that he intentionally caused the patient's death by withdrawing the supportive therapy. Criminal liability would be based on the necessary finding that the doctor had the intent to kill his patient.

If the brain death test is accepted as the criterion for determination of death, it would be difficult to sustain a civil action for wrongful death or a criminal indictment for homicide against a physician who terminates supportive measures on a patient who has undergone an irreversible cessation of spontaneous respiratory and circulatory functions. One observer has addressed the issue in terms of euthanasia (16):

> The importance of these statutes (brain death criteria) to the physician in respect to the euthanasia situation is significant. If the patient's EEG is no longer active, indicating a cessation of brain functioning, the patient may be pronounced legally dead, even though his heart is still beating. In this situation, the physician who unplugs the patient's respirator (which may be allowing his heart and lungs to continue functioning) and thereby hasten death, will escape criminal liability for his actions.

Without a set of statutory or common law criteria for brain death, criminal liability may exist when a physician fails to take extraordinary measures to support life. Ordinary measures have been said to be those that offer a reasonable hope of benefit and that can be obtained and used without excessive expense, pain, or other inconvenience. Extraordinary measures are considered to be those that do not involve these factors or that, if used, would offer no reasonable hope of benefit. The nationally prominent criminal lawyer Percy Foreman addressed this issue (*In Re Karen Quinlan*, 70 N.J. 10, 355 A.2d 647, 1976):

> The distinction between involuntary euthanasia by a positive act and involuntary euthanasia by omission is not always easy to discern. Suppose a patient is alive only because he is connected to a mechanical respirator. Without the machine, he would die. Attempts are made by the physician to revive him to a self-sufficient state, while the machine artifically keeps him breathing. After a period of time, the doctor concludes his efforts are futile and decides to unplug the machine. The patient dies. Is the doctor's act of unplugging the life-supporting machine an 'external manifestation of the doctor's will,' that is a positive act? Or is the act to be considered an omission by the doctor in that he is omitting to provide further life saving medical care? If it is an affirmative act, and without the patient's consent, theoretically, the doctor would be liable for murder. On the other hand, if it is deemed an omission, then the criminal liability of the doctor would turn on the question of duty. Although the doctor has a duty to administer ordinary means to preserve life, there is not a duty to administer 'extraordinary' means.

Termination of artificial life support for a brain-dead patient, however, would probably not give rise to civil or criminal liability because the ensuing death would be said to be due to existing natural causes. That is, the patient will be said to have died from his underlying medical problem and not from the rather perfunctory act of disconnecting a life support modality. The *Quinlan* case is of significance in this regard. In that case the court appointed Karen's father to be her guardian and authorized him to disconnect her respirator if (a) the family concurred in the decision, (b) the attending physician concluded that there was no reasonable expectation of her recovery, and (c) a hospital "ethics committee" agreed with the grim prognosis.

With respect to a deviation from accepted medical standards—the keystone of liability for malpractice—the court in the *Quinlan* case specifically made note that physicians do not artificially breathe terminal patients where this would be of no benefit. In eschewing the fastening of liability on a physician under these circumstances, the court ruled:

> If that consultative body (ethics committee) agrees that there is no reasonable possibility of Karen's ever emerging from her present comatose condition to a cognitive, sapient state, the present life-support system may be withdrawn and said action shall be without any civil liability therefore, on the part of any participant, whether guardian, physician, hospital or other.

(It is an interesting and provocative aspect of the *Quinlan* case that Karen was ultimately removed from the respirator and did not die, but remained in a vegetative state breathing spontaneously.)

Closely related to the concept of brain death, and in certain circumstances inextricably intertwined with it, is the "right to die," as that term has been defined by several courts and legislatures. There would appear to be no constitutional right to die, but it is clear that a competent person of the age of majority has the right to refuse even life-saving medical treatment (17). This right is perhaps more aptly described as the option to determine what is to be done with one's body and the right to acquiesce in an imminent and inevitable death (Am. Jur. 2d, New Topic Service, "Right to Die; Wrongful Life," Section 7, p. 8). The right of a competent adult to choose life over death, however, is not absolute and in no way legitimizes or justifies suicide. But the right to reject potentially life-saving therapy is high in the constellation of civil rights and may not be overridden without a compelling state interest. Courts have even held bedside hearings to make this determination. In the *Osborne* case (*In Re Osborne*, 294 A.2d 372, D.C. App. 1972), the court stated that in cases of a patient wishing to reject life-saving therapy it is better, if possible, "for the judge to make a first-hand appraisal of the patient's personal desires and ability for rational choice."

While it is relatively simple for a competent adult to choose, in effect, to die, the issue becomes clouded where a comatose patient who meets the criteria for brain death is being kept "alive" only by artificial means of life support. Under these circumstances, the focal point of the decision whether to discontinue such means of life support is the prognosis as to the reasonable possibility of return to cognitive and sapient life, as distinguished from the forced continuance of that biological vegetative existence to which the patient seems to be doomed.

The right to be free of a hopeless and vegetative existence also implies the right of privacy, or the right to be left alone. This right includes the choice of a mature, competent adult to refuse to accept therapeutic modalities that may prolong his life. This right is but an expression of the sanctity of individual free choice and self-determination (Am. Jur. 2d, *supra* at Section 26, pp. 25–26). This thought has been eloquently expressed as follows:

> It may be convenient for hospitals and/or physicians to insist on continuing the patient's life so that there can be no question of foul play, no resulting civil liability, and no possible trespass on medical ethics. But it is quite another matter to do so at the patient's sole expense and against his competent will, thus inflicting never-ending physical torture on his body until the inevitable but artificially suspended moment of death. Such a course of conduct invades the patient's constitutional right of privacy, removes his freedom of choice and invades his right of self-determination.

Consistent with an individual's right of self-determination, a person may draft what has come to be known as a "living will." This is usually a written directive that life-sustaining measures be withheld or withdrawn in the event of a terminal condition. The concept behind a living will is that a person, in full grasp of his faculties, may direct that artificial life support measures not be used if he ever becomes incapable of expressing such a desire in the future. California has recognized the right to draft a living will in the California Natural Death Act. The reason for its enactment by the legislature was that adult persons have the basic right to control the decisions relating to the rendering of their medical care, including the decision to embrace or reject life-sustaining procedures. The act also provides that modern medical technology has made possible the artificial extension of life beyond natural limits and that this, in hopeless cases, may result in the loss of patient dignity and unnecessary pain and suffering, while providing nothing medically beneficial to the patient.

Whether a patient is brain dead may have great significance in "no code" or "do not resuscitate" (DNR) situations. In 1974, the American Medical Association determined that cardiopulmonary resuscitation (CPR) was not indicated in situations of terminal, irreversible illness where death is not unexpected or where prolonged cardiac arrest dictates the futility of resuscitation efforts (18). In 1976, Rabkin, Gillerman and Rice (19) authored an extensive article designed to be a guide as to how hospitals could implement "no code" orders.

The most common instance in which to withhold resuscitation efforts is when the patient is irreversibly and terminally ill, with death imminent. If a patient is brain dead and is being artificially kept alive, the implementation of DNR or "no code" orders seems singularly appropriate and not open to much dispute. The procedural guidelines for the implementation of these orders must be scrupulously followed, however. The American Medical Association National Conference on CPR has confirmed that the following protocol (summarized here) must be followed (20):

The 'no code' order should be entered clearly on the patient's chart. The entire medical team responsible for care of the patient should concur with the advisability of the order. The patient must give an informed consent before the order should be written if he is competent. While the family should be informed of the decision, understand the reason for it, and be in agreement, their consent is not controlling. This is as it should be.

The time of death is peculiarly relevant to a prosecution for homicide, or the wrongful killing of one human being by another. A charge of homicide implies that the deceased was living at the time of the mortal blow. If a comatose, persistently vegetative patient, who is being kept alive only by the use of a mechanical respirator, is assaulted or wounded and later dies, the assailant may claim that he should not be guilty of homicide. This contention was made in the Massachusetts case of *Commonwealth v. Golston* (366 N.E.2d 744, Supreme Judicial Court of Massachusetts 1977).

In the *Golston* case, the defendant was charged with homicide. He had struck his victim on the head with a baseball bat and a craniotomy was performed to relieve the cerebral pressure. The victim was being ventilated with a respirator and when he was removed from ventilatory support he failed to breathe spontaneously. Moreover, an EEG showed no evidence of brain-wave activity. After consultation with the family of the victim, the respirator was removed when the victim's heart stopped. In appealing his conviction of murder, the defendant claimed that the death of the victim had not been properly established. The court rejected this contention, adopting the brain death criteria of the Harvard Medical School Ad Hoc Committee.

The Supreme Judicial Court of Massachusetts approved the following instructions on the law which the trial judge had given to the jury:

Brain death occurs when, in the opinion of a licensed physician, based on ordinary and accepted standards of medical practice, there has been a total and irreversible cessation of spontaneous brain functions and further attempts at resuscitation or continued supportive maintenance would not be successful in restoring such functions.

The determination of the moment of death has particular relevance to the transplantations of vital organs, especially the heart. The issue has been raised but not resolved (21):

Obviously, for a heart to be transplanted to a recipient, the donor must be dead or the surgical team has committed homicide. The dilemma faced by medicine in this area is that if the surgical team is forced to wait until the donor is quite legally dead, that is, until the heart is stopped, the operation is useless.

The time of death may be a determination of crucial significance in the law of real property. Aside from sales of real estate, the major way in which ownership or interest in real property changes is through the death of the current owner or possessor.

The question of apparent simultaneous death has been treated by a statute that has solved certain obvious problems but has raised others in determining survivorship. The Uniform Simultaneous Death Law, adopted in almost all of the states, provides:

> Where the title of property or the devolution thereof depends upon priority of death and there is no sufficient evidence that the persons have died otherwise than simultaneously, the property of each person shall be disposed of as if he had survived . . .

The obvious difficulty is the provision dealing with "no sufficient evidence that the persons have died other than simultaneously." There is no difficulty where both persons are pronounced dead at the scene of a common disaster. But where one immediately is resuscitated and the other is pronounced dead, and the one who is resuscitated is sustained thereafter mechanically but in a chronic, vegetative state and later "dies," the issue of who survived or outlived whom very well may be questioned.

Frequently, a testator, or a person making a will, will direct that his property be distributed to several different individuals over several different periods of time. These future interests are known as "remainders." A precise time of death is critical in determination of whether attempts to establish remainders are successful. Similarly, antilapse statutes, which may radically affect the distribution of a testator's estate, also hinge upon whether a beneficiary of a will "dies" before the testator.

Determination of time of death also may be of crucial significance in determining who will benefit from a will because of the Rule Against Perpetuities. This rule draws a line at a certain period of time after a person's death beyond which he may not control his wealth. The rule generally denies effect to any interest that a person may attempt to establish approximately 21 years after a life or lives in being at the time of the creation of the interest. Consequently, the application of this denial may depend upon a definition of death.

A determination of the time of death has important implications in deciding whether the statute of limitations has run and may be significant in the law of evidence. A major principle of evidence is the hearsay rule, which provides generally that an out-of-court statement is not admissible at a trial. The dying declaration rule provides that in a criminal proceeding, a statement made by a victim unavailable as a witness because of his death is admissible, if it was made voluntarily and in good faith and while the declarant was conscious of his impending death. Another rule of evidence provides that a statement of a witness unavailable because of death is admissible if several similar conditions are met. Thus, the hearsay rule unjustly may bar the admission of evidence at trial if at the time of trial the declarant is dead according to one definition of death, but not according to another definition.

An accurate definition of death also has implications in the area of financial transactions and may be important to the disposition of jointly owned property.

It now seems that the diagnosis of brain death requires a combination of clinical findings that include unresponsive coma, apnea, unreactive dilated pupils, and absent brain-stem reflexes, such as oculocephalic, corneal, and vestibular. Additional laboratory studies, including at least an isoelectric EEG and perhaps some index of absent cerebral flow, are confirmatory. Persistence of clinical findings and an isoelectric EEG for more than three hours should establish the diagnosis. In the presence of drug intoxication, indicators of cerebral blood flow are most helpful.

Despite the recognition of cerebral death as opposed to cardiac death and the availability of a workable set of criteria to make this diagnosis, it should be remembered that cardiovascular collapse will follow cerebral death. The distinction is meaningful only when the acquisition of organs, legal ramifications, or economic costs are involved. Those instances of prolonged survival without meaningful cerebral function and without an optimistic prognosis, such as the case of Karen Quinlan, often do not meet the criteria for cerebral death. Such cases require individual analysis and subsequent judicial or legislative guidelines. It is probable that the outcome of such cases will be determined along guidelines relating to the patient's and the family's right to privacy. This will involve the right to consent to further care and considerations of what constitutes ordinary and what constitutes extraordinary care.

Paramount to the issues is the question of who is to make the decision. The doctor, family, or a collegiate group, such as an "ethics committee" all may be involved.

The medicolegal concept of brain death, while no longer in its infancy, has still not matured into established doctrine in all of the several states. It is a certainty, however, that it will become an accepted part of our jurisprudence in the years to come. At the present time one author has taken a broad look and has reached, among others, the following conclusions (22):

1. Brain death has become an accepted alternate means of defining death replacing the traditional definition relying solely on absence of cardiac and respiratory function.
2. A clear medical consensus exists that brain death may only be found where there has been a total, irreversible cessation of all brain functions, that is, where all parts of the brain, including the stem, have permanently ceased any functioning.
3. The 'Harvard' criteria are the most widely accepted criteria for ascertaining brain death. However, other criteria promulgated by equally prestigious sources are accepted and followed by substantial segments of the medical community.
4. A clear medical consensus does not yet exist as to exactly what criteria must be met before a patient may be considered brain dead, nor as to whether brain death can properly be diagnosed based on clinical findings alone.

For years it was the cessation of heartbeat and breathing that signaled the end of human life. While these criteria are time-honored and certainly of great value, they will inevitably yield to the more precise and specific criteria of brain death for determining whether a human being has died.

REFERENCES

1. Plum R, Posner JR: The diagnosis of stupor and coma, ed 3. Philadelphia, FA Davis, 1980.
2. Ad Hoc Committee, Harvard Medical School. A definition of irreversible coma. JAMA 1968;205:337-340.
3. Cranford R: Brain death, concepts and criteria. Parts I and II. Minn Med 1968; 61:561, 600.
4. Beecher HK: After the definition of irreversible coma. N Engl J Med 1968;281:1070.
5. Jennett B: Brain death. Br J Anaesth 1981;53:1111-1119.
6. Taub S: Brain death: A re-evaluation of the Harvard criteria. Conn Med 1981;45:587-599.
7. Proceedings, Conference of Medical Royal Colleges: Diagnosis of brain death. Br Med J 1976;2:1187-1188.
8. Ivan LP: Spinal reflexes in cerebral death. Neurology 1973;23:650.
9. Walker AE: Ancillary studies in the diagnosis of brain death. Am NY Acad Sci 1978;315:228-240.
10. The International Federation of EEG Societies report. Electroencephalogr Clin Neurophysiol 1975;38:536.
11. Mishkin F: Determination of cerebral death by radionuclide angiography. Radiology 1975;115:135-137.
12. Arnold H, Kuhne D, Rohr W, et al.: Contrast bolus technique with rapid CT scanning. Neuroradiology 1981;22:129-132.
13. Quakine G, Kosary I, Brakan J, et al.: Laboratory criteria of brain death. J Neurosurg 1973;39:429-433.
14. Goldie WD, Chiappa KH, Young RR, et al.: Brainstem auditory and short latency somatosensory and evoked responses in brain death. Neurology 1981;32:248-256.
15. Drory I, Quakine G, Kosary I, et al.: EKG findings in brain death. Chest 1975;67:425-432.
16. Foreman S: The physician's criminal liability for the practice of euthanasia. Baylor Law Review 1975;27:54.
17. Bok S: Personal directions for care at the end of life. N Engl J Med 1976;295:367-369.
18. Standards for cardiopulmonary resuscitation and emergency cardiac care. Part V. Medicolegal considerations and recommendations. JAMA 1974;277:864-866.
19. Rabkin MT, Gillerman GG, Rice NR: Orders not to resuscitate. N Engl J Med 1976; 295:364-366.
20. Meyers DW: Medico-legal implications of death and dying. Section 9.3, Lawyers Cooperative Publishing Co, 1981, p 190.
21. The time of death—a legal, ethical and medical dilemma. Catholic Lawyer 1972; 18:242.
22. Meyers DW: Medico-legal implications of death and dying. Section 4.10, Lawyers Cooperative Publishing Co, 1981, p. 57.

INDEX

469